LEISHMANIASIS

Biology, Control and New Approaches for Its Treatment

LEISHMANIASIS

Biology, Control and New Approaches for Its Treatment

Saurabh Bhatia, PhD

Divakar Goli, PhD

AAP APPLE ACADEMIC PRESS

Apple Academic Press Inc.
3333 Mistwell Crescent
Oakville, ON L6L 0A2
Canada

Apple Academic Press Inc.
9 Spinnaker Way
Waretown, NJ 08758
USA

Exclusive worldwide distribution by CRC Press, a member of Taylor & Francis Group

International Standard Book Number-13: 978-1-77188-419-8 (Hardcover)

International Standard Book Number-13: 978-1-77188-420-4 (eBook)

Library and Archives Canada Cataloguing in Publication

Bhatia, Saurabh, author
Leishmaniasis : biology, control and new approaches for its treatment / Saurabh Bhatia, PhD, Divakar Goli, PhD.

Includes bibliographical references and index.
Issued in print and electronic formats.
ISBN 978-1-77188-419-8 (hardcover).--ISBN 978-1-77188-420-4 (pdf)
1. Leishmaniasis. 2. Leishmaniasis--Prevention. 3. Leishmaniasis--Treatment. I. Goli, Divakar, author II. Title.

RC153.B43 2016   616.9'364   C2016-904971-X   C2016-904972-8

Library of Congress Cataloging-in-Publication Data

Names: Bhatia, Saurabh, author. | Goli, Divakar, author.
Title: Leishmaniasis: biology, control and new approaches for its treatment/Saurabh Bhatia, PhD, Divakar Goli, PhD.
Description: New Jersey : Apple Academic Press, Inc., [2017] | Includes bibliographical references and index. | Description based on print version record and CIP data provided by publisher; resource not viewed.
Identifiers: LCCN 2016033113 (print) | LCCN 2016032864 (ebook) | ISBN 9781771884198 (hardcover : alk. paper) | ISBN 9781771884204 (eBook)
Subjects: LCSH: Leishmaniasis.
Classification: LCC RC153 (print) | LCC RC153 .B43 2017 (ebook) | DDC 616.9/364--dc23
LC record available at https://lccn.loc.gov/2016033113

Apple Academic Press also publishes its books in a variety of electronic formats. Some content that appears in print may not be available in electronic format. For information about Apple Academic Press products, visit our website at **www.appleacademicpress.com** and the CRC Press website at **www.crcpress.com**

MIX
Paper from responsible sources
FSC www.fsc.org FSC® C013056

Printed and bound in Great Britain by
TJ International Ltd, Padstow, Cornwall

ABOUT THE AUTHORS

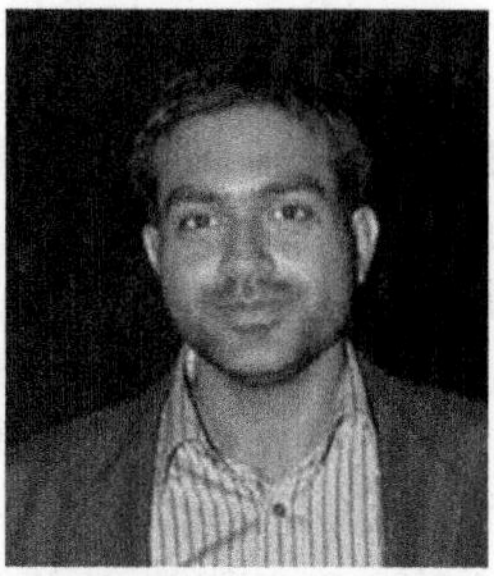

Saurabh Bhatia, PhD

Saurabh Bhatia, PhD, is currently working as an Assistant Professor at the School of Medical and Allied Sciences, GD Goenka University, Gurgaon, Haryana, India. He has several years of academic experience, teaching such specialized subjects as natural product science, nanotechnology, biotechnology, parasitology, polymeric sciences, and biomaterials. He has promoted several marine algae and their derived polymers throughout India. He has written more than 30 international publications in these areas and has been an active participant of more than 35 national and international conferences. So far he has successfully finished nine books in pharma and its allied sciences. His published books include *Modern Applications of Plant Biotechnology in Pharmaceutical Sciences* (Academic Press, Elsevier, 2015); *Nanotechnology in Drug Delivery: Fundamentals, Design, and Applications* (Apple Academic Press, 2016); *Leishmaniasis: Biology, Control and New Approaches for Its Treatment* (Apple Academic Press, 2016); *Natural Polymer Drug Delivery Systems: Nanoparticles, Plants, and Algae* (Springer, 2016); and *Natural Polymer Drug Delivery Systems: Nanoparticles, Mammals and Microbes* (Springer, 2016). Dr. Bhatia graduated from Kurushetra University followed by earning his MPharm from Bharati Vidyapeeth University, Pune, India. He received his PhD degree from Jadavpur University, Kolkata, India.

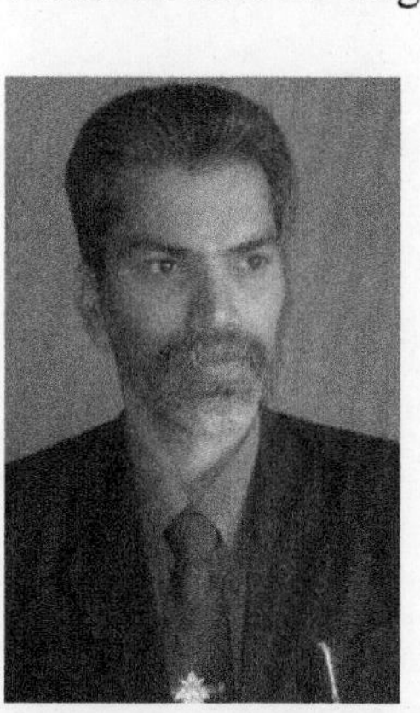

Divakar Goli, PhD

Divakar Goli, PhD, is currently a Professor and Principal at the Acharya & B M Reddy College of Pharmacy in Karnataka, India. He is the Editor of the *Indian Journal of Pharmaceutical Sciences*, the official scientific publication of the Indian Pharmaceutical Association from 2014-2016-2018 as well as the regional *RGUHS Journal of Pharmaceutical Sciences.* He holds or has held many prestigious roles, including Honorary President and Director at Iphar

Pharmaceuticals Limited and at Du Laboratories Limited; Secretary of the Education Division and Associate Secretary of the Indian Pharmaceutical Association; Chairman of the 50th Golden Jubilee Celebration Committee of National Pharmacy Week in 2011; Secretary of the International Society of Pharmaceutical Engineering (ISPE), Bangalore chapter; and member of many academic bodies. In 2014, Dr. Goli received the coveted Principal of the Year award from the Association of Pharmaceutical Teachers of India. He is also the recipient of the prestigious fellowship of the Indian Pharmaceutical Association, and fellow of the Association of Biotechnology and Pharmacy, and the Institution of Chemists (India). Active in his field of specialization, pharmaceutical biotechnology and management studies, he is a member of many professional organizations and has presented at numerous national and international conferences. Dr. Goli has published almost 100 research articles in peer-reviewed professional publications and is also coauthor of the book *Pharmaceutical Marketing Management*. Dr. Goli has earned PhDs in both Pharmaceutical Sciences and also in Commerce and Management Studies from Andhra University, Visakhapatnam, and as well as a degree in computer applications.

CONTENTS

LIST OF ABBREVIATIONS

SETS	4-acetamido-4'-isothiocyanato-2-2'stilbenedisulfonic acid disodium salt hydrate
AC	acidocalcisomes
AIDS	acquired immunodeficiency syndrome
ATP	adenosine 5′-triphosphate
ATPase	adenosinetriphosphatase
AG	aggregated
AGE	aqueous garlic extract
AAMos	alternatively activated macrophages
AmB	amphotericin B
APCs	antigen-presenting cells
Ags	antigens
AIA	anti-inflammatory activity
AMP	antimicrobial peptide
Sb(V)	antimonials
AAL	*A. annua* leaves
AAS	*A. annua* seeds
BPS	bathophenanthroline disulfonate
CMI	cell-mediated immune
cMO	classically activated macrophages
CRH	corticotropin-releasing hormone
CpG ODN	CpG oligodeoxynucleotide
CMC	critical micellar concentration
CL	cutaneous leishmaniasis
cAMP	cyclic adenosine 5′-monophosphate
Cox-2	cyclooxygenase-2
DTH	delayed type hypersensitivity
DS	delivery system
DCs	dendritic cells
DNA	deoxyribonucleic acid
DAG	diacylglycerol
DDT	dichlorodiphenyltrichloroethane
DIDS	4,4'-diisothiocyanatostilbene-2,2'-disulfonic acid
DAT	direct agglutination test

DDSs	drug delivery systems
EA	electroacupuncture
	endothelial or eNOS/NOS_3
EHP	Environmental Health Project
ELISA	enzyme-linked immunosorbent assay
VAEO	EO of *Vanillosmopsis arborea*
EOs	essential oils
EDTA	ethylenediaminetetraacetic acid
FO	fish oil
FMN	flavin mononucleotide
FML	fructose mannose ligand
g-GCS	*gamma-glutamylcysteine synthetase*
GIT	gastrointestinal tract
GSTs	glutathione S-transferases
GRP	glycine-rich proteins
GLY	glycosomes
GIPLs	glycosylinositol phospholipids
GRA	glycyrrhetinic acid
GA	glycyrrhizic acid
HSP 70	heat shock protein 70
HIV	human immunodeficiency virus
HASPB1	hydrophilic acylated surface protein B1
IFN-γR	IFN-γ receptor
iNOS or NOS_2	inducible nitric oxide synthase
IP-10	inducible protein-10
IC_{50}	50% inhibitory concentration
IFN	interferon
IL	interleukin
JAK-STAT	Janus kinase/signal transducers and activators of transcription
KA	kala-azar
kDNA	kinetoplast DNA
LRV1	*Leishmania* RNA virus
LAP	leucyl aminopeptidase
LPG	lipophosphoglycan
LPS	lipopolysaccharide
LIT1	*Leishmania* Fe transporter 1
LDLs	low density lipoproteins
MCP-1	macrophage chemotactic protein 1
MIP-1α	macrophage inflammatory protein 1α

Mg	magnesium
MHC	major histocompatibility complex
MI	micellar
MILT	miltefosine
M	mitochondrial
MAPK	mitogen-activated protein kinase
MAPKs	mitogen-activated protein kinases
MPS	monocyte phagocyte system
M	monomers
MPEO–PLA	monomethoxypoly(ethylene oxide)–poly(lactic acid)
MCL	mucocutaneous leishmaniasis
MyD88	myeloid differentiation protein 88
NK	natural killer
nNOS/NOS_1	neuronal or
NADH	nicotinamide adenine dinucleotide
NADPH	nicotinamide adenine dinucleotide phosphate
NO	nitric oxide
NSAO	nonsoluble aggregation of oligomers
$NSAID_s$	nonsteroidal anti-inflammatory drugs
NF-κB	nuclear factor-kappaB
ODN	oligonucleotides
ODC	ornithine decarboxylase
PAR	paromomycin
As(V)	pentavalent arsenate
PXNs	peroxidoxins
PRX	peroxiredoxin
PACA	polyalkylcyanoacrylate
PEG	polyethylene glycol
PCR	polymerase chain reaction
PMNs	polymorphonuclear neutrophils
PKDL	post-kala-azar dermal leishmaniasis
KCl	potassium chloride
PKC	protein kinase C
PGE2	prostaglandin E2
PPG	proteophosphoglycan
RNS	reactive nitrogen species
ROS	reactive oxygen species
GSH	reduced glutathione
RSV	respiratory syncytial virus
RES	reticuloendothelial system

sAP	secreted acid phosphatase
Se	selenium
Sec or U	selenocysteine
SASO	self-associated soluble oligomers
SRES	slow release emulsified suspension
siRNA	small interfering RNA
SLNs and NLPs	solid and nanostructured lipid nanoparticles
SAARC	South Asian Association for Regional Cooperation
T[SH2]	specific trypanothione
SAG	super antigens
SOD	superoxide dismutase
TTO	tea tree oil
TDR1	thiol-dependent reductase
Th1	T-helper 1
TLRs	toll-like receptors
TLR3	toll-like receptor 3
TGF	Transforming growth factor
TCA	tricarboxylic acid
TryR	trypanothione reductase
TXN	tryparedoxin
TryP	tryparedoxin peroxidase
TNF	tumor necrosis factor
TNFα	tumor necrosis factor
VEGF	vascular endothelial growth factor
V-P-K	*vata-pitta-kapha*
VL	visceral leishmaniasis
WRAIR	Walter Reed Army Institute for Research
WT	wild-type
WBCs	white blood cells
WHO	World Health Organization

PREFACE

Diseases caused by insect-borne trypanosomatid parasites are significant, yet remain a neglected public health problem. *Leishmania*, a genus of unicellular protozoan parasite is the causative organism of leishmaniasis and is transmitted by female phlebotamine sandflies affecting millions of people worldwide. Infections caused by genus *Leishmania* is a major health problem worldwide, with high endemicity in developing countries. The disease currently threatens about 350 million women, men, and children in 88 countries around the world, with about 2 million affected annually. Using an overall case-fatality rate of 10%, a tentative estimate of 20,000 to 40,000 leishmaniasis deaths per year. Leishmaniasis is one of the most important parasitic infections, but current treatments are unsatisfactory due to their toxicity, cost, and resistance. Therefore, the development of new antileishmanial compounds is imperative. In the absence of a vaccine and wake of resistance to pentavalent antimonial drugs, there is an urgent need for effective drugs to replace/supplement those in current use.

Here in this book, we are introducing various natural remedies to prevent or cure leishmaniasis. In addition, current pharmacological status including etiology, molecular epidemiology, steps involved in transmission including sandfly-*Leishmania* and *Leishmania*-macrophage interactions, glycobiology and genetics of *Leishmania donovani*, new biochemical targets for therapy in contrast with mode of action of recent chemotherapeutic agents, vaccines and adjuvants for vaccine candidates, drug resistance, pathophysiology with clinical manifestations, and development in diagnostic procedures, are also discussed. However, the primary projection of the book is toward the treatment of leishmaniasis.

The plant kingdom is undoubtedly valuable as a source of new medicinal agents. A series of ethnopharmacological surveys and reports suggested the traditional use of plants against different pathologies and interestingly, some of them presented antileishmanial activity *in vitro* and *in vivo*, possibly due to their immunostimulatory, healing, and microbicidal properties. Therefore, the selection of a single or multiple plants against the *Leishmania* parasite can be proved to be a successful approach to obtain new antileishmanial alternatives. The plant kingdom has in the past provided several affordable compounds, and therefore our book's main aim is to provide an overview of the current status of available leishmanicidal plant-derived compounds that are effective singly or in combination with conventional anti-leishmanial drugs yet are nontoxic to mammalian host cells. In addition, the book also discusses reports of the anti-leishmanian products that are obtained from marine, fresh water, bacterial, fungal, and animal sources. Furthermore alternative therapies, such as the role of traditional systems (Ayurveda, Sidha, Unani, and Tibi recommendations and prescriptions suitable for *Leishmania*), homeopathy, dietary supplementation (especially metals and vitamins intake), chelation therapy, oil therapy, acupuncture, and naturopathy are comphehensively discussed. In addition to current pharmacological update of leishmaniasis, this book covers the vast literature on natural extracts, isolated compounds, and alternative natural therapies to combat against the *Leishmania* parasite.

There is dire need to have a book on therapy of *Leishmania* that especially focuses on the natural treatments and precautions adopted to treat and prevent *Leishmania*. Students always feel the unavailability of book on such topics, hence this attempt is to fill the void of such necessity.

In addition to its focus on natural remedies, this book also deals with the comprehensive pharmacology and the current chemotherapeutic agents used against leishmaniasis. I am sure this book will serve as an important primer for students, researchers, and teachers who wish to learn traditional concepts to treat *Leishmania* in a simple way. It is my hope that this book will be useful for all undergraduate, graduate, postgraduate students, researchers, and industrialist.

We wrote this book, *Leishmaniasis: Biology, Control and New Approaches for Its Treatment*, primarily to share the up-to-date available knowledge with students, professors, researchers, and industrialists. The book has 14 chapters. All the chapters are written in a lucid way with necessary illustrations and up-to-date information so that our students become familiar with the relationship between holistic concepts and modern therapies for leishmaniasis. Errors and inaccuracies, if any, will be corrected in future editions through feedback and suggestion from readers. We earnestly believe that the book will be a valuable resource for undergraduate and postgraduate students. We are sure that the readers of this book will find it interesting.

We wish to thank Ms. Kiran Sharma for her motivation and support. We are thankful to the School of Medical and Allied Sciences, GD Goenka University,Gurgaon, India, for providing a platform to work day and night for this book to finish this book project successfully. The publication of this book would not have been possible without the valuable work of earlier researchers. This book would not have seen the light of the day without the moral support and patience of my parents. I am highly thankful to my parents and my dearest brother, Sanjay Bhatia, for his valuable suggestions and timely input.

We also thank the Publisher and President of Apple Academic Press, Ashish Kumar, for the active work and support in our effort from him and his team.

FOREWORD

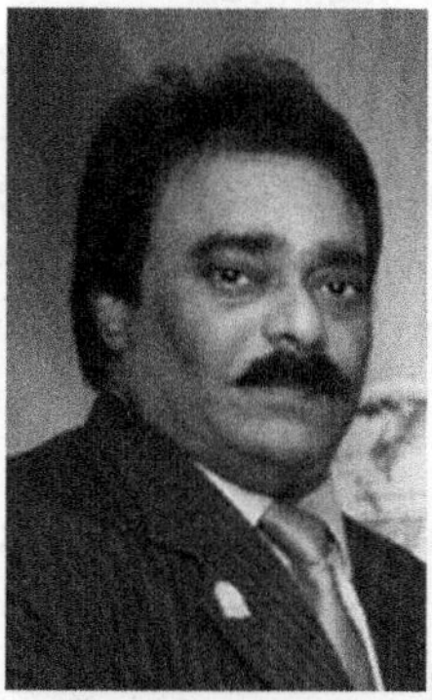

Leishmania-related illnesses remain among the world's deadliest neglected tropical diseases, affecting approximately 12 million people in 88 countries. Recent advancements have led to certain preventive treatments and cures for this disease. To add to the existing resources of information on parasitic disease, Dr. Bhatia and Dr. Divakar have conceptualized this book, titled *Leishmaniasis: Biology, Control and New Approaches for Its Treatment.* It contains a detailed account of insightful information required by a medical graduate to help one to understand the entire life cycle of the *Leishmania* parasite and its potential treatments. The content of this book helps in keeping abreast with latest developments in this field.

This book contains nine chapters that deal with Ayurveda and leishmaniasis, pharmacology of leishmaniasis, diagnosis and strategies to control leishmaniasis, immunomodulatory agents for leishmaniasis, Ayurvedic treatments for leishmaniasis, phytotherapy for leishmaniasis, elements supplementation in leishmaniasism alternative therapies for leishmaniasis, inflammation and leishmaniasis, and modern treatment for leishmaniasis. Every chapter is designed in a thematic manner with a brief classification based on habitat and site of infection. This is followed by the description of the parasite morphology, epidemiology of the disease, and pathogenesis. The clinical spectrum of the disease is described with emphasis on pathology, clinical features, and stages of the parasite that are encountered in the human host.

The book starts with Ayurvedic concepts, including various dosage forms, extraction methods, basic therapies used for the improvement of health, and various disease ailments, especially leishmaniasis, followed by an overview of the pharmacology and effective therapies used for leishmaniasis worldwide. It also has information related with diagnostic procedures for leishmaniasis, various noninvasive tests, with different specificities and sensitivities. Certain key topics, such as potential immunomodulatory agents for leishmaniasis, antimicrobial peptides with *Leishmania* and their functional role in host parasitism, visceral leishmaniasis and amphoterecin b with insight knowledge of *Leishmania*-macrophage interactions, make this book more interesting. This book is an additional source of information related with phagocytosis and potential drug delivery systems and recent advances in the development of novel chemotherapies against leishmaniasis. Key, unique, and burning topics such as Ayurvedic, acupuncture, chelation, oil therapies in leishmaniasis offer the next level of curative measures.

The discussion of treatments and control are suitably detailed for the target audience, and their rationales are thoroughly explained. This book fills an important niche and is usefully written in the broadest sense of the subject. The authors are immensely experienced and knowledgeable university teachers. This book is a valuable addition to the literature on veterinary parasitology. It will be useful to the students of the subject throughout the world.

Despite the explosion of online information available with the click of mouse, this is a handy and easy-to-read book that has been carefully conceived and crafted by experts; it will become indispensable. I congratulate Dr. Bhatia and Dr. Divakar for bringing out this reference book on leishmaniasis, and I am sure the book will find respectable space in the bookshelves of academicians, busy practitioners, and students alike.

— Professor T. V. Narayana
Secretary, Indian Pharmaceutical Congress Association;
Vice President, Indian Pharmaceutical Association

CHAPTER 1

AYURVEDA AND LEISHMANIASIS

CONTENTS

PART I AYURVEDA AND ITS POTENTIAL THERAPIES USED FOR HEALTH CARE AND DISEASE MANAGEMENT

ABSTRACT

Ayurveda's origin is critical to the development of its medical assumption. India has a rich scientific history, Ayurveda in particular dates 3500 to 5000 years ago. It is the most ancient form of medicine in India and traces back to *Lord Brahma* (the Hindu God of Creation), according to Hindu mythology. Medicinal plants forms a dominant part of Ayurvedic pharmacopoeia. Earliest references to such medicinal plants are to be found in the *Rig Veda* and *Atharva Veda*. Medicine derived from these plant drugs have been classified as per their pharmacological/therapeutic action. Various dosage forms and its preparation methods are available in Ayurvedic system of medicine. From decades, Ayurveda emphasizes on preventative and healing therapies along with various methods of purification and rejuvenation. *Panchakarma* is the cornerstone to Ayurvedic management of disease, having the potential to re-establishes the essential balance of "*Tridosha*" (three doshas: *vata, pitta,* and *kapha*) in body. Many other therapies such as *rasnaya*, yoga, and massage therapies provide positive health and improve the general health and vitality. This chapter covers the brief overview of Ayurveda, including various dosage forms, extraction methods, and basic therapies used for the improvement of health and various disease ailment especially *Leishmania.*

1.1 INTRODUCTION TO AYURVEDA

Ayurveda is derived from Ayus(r), meaning life, and Veda meaning knowledge. Combining together Ayurveda literally means the science of life, which has been utilized from ancient time by Indians for health care and longevity. It is the chief of Indian medicine originated from *Brahma.* Ayurveda aim toward the positive functioning of human system, which has been defined as well-balanced metabolism, coupled with a healthy state of being. According to Ayurveda, disease can arise from the body and mind due to external factors and intrinsic causes. Ayurveda potentially improves the human health by providing treatment in form of natural drugs, diet, and various therapies. The vast literature of Ayurveda is available in Sanskrit and other Indian languages. This literature includes all aspects of diseases, therapeutics, and pharmacy. It is a traditional system of medicine, thus difficult to comprehend in terms of modern scientific concepts.

Health plays an important role in human development. According to Ayurveda, health is defined as the state where physical body, senses, and psyche are in original or natural state with respect to body and function. All needs of the body and senses must be in balance to avoid illness and maintain good health. In Ayurveda, it is widely believed that the world is made up of five elements called *Panch mahabhuta.* These five elements are in devisable therefore designated as Panchmahabhuta. According to Ayurveda, human body is made up of somatic dosas (*vata, pita, and kapha*), body tissue (*dhatus*), psychic components (*dosas*), and waste products (*malas*). Ayurvedic concept of good health is based on the dynamic equilibrium of *doshas* (humor), *agni* (digestive fire), *dhatu* (seven body tissue: lymph, blood, muscle, adipose tissue, bone, bone marrow, and semen), and *male* (feces, urine, and other waste products). The imbalance of *vata, pitta,* or *kapha* is considered as major factor in the causation of a disease.

Vata is considered as wind that corresponds to mind and nervous system. It is regarded as the prime sustainer of life and responsible for the communication in the body. The modern Ayurvedic reports suggested that *vata* indicates the nervous system. The activity of *vata* is dependent on the transmission of acetylcholine and also in whole body at the nerve endings of the parasympathetic nerves and the peripheral nerves or voluntary muscles. Second element is *pitta,* which is considered as the fire or bile. It is also responsible for all metabolic activities and transformation including the digestion and assimilation of food as well as the clarity of thought and understanding. Its activities are closely related to sympathetic nervous system. Thus perhaps its main seat is hypothalamus, while its neuro-humor is catecholamine (adrenaline, noradrenaline, and dopamine)

1.2 MEDICINAL PLANTS IN AYURVEDA

Medicinal plants forms a dominant part of Ayurvedic pharmacopoeia. Earliest reference to such medicinal plants are to be found in the *Rig Veda* and *Atharva Veda*, dating back to second millennium B.C. *Chakra Samhita* (900 B.C.) is the first recorded treatise fully devoted to the concepts and practices of Ayurveda. Its hallmark is kayachikitsa (therapeutics).[1] This work contains 341plants and its products for use in medicine. Next is *Sushruta Samhita* (600 B.C.), who has special emphasis on surgery. It includes 395 plants, 57 drugs of animal origin, and 64 minerals and metals as therapeutic agents.

Sushruta is the father of surgery, lives, and practiced surgery in Varanasi some 2500 years ago.[2] In another words, *Charaka Samhita* deals with the etiology, symptomatology, pathology, prognosis, and medical management of disease and *Sushruta Samhita* deals with various surgical instruments and procedures.

Other mile stones of Ayurvedic medicine are mentioned as follows:

- *Vagbhatta of Sindh*: Practiced around seventh century A.D. His work *Asthnga hridya* is considered as the most popular practice of medicine. Chakra, Sushruta, and Vagbhatta are known to be the powerful triad of Ayurveda and their period of practice is considered as the golden age of Ayurveda.
- *Sarangdhara*: It is the systematic Ayurvedic *materia medica* of 14th century. His work (Sarangdhara samhita) consists of 3 parts, 32 chapters, and 2500 verses.
- *Bhava mishra of Magadha*: *Bhava prakasha* contains 10,831 verses and approximately 470 medicinal plants.
- *Nighantu Granthas* (pharmacy lexicons): *Raj Nighantu* by Nirali Pandita and *Madanpala Nighantu* by Madanpala are acknowledged as the masterpiece on medicinal plants.

1.3 AYURVEDIC CLASSIFICATION OF PLANT-BASED DRUGS

In Ayurvedic system of medicine, plant drugs have been classified as per their pharmacological/therapeutic action. The classification of plant drugs introduced by chakra is listed in Table 1-1. Various traditional drugs that are widely utilized by Ayurveda are listed in Table 1-1.

1.4 DIFFERENT TYPES OF AYURVEDIC DOSAGE FORMS

While dealing with allopathic or modern system of medicine, it is essential that a pharmacist must be familiar with current Ayurvedic dosage forms and preparation methodologies. Since large proportion of Indians (especially in rural areas) is dependent on Ayurvedic drugs, all of the Ayurvedic practitioner should be familiar with the knowledge of medicines and healing art introduced by Ayurveda. From ancient times, various pharmaceutical dosage forms have been used in Ayurvedic system of medicine and some of them are in practice even today. A simplified form of classification is mentioned in Tables 1-1 and 1-2.

TABLE 1-1 Prominent Ayurvedic classification of plant based drugs introduced by Chakra

Sanskrit name	Remarks
Balya	Promoting strength
Dipaniya	Promoting digestion
Javarahara	Febrifuge
Jivaniya	Promoting longetivity
Kasahara	Antitussive
Krmighna	Anthelmintic
Lekhaniya	Anti-obesity
Mutravirechaniya	Diuretic
Stanyajanana	Galactagogue
Svayathuhara	Anti-inflammatory
Vamaanopaga	Emetic
Vamanopaga	Purgative
Varnya	Complexion promoting
Vayahsthapana	Anti-aging
Vedansthapana	Analgesic

TABLE 1-2 Classification of different types of dosage forms available in Ayurveda

Solid	Semisolids	Liquids
Churna (powders)	*Kalka* (ointment and pastes)	Aqueous
		Swarasa (fruit juices)
		Kasaya (extracts)
		Shita kasaya (cold infusion)
		Phanta kasaya (hot infusion)
		Kwatha (decoction)
		Paniya (weak decoctions)
		Kshira-paka (milk decoctions)
		Vasti (enemas)
		Sugandhgita jala (perfumed waters)
Dhumapana (inhalations)	*Yavagu* (gruels)	Oily
		Taila (medicated oils)
		Ghrita (medicated clarified butter)
		Mantha (a kind of emulsion)

TABLE 1-2 *(Continued)*

Solid	Semisolids	Liquids
Guggulu (plant exudations)	*Avaleha* (soft extract)	Liquids
		Acetus
		Kanjika (vinegars)
		Samkhadrav (mineral acids)
		Swalpadravaka (mineral acids)
Kshara (alkalis)		Spiritous
		Sura (wines)
		Asava (tinctures)
		Arishta (tinctures)
Modaka (boluses)		
Nasua (snuff)		
Netranjan (collyria)		
Phalavarti (suppositories)		
Vatika (pills)		

1.5 EXTRACTION PROCEDURES USED TO PREPARE THESE PREPARATIONS

Most of the Ayurvedic preparations composed of two words. The first initial word indicates the diseases for which the preparation is used, the property of preparation, the drug contained, or the name of god or saint. The second word signifies the type of preparation. There are various processes used for preparations. These processes are divided in to two parts, that is, extraction and fermentation. In addition, there are various types of apparatus and procedures used for the preparation of Ayurvedic dosage forms (Table 1-3).

TABLE 1-3 Various types of apparatus and procedures used for the preparation of Ayurvedic dosage forms

Procedures	Sanskrit name	Preparation composition
Simple expression	*Swarasa*	Juice of fresh vegetable drugs
Infusion	*Kasaya*	Drug + 8 parts of cold water
	Shita kasaya (cold infusion)	
	Phanta kasaya (cold infusion)	

TABLE 1-3 *(Continued)*

Procedures	Sanskrit name	Preparation composition
Decoction	*Kwatha*	Drug + 16 parts of cold water
	Paniya (weaker decoction)	
Digestion	Similar to decoction	
Soft extract or avaleha	Concentrated decoction	
Maceration	*Bhawana*	Mineral + fresh juice decoction of several drugs = solid residue
Hot extraction	*Putapaka* (roasting method)	Drugs are coated with leaves followed by thick layer of clay and roasted in to fire
Milk decoction	*Kshirapaka*	Drug + 8 parts of milk + 32 parts of water
Medicated oils and clarified butter	*Ghee*	Drug + ghee or oil
Acetous fermentation	Method of preparation of *kanjika* (vinegar)	Fermentation of sugarcane juice
Spirituous fermentation	*Asavas* and *aristas* are prepared by this method	*Suras* or wine are prepared by this method
Confection	*Khandapaka* making	Drugs + syrup + milk or water + honey
Gruel	*Yavagu*	Drug + cereals

1.6 NATURAL THERAPIES USED TO TREAT DISEASE

Ayurveda emphasizes preventative and healing therapies along with various methods of purification and rejuvenation. Ayurveda is more than a mere healing system, it is a science and an art of appropriate living that helps to achieve longevity. It can guide every individual in the proper choice of diet, living habits, and exercise to restore balance in the body, mind, and consciousness; thus preventing disease from gaining a foothold in the system.

According to Ayurveda, every human being is a unique phenomenon (manifested through the five basic elements (ether, air, fire, water, and earth) of cosmic consciousness. *Vata* (ether plus air), *pitta* (fire plus water), and *kapha* (water plus earth) are called the *tridosha*, meaning the three humors or the three organizations of the body, which are also derived from consciousness. Every individual psycho-somatic temperament or constitution is determined by these three *doshas* at the time of fertilization. When the embryo is formed, the constitution is determined. There are seven basic constitutions according to Ayurveda: *vata, pitta, kapha, vata-pitta, pitta-kapha, kapha-vata, and vata-pitta-kapha*. Every individual constitution has its own unique balance of V-P-K according to its own nature. The balance of V-P-K is the natural order, thus when this doshic balance is disturbed, it creates imbalance, which is disorder. Health is order; disease is disorder. Within the body there is a constant interaction between order and disorder, thus once one understands the nature and structure of disorder, one can reestablish order. Ayurveda believes that order lies within disorder.

Order is the state of health, as defined by Ayurveda, which exists when the digestive fire (agni) is in a balanced condition; the bodily humors (*vata, pitta,* and *kapha*) are in equilibrium, the three waste products (urine, feces, and sweat) are produced and eliminated normally, the seven bodily tissues (*rasa, rakta, mamsa, meda, asthi, majja, and shukra*) are functioning normally, and the mind, senses, and consciousness are working harmoniously together. When the balance of these systems is disturbed, the disease (disorder) process begins.

The internal environment is governed by V-P-K, which is constantly reacting to the external environment. The wrong diet, habits, lifestyle, incompatible food combinations (e.g., milk and fish, melons and grain, yogurt and meat, or cooked honey etc.), seasonal changes, repressed emotions, and stress factors can all act either together or separately to change the balance of V-P-K. According to the nature of the cause, either *vata, pitta, or kapha* undergo aggravation or derangement that affects the *agni* (gastric fire), and produces *ama* (toxins). This *ama* enters the blood stream and is circulated throughout the body clogging the channels. Retention of toxins in the blood results in toxemia. This accumulated toxicity, once well established, will slowly affect *prana* (vital life energy), *ojas* (immunity), and *tejas* (cell metabolic energy) and result in disease. This can be nature's effort at eliminating the toxicity from the body. Every so-called disease is a crisis of *ama* toxicity. *Ama* is the basic internal cause of all disease, due to the aggravated doshas. Herein lies the key to the prevention of disease that is to help the body eliminate the toxins. To stop the further production of *ama,* Ayurvedic literature suggests putting the person on a proper diet with appropriate lifestyle, habits, and exercise, and administering a proper cleansing program such as *panchakarma*.

1.6.1 PANCHAKARMA THERAPY

Panchakarma therapy is known to be the most successful therapy in eliminating toxic materials (vitiated dosas) from the body in order to cure a disease. It was suggested in Ayurveda that the toxic materials of the body need to be eliminated radically before a palliative therapy is given. This was postulated on the basis that the palliative therapy in the form of drugs and digests may not be effective unless the body channels are properly cleansed and toxic materials are eliminated. This therapy purifies the body tissue and brings harmony of neurohumors (*tridosas*) and *mansas dosas*. *Panchakarma* therapy is widely utilized by Ayurvedic practitioners for internal purification of the body through emesis, purgation, enema, errhines, and bloodletting.[3,4] Classical procedures of panchakarma therapy involve various stages such as the following:

- Preparatory procedure: This procedure is adopted to prepare the body to undergo a proper and thorough cleansing. These are done by applying as well as ingesting oils and fats, sweating and also advising which herbs to be used to improve the digestion and metabolism in tissues.
- Main cleansing procedures: These procedures include five purification procedures (emesis, purgation, enema, errhines, and bloodletting) especially designed to eliminate toxic materials from the imbalance dosas of the body.
- Post procedures (*pashchata karma*): These procedures consists mainly recuperative measures in the form of diet, lifestyle changes, and rejuvenating herbs.

Panchkarma involves a prepurification measure called as *Purvakarma*, preparing the body to encourage the body to let go of the toxins. This procedure is applied before the actual operation of purification begins.[3,4] The two procedures are *snehan* and *swedan*. *Snehan* is the oil massage. Oil is applied to the entire body with a particular type of massage that helps the toxins to move toward the gastrointestinal tract. Oil massage also makes the superficial and deep tissues soft and supple, thus helping to remove stress and to nourish the nervous system. *Snehan* is given daily for three to seven days, as indicated.[3,4] *Swedan* is sudation or sweating and is given every day immediately following the *snehan*. An herbal concoction may be added to the steam to further loosen the toxins from the individual. *Swedan* liquefies the toxins and increases the movement of toxins into the gastrointestinal tract.[3,4] After three to seven days of *snehan* and *swedan*, the doshas become well "ripened." A particular *panchakarma* method is then given according to the individual's constitution and disorder, *prakruti* and *vikruti,* respectively. After preparatory procedure, panchakarma method involves five basic cleansing methods:

- *Vaman:* therapeutic vomiting or emesis
- *Virechan*: purgation
- *Basti*: enema
- *Nasya*: elimination of toxins through the nose
- *Raktalmoksha*: detoxification of the blood

1.6.1.1 VAMAN: EMESIS THERAPY

When there is congestion in the lungs causing repeated attacks of bronchitis, colds, cough, or asthma, the Ayurvedic treatment is therapeutic vomiting, *vaman*, to eliminate the *kapha* causing the excess mucus. First, after the *snehan* and *swedan*, three to four glasses of licorice or salt water is administered, then vomiting is stimulated by rubbing the tongue that triggers the vomiting center through the gag reflex.[3,4] Often times, this also releases repressed emotions which have been held in the *kapha* areas of the lungs and stomach along with the accumulated *dosha*. One may alternatively take two to three glasses of salt water which will also aggravate *kapha* and then rub the tongue to induce vomiting. Once the mucus is released, the patient will feel instantly relieved. It is likely that congestion, wheezing, and breathlessness will disappear and that the sinuses will become clear. Therapeutic vomiting is also indicated in chronic asthma, diabetes, chronic cold, lymphatic congestion, chronic indigestion, and edema.

1.6.1.2 EMETIC SUBSTANCES

Emetic substances madan—emetic nut, madhuka-yastimadhu—licorice, neem—bitter leaf, bimbi, kutaj-kurchi—conessi bark, murva—clematis, triloba-devdaru—deodar, *Cedrus deodara*, Salt—NaCl, ela—cardamom, nux vomica.[3,4]

After *vaman*, resting, fasting, smoking certain herbal cigarettes, and not suppressing natural urges (i.e., urination, defecation, gas, sneezing, coughing) is recommended. If *vaman* is administered properly, the person should feel relaxation in the lungs, will be able to breathe freely, will have lightness in the chest, clear thinking, clear voice, a good appetite, and all symptoms of congestion disappear.

1.6.1.3 VIRECHAN: PURGATION THERAPY

When excess bile, *pitta*, is secreted and accumulated in the gall bladder, liver, and small intestine; it tends to result in rashes, skin inflammation, acne, chronic attacks of fever, biliary vomiting, nausea, and jaundice. In these conditions, Ayurvedic literature suggests the administration of therapeutic purgation or a therapeutic laxative. *Virechan* is facilitated with senna leaves, flax seeds, psyllium husks, or *triphala* in a combination that is appropriate for the individual person.[3,4]

Senna leaf tea is a mild laxative, but in people of *vata* constitution, this might create griping pain, since its action aggravates peristaltic movement in the large intestine.

An effective laxative for *vata* or *pitta* constitutions is a glass of hot milk to which two teaspoons of ghee have been added. This laxative, taken at bedtime will help to relieve the excess *pitta* causing the bile disturbance in the body. In fact, purgatives can completely cure the problem of excess *pitta*.

When purgatives are used, it is important to check the diet. The patient should not eat foods that will aggravate the predominant humor or cause the three humors to become unbalanced.

1.6.1.4 BASTI: ENEMA THERAPY

Vata's predominant site is the colon.[3,4] Ayurvedic *basti* involves the introduction into the rectum of herbal concoctions of sesame oil, and certain herbal preparations in a liquid medium. *Basti* is the most effective treatment of *vata* disorders, although many enemas over a prescribed period of time are usually required. It relieves constipation, distention, chronic fever, cold, sexual disorders, kidney stones, heart pain, backache, sciatica, and other pains in the joints. Many other *vata* disorders such as arthritis, rheumatism, gout, muscle spasms, and headaches may also be treated with *basti*. *Vata* is a very active principle in pathogenesis. If we can control *vata* through the use of *basti*, we have gone a long way in going to the root cause of the vast majority of diseases. *Vata* is the main etiological factor in the manifestation of diseases. It is the motive force behind the elimination and retention of feces, urine, bile, and other excreta. *Vata* is mainly located in the large intestine, but bone tissue (*asthi dhatu*) is also a site for *vata*. Hence, the medication administered rectally effects *asthi dhatu*. The mucus membrane of the colon is related to the outer covering of the bones (*periosteum*), which nourishes the bones. Therefore, any medication given rectally goes into the deeper tissues, such as bones, and corrects *vata* disorders.

1.6.1.5 NASYA: NASAL ADMINISTRATION

The nose is the doorway to the brain and it is also the doorway to consciousness. The nasal administration of medication is called *nasya*.[3,4] An excess of bodily humors accumulated in the sinus, throat, nose, or head areas is eliminated by means of the nearest possible opening, the nose.

Prana, life force as nerve energy, enters the body through the breath taken in through the nose. *Prana* is in the brain and maintains sensory and motor functions. *Prana* also governs mental activities, memory, concentration, and intellectual activities. Deranged *prana* creates defective functioning of all these activities and produces headaches, convulsions, loss of memory, and reduced sensory perception. Thus nasal administration, *nasya* is indicated for *prana* disorders, sinus congestion, migraine headaches, convulsions, and certain eye and ear problems.

Breathing also can be improved through nasal massage. For this treatment, the little finger is dipped into ghee and inserted into the nose. The inner walls of the nose are slowly massaged, going as deeply as possible. This treatment will help to open the emotions. (Nose tissue is tender and for this application the fingernail must be kept short to avoid injuring the delicate mucus membranes.) Since most people have deviated nasal septums, one side of the nose will be easier to penetrate and massage than the other. The finger should not be inserted forcibly. The massage should proceed by slow penetration, the finger moving first in a clockwise, then counterclockwise direction. By this means, the emotions that are blocked in the respiratory tract will be released. One may use this treatment each morning and evening. In this way, breathing patterns will change as the emotions are released and the eyesight also will improve.

1.6.1.6 RAKTAMOKSHA

Raktamoksha is the traditional Ayurvedic method for the purification and cleansing of the blood.[3,4] Toxins present in the gastrointestinal tract are absorbed into the blood and circulated throughout the body. This condition is called toxemia, which is the basic cause of repeated infections, hypertension, and certain other circulatory conditions. This includes repeated attacks of skin disorders such as urticaria, rashes, herpes, eczema, acne, scabies, leukoderma, chronic itching, or hives. In such conditions, along with internal medication, the elimination of toxins and purification of the blood are necessary. *Raktamoksha* is also indicated for the cases of enlarged liver, spleen, and gout.

Pitta is produced from the disintegrated red blood cells in the liver. So *pitta* and blood have a very close relationship. An increase in *pitta* may go into the blood causing toxicity resulting in many *pittagenic* disorders.

Extracting a small amount of blood from a vein relieves the tension created by the *pittagenic* toxins in the blood. Bloodletting also stimulates the spleen to produce antitoxic substances that helps to stimulate the immune system. Toxins are neutralized enabling radical cures in many blood-born disorders.

Bloodletting is contraindicated in cases of anemia, edema, extreme weakness, diabetes, and in children and elderly persons. It is also an illegal procedure within the United States.

Certain substances such as sugar, salt, yogurt, sour tasting foods, and alcohol are toxic to the blood. In certain blood disorders, these substances should be avoided to keep the blood pure. Burdock root tea, sandalwood, saffron, manjista, guduchi, rose, and lotus are herbs that help to purify the blood. Turmeric, goldenseal, pomegranate juice, neem, oranges, beets, and raisins can also be beneficial for blood disorders.

For *raktamoksha* treatment other than bloodletting, there are blood-purifying practices involving herbs, gem therapy, or color water therapy.

For blood-purifying therapy, look for substances that are bitter and astringent and have blood thinning properties. Burdock root tea is the best blood purifier. For blood carried disorders such as allergy, rash, or acne; the patient should take a milk laxative and the next evening begin burdock root tea therapy. The tea is made from one teaspoon of powder in one cup of hot water. If taken every night, the action of the herb will begin to purify the blood.

1.6.2 RASNAYA THERAPY

Rasnaya (rasa: nutrition; ayana: transportation in the body) therapy provides a positive health by improving the transportation of nutritional materials to the body tissue.[5] This therapy is based on the providing optimum nutritional value or overall balanced diet to improve the vitality, rejuvenate body tissues, improve immunity, and prevent aging. They refer to compound preparations containing multiple herbs and minerals that act by improving the nutritional value of the food, digestion, absorption of nutrients, transportation of nutrients to tissues, bioavailability, and metabolism of nutrients, immunity and clean the microcirculatory channels or pores. In modern Ayurveda, they are referred as dietary supplements.

1.6.3 YOGA THERAPY

Yoga is not only used as a therapy but also to improve the general health and vitality. Yoga defined as the inhibition of fluctuations of consciousness. In effect, it has the potential to restrains the mental activity. Mind in total is composed of three faculties: brain, intellect, and ego. Yoga teaches the means by which the mind is controlled and redirected in to constructive channels. It is a psycho-somatic-spiritual discipline for achieving union and harmony between our mind, body, and soul and the ultimate union of our individual consciousness with the universal consciousness.[6] *Pranayama* is derived from two Sanskrit words, namely, *prana* that means vital force or life energy, *ayama* means to prolong.[7]

1.6.4 MASSAGE THERAPY

Vital points exist where muscle, cartilage, nerves, and bones join each other. The life energies are believed to be concentrated at these points.[8] Manipulation and massage of these points have been used in Ayurveda to treat diseases and strengthen the body. Ayurvedic massage is the combination of massage with medicinal oils and acupressure. Since lipohillic materials can be easily absorbed through skin, medicated oil can be very effective therapy. Specific medicated oils and types of strokes are chosen based on the disturbed dosas, body constitution, injury, and disease condition. Contraindications for massage therapy are fever, indigestion, and patients undergoing cleansing processes. Massage is also advised for healthy people to maintain their health and relative muscular fatigue.

1.6.5 DIETARY MANAGEMENT AND LIFESTYLE CHANGES

These interventions can be initiated according to the disturbed doses and the physical and mental constitution of a person. This may include yoga, exercise, removing of stress, worries, and by spiritual nurturing. If *vata* is disturbed, then diet would include oils, butter, and sweet food.[8] If *kapha* disturbed, the diet would include bitter, sour, vinegary, spicy, and dry food. If *kapha* were disturbed, the diet would include mild tasting food grains, lentils and moderate amount of sweet and oils. Healthy life style is very important to maximize the effect of pallitative treatment. Ayurveda strongly recommends the patient to do regular sleeping schedule (8 hours), do regular exercise, and eat breakfast. Exercise is likely to create a need for nutrients inside the cells. It is believed to open up the microchannels (shrotas) in the body cell for nutrients and for medicine to enter.

1.7 FORMULAS AND VARIOUS DOSAGE FORMS

The drug treatment in Ayurveda primarily consists of herbal formulas. A single herb is rarely administered to a patient. Usually an herbal formula is made up of several herbs. These herbs are prescribed with various minerals and food articles such as milk, ghee, honey, etc. these formulas are designed to mitigate the toxicity, to increase the absorption of certain ingredients, synergistic affect, and counterbalancing effects of drug. Sometime none of the herbs in a formula exhibit therapeutic affects individually, but the formula could nevertheless be effective. Various Ayurvedic preparations are mentioned in Ayurvedic formulary of India. These preparations are prepared by using various classical protocols. Various apparatus such as *Dolayantrum (or dolo or doli), svedaniyantrum, dhupayantram, patanayantram, adhaspatanayantram, tiryakapathanyantram, vidyadharyaantram, putas, mahaputa, musha,* and *hamspakayantram* are used in Ayurvedic pharmacy from ancient time. Various types of dosage forms are briefly described as follows[9,10]:

- *Asava* and *arista*: These are medical preparations made by soaking the drugs either in powder form or in the form of decoction (*kasaya*), in a solution of sugar or jiggery, for a specified period of time. During this proves, fermentation takes place and alcohol is generated that facilitates the extraction of active principles contained in the drugs. The alcohol so generated serves as a preservative.

- *Arka*: It is a liquid preparation obtained by the distillation of certain liquids or drugs soaked in water using any convenient distillation apparatus.
- *Avaleha*: It is a semisolid preparation of drugs prepared with the addition of jiggery or sugar candy and boiled with prescribed drug juice or decoction.
- *Kwatha churna*: Certain drugs or combination of drugs are made in to coarse powder (*javkuf*) and kept for preparation of *kasaya*.
- *Guggulu*: It is an exudates obtained from the plant *Commiphora mukul.*
- *Ghrita*: It is a preparation in which ghee is boiled with prescribed *kasayas* (decoction) and *kalkas* of drugs according to the formula.
- *Churna*: It is a fine powder of drug or combination of drugs.
- *Taila:* It is the preparations in which tail is boiled with prescribed *kasayas* and *kalkas* of drugs according to the formula.
- *Dravaka*: They are liquid preparations obtained from *lavanas* and *ksharas* by *tiryakapatna* (distillation) process with or without addition of any fluids.
- *Lavana-kshara: Ksharas* are alkaline substances obtained from the ash of the drugs.
- *Lepa*: medicines in the form of a paste used for external application are called as *Lepas.*
- *Vati* and *gutika*: Medicine prepared in the form of tablets or pills are known as *vati* and *gutika*. These are made from one or more drugs of plant, animal, or mineral origin.
- *Vartti-netrabindu* and *anjana*: Medicines used externally for the eye fall under the category of *vartii, netrabindu, and anjana.*
- *Sattva*: It is a water extractable solid substance collected from a plant.
- *Kupipakva rasayana*: Drugs of mineral.

Ayurvedic therapeutics is based on the five pharmacological principles (*panchsheel*) of the drug. These principles are the following[9,10]:

- *Rasa*: It gives only taste (*dravya*), but may indicate the properties and actions of drug.
- *Guna*: They are certain physical attributes of drug that affect the *tridosha*. Effect of *guna* of drug supersedes in *rasa.*
- *Vipaka*: The end product of all digestive transformations of drug is *vipaka*. It is also called as *nisthapaka.*

- *Virya*: It indicates potency of drug and shows two intrinsic properties, including *Sita virya* and *Ushna virya. Virya* influences the balance of *tridosha*.
- *Prabhava*: The pharmacological principle indicates specific power of a drug. It is characterized by chemical composition and site of action of a drug. *Prabhava* can be compared with pharmaco-therapeutic action of the drug.

1.8 NATURAL REMEDIES FOR *LEISHMANIA*

Leishmaniasis, a vector-borne disease caused by an intramacrophage protozoa, *Leishmania* (Order: Kinetoplastidae, Family: Trypanosomatidae, Genus: *Leishmania*) is generally transmitted by sandflies, either *Phlebotomus* (old world). It comprises a group of diseases caused by several species of *Leishmania* and expresses a variety of clinical symptoms.[11,12] It is regarded as a major public health problem, causing significant morbidity and mortality in Africa, Asia, and Latin America. In addition, this group of diseases is the third largest among infectious diseases transmitted by vectors, behind malaria and filariasis. World Health Organization (WHO) classified leishmaniasis as a category 1 disease, that is, emerging and uncontrollable disease. The disease endemicity extends to over 88 countries, the major group (n = 72) belonging to the developing world while 13 belongs to the category of least developed countries; sadly, its public health impact remains grossly neglected.[11,12] The disease currently threatens about 350 million women, men, and children in 88 countries around the world, with about 2 million affected annually. In Brazil, studies report the occurrence of about 20,000 new cases of the illness annually. An increase in the incidence of leishmaniasis can be associated with urban development, forest devastation, environmental changes, and migrations of people to areas where the disease is endemic. Leishmaniasis occurs mainly in three clinical forms, of which visceral leishmaniasis (VL) or kala-azar caused by *Leishmania donovani* is the most severe form. The estimated annual incidence of VL is around 500,000 in 61 countries with 90% of these cases confined to five countries namely India, Bangladesh, Nepal, Sudan, and North Eastern Brazil. Species of the genus *Leishmania*, a protozoan member of the hemoflagellate group, are the causative agents of human leishmaniasis, which has a reservoir in rodents, dogs, saguins, marsupials, and others in the wild animal population, and is transmitted by mosquitoes of the genera *Lutzomia* and *Phlebotomus*. The term leishmaniasis comprises three clearly distinguishable clinical manifestations: generalized visceral infection (visceral leishmaniasis or "'*Kala-azar*"), cutaneous leishmaniasis (Oriental button), and mucocutaneous leishmaniasis (ulceration of the skin and hyperdevelopment of the mucous membranes).[11,12] Members of the genus *Leishmania* differentiate from proliferative promastigotes in the sandfly vector gut to infective metacyclic promastigotes in the insect foregut. Parasites are inoculated by the vector as the flagellate promastigotes enter the mammalian host, where they infect macrophages, differentiating into nonmotile. The mechanisms by which visceral and cutaneous manifestations develop have not been fully clarified. The life cycle of *Leishmania* begins with a bite of the female sandfly that feeds on the vertebrate host and imbibes blood; once in the host, promastigotes are transformed into amastigotes within phagocytic cells. While in the mammalian system, amastigotes multiply such that phagocytic cells eventually rupture to further infect other cells, thus sustaining their survival. *Leishmania* have the capability to withstand, inhibit or circumvent the microbicidal activity of host macrophages, by subverting induction of both innate and adaptive immune responses by mediating an imbalance of T helper cells. The treatment of leishmaniasis is difficult because of the intramacrophagic location of the infectious form. Victims of this illness present an immune deficiency and are not able to eliminate the parasites through a natural mechanism of defense. Moreover, malnutrition is associated with certain cases of leishmaniasis. Parallel infection with diseases such as malaria and pneumonia increases the fatality of the illness if it is not diagnosed and treated in time. The problem of leishmaniasis has been worsened by the evolution of AIDS due to parallel infections in AIDS patients, as well as by the development of drug resistance by parasites. In the absence of a vaccine, there is an urgent need for effective drugs to replace/supplement those in current use. The clinically used drugs, many of which are based on pentavalent antimony compounds, were developed before 1959. The toxicity of these agents and the persistence of side effects even after modification of the dose level and duration of treatment are, however, severe drawbacks. The search for antileishmanial agents has been exhaustive. Alternative drugs, such as amphotericin B and pentamidine, also have unpleasant side effects.[11,12] On the other hand, plant extracts or plant-derived compounds are likely to provide a valuable source of new medicinal agents and the urgent need for alternative treatments has led to a program to screen natural products for potential use in the therapy of leishmaniasis.[11,12] Therefore, there is an urgent need for new, less toxic, safe, effective, and economically feasible drugs for the treatment of leishmaniasis. The researchers therefore have diverted their attention toward plant kingdom, which are ecofriendly and cost-effective. The use of secondary metabolites from certain plants were effective in in vitro studies on different forms of *Leishmania sp*., demonstrating the feasibility of obtaining new combating compounds against the parasite. Plants and their extracts have been used traditionally against different pathologies; and in some poor regions, they are the only therapeutic source for treatments and the presence of specific active secondary metabolites can be accounted for the amelioration of clinical status of suffering individual. Furthermore alternative therapies, such as role of traditional systems (*Ayurveda, sidha, unani,* and *tibi* recommendations and prescriptions suitable for leishmania), homeopathy, dietary supplementation (especially metals and vitamins intake), chelationa therapy, oil therapy, acupuncture, and naturopathy are comprehensively discussed (Figure 1-1). A series of ethnopharmacological surveys and reports suggested the traditional use of plants against different pathologies and interestingly, some of them presented antileishmanial activity *in vitro* and *in vivo*, possibly due to their immunostimulatory, healing and microbicidal properties. However, holistic concepts based alternative therapies, such as role of traditional systems (*Ayurveda, sidha, unani,* and *tibi* recommendations and prescriptions suitable for leishmania), homeopathy, dietary supplementation (especially

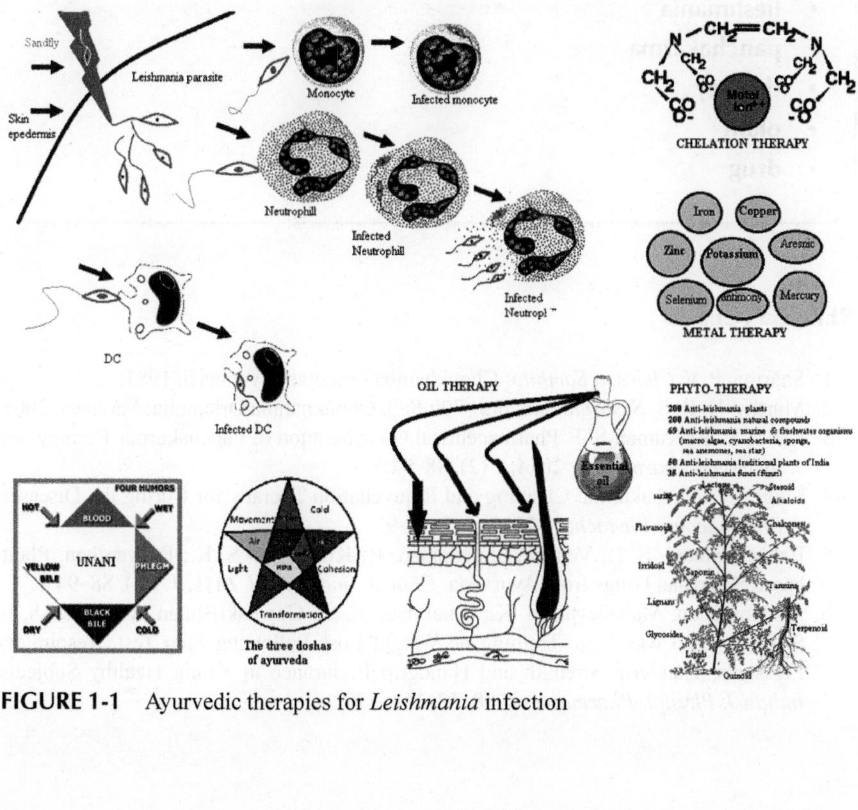

FIGURE 1-1 Ayurvedic therapies for *Leishmania* infection

metals and vitamins intake), chelation therapy, oil therapy, acupuncture, and naturopathy. The extracts or secondary metabolites presented in plants and role of alternative therapies that might be capable of modifying these pathological conditions can be attractive candidates in the development of new chemo-therapeuticals against leishmaniasis. In fact, the WHO advocated the use of traditional medicine where appropriate health services are inaccessible. Furthermore, the leads obtained from the search for natural products with antileshmanial activity give new impetus for obtaining valuable synthetic compounds. With the objective of contributing to these studies, a literature search on the use of natural products (crude plant extracts, semi-purified fractions, and chemically defined molecules), which have already been evaluated particularly for leishmaniasis, has been carried out.

KEYWORDS

- **Ayurveda**
- **dosage forms**
- **lieshmania**
- **panchakarma**
- **therapy**
- **plant**
- **drug**

REFERENCES

1. Sharma, P. V. *Charaka Samhita*; Choukhamba Orientalia: Varanasi, 1981.
2. Murthy, K. R. S. *Sushruta Samhita (700 BC)*. Choukhamba Orientalia: Varanasi, 2005.
3. Kanti, K. P.; Kumar, S. P. Pharmaceutical Consideration of Panchakarma Therapy. *Int. J. Ayurveda Pharma Res.* **2014,** *2* (2), 88–94.
4. Singh, N. Panchakarma: Cleaning and Rejuvenation Therapy for Curing the Diseases. *J. Pharmacogn. Phytochem.* **2012,** *1* (2), 1–9.
5. Balasubramani, S. P.; Venkatasubramanian, P.; Kukkupuni S. K.; Patwardhan. Plant-based Rasayana Drugs from Ayurveda. *Chin. J. Integr. Med.* **2011,** *17* (2), 88–94.
6. Madanmohan; Mahadevan, S. K.; Balakrishnan, S.; Gopalakrishnan, M.; Prakash, E. S. Effect of 6 wks Yoga Training on Weight Loss Following Step Test, Respiratory Pressures, Handgrip Strength and Handgrip Endurance in Young Healthy Subjects. *Indian J. Physiol. Pharmacol.* **2008,** *52*, 164–170.

7. Tandon, O. P. Yoga and its applications. In *Best and Taylor's Physiological Basis of Medical Practice*; Tandon, O. P., Tripathi, Y., Eds. Wolters Kluwer health/Lippincott Williams and Wilkins publishers: Gurgaon, 2012; 13th ed.; pp 1217–1230.
8. Tabish, S. A. Complementary and Alternative Healthcare: Is it Evidence-based? *Int. J. Health Sci. (Qassim)*. **2008,** *2* (1), V–IX.
9. Mallick, A.; Kaur, A.; Das, M. Shelf Life Period of Ayurvedic Medicine in Context to Ancient and Modern Literature. *Int. J. Pharm.* **2013,** *2* (3), 43–46.
10. Arun, N.; Kadibagil, V. R.; Ganti, B. Y. Various Dosage forms of Ayurveda. *Unique J. Ayurvedic Herbal Med.* **2014,** *02* (04), 20-23.
11. Passero, L. F. D.; Laurenti, M. D.; Santos-Gomes, G.; Campos, B. L. S.; Sartorelli, P.; Lago, J. H. G. Plants Used in Traditional Medicine: Extracts and Secondary Metabolites Exhibiting Antileishmanial Activity. *Curr. Clin. Pharmacol.* **2014,** *9* (3),1–17.
12. Sonika; Mahor S.; Chadha, H.; Tripathi, S.; Vaibhav, P. S.; Upadhyay, M. Leishmaniasis: An Appraisal of Current Medications and Potential Natural Sources. *IJCPS*. **2013,** *1* (7), 473–481.

CHAPTER 2

PHARMACOLOGY OF LEISHMANIASIS

CONTENTS

PART II PHARMACOLOGY OF LEISHMANIASIS

ABSTRACT

Current *Leishmania* research attracts drug candidates, delivery systems, and vaccines to explore the more reliable therapy without inducing any side effects and resistance. Clinical manifestation and early diagnosis can prevent the progression of *Leishmania*. For such an effective treatment, profound understanding related with pathogen genetics, etiology, epidemiology, glycobiology, transmission, fly–*Leishmania*, and *Leishmania*–macrophage interactions is required. In addition, an exploration of biochemical targets and mechanism of action of antileishmanian drugs provide more clarity for an effective therapy. Covering these issues, this chapter overviews the pharmacology and effective therapies used for *Leishmania* worldwide.

2.1 INTRODUCTION

An exploration of effective therapy against *Leishmania* is still in pipeline. Apart from the classic treatments of leishmaniasis (pentavalent antimony), only a few new drugs have been introduced over the years as second-line therapy in the case of antimonial failure. Complete knowledge of genome sequences and metabolomics of prominent strains such as *Leishmania major*, and *Leishmania infantum*, and *L. brasiliensis* genomes, facilitate the identification of suitable drug targets. This chapter describes the etiology and molecular epidemiology of deadliest infection caused by the pathogen known as *Leishmania*. In addition, this chapter also describes the transmission mode and glycobiology of *Leishmania* pathogen. Interactions of *Leishmania* with vector called as sandfly and host macrophage were also described. For developing the suitable therapy, it is essential to explore biochemical targets of the pathogen. Various biochemical targets were explored with a brief outlook of current therapies and their respective drug delivery systems (DDSs) used for the treatment against *Leishmania*. Chemotherapeutic treatments for leishmaniasis exist but are expensive, toxic, and ineffective against resistant strains. This requires the development of vaccines against several pathogenic *Leishmania* strains. According to various reports, vaccines can also known to be an effective therapy against leishmaniasis especially among those individuals that were once infected become resistant to clinical infection when later exposed. There is still no antileishmanial vaccine and despite the identification of a multitude of novel drug candidates, none of these are currently undergoing clinical evaluation. Recent advances in our understanding of parasite biology and immunity have not translated to measurable clinical outcomes. Evaluation of clinical features of a patients suffering from *Leishmania* by history and physical examination can also proved to be good strategy to discover effective therapy at particular stage of infection. The clinical manifestations of *Leishmania* vary with geography, epidemiology, immunity, and age. Evaluation of clinical factors can prevent the progression of disease and allows the selection of effective therapy against leishmaniansis.

2.2 ETIOLOGY

Leishmaniasis is a group of infectious diseases caused by species of *Leishmania* genus. Various species of *Leishmania* parasite are reported that are transmitted by mosquito bites. This transmission can cause cutaneous leishmaniasis (CL); mucocutaneous leishmaniasis (MCL; also known as espundia); visceral leishmaniasis (VL; also known as kala-azar); and diffuse leishmaniasis in humans, dogs, and various wild vertebrate hosts. Transmission of this parasite is achieved by 30 species of sandfly and essentially requires two different hosts: an invertebrate insect vector, *Phlebotomus* (in the Old World) or Luztomiya (in the New World) sandfly-mosquito and a vertebrate host (human, dog, or even a wild vertebrate).[1] Leishmaniasis continues to be one of the six entities on the World Health Organization (WHO)tropical disease list affecting more than 12 million people with more than 400,000 (300,000 of CL and 100,000 of VL) new cases worldwide per year and with growing tendency.[2] Leishmaniasis is prevalent in tropical and temperate regions of world, ranging from rainforests in Central and South America to deserts in West Asia and the Middle East. It is prevalent in 88 countries throughout the world (21 in the New World and 66 in the Old World; 16 of them are developed countries and the other 72 are developing countries).[3] More than 90% of the visceral conditions produced by *Leishmania donovani* are registered in India, Bangladesh, Indonesia, and Sudan. The VL has an estimated incidence of 500,000 new cases and 60,000 deaths each year with more than 90 % of cases are centralized to India, Bangladesh, Nepal, Sudan, and Brazil.[4] *Leishmania* and its prevalence in various countries are highlighted in Table 2-1.

TABLE 2-1 Affected nations and their respective Leismania strains[1]

Sr. No.	Parasite	Affected countries	References
1	*Leishmania donovani*	India, Bangladesh, Indonesia, and Sudan	Anonymous 1997
2	*Leishmania majoris*	Iran, Saudi Arabia, Syria, and Afghanistan	Anonymous 1997
3	*Leishmania mexicanais*	Brazil and Peru	Anonymous 1997
4	*Leishmania tropica* and *Leishmania infantum*	Southern European countries, including France, Italy, Portugal, and Spain	Anonymous 1997
5	*Leishmania panamiensis* and *Leishmania braziliensis*	Central and South American countries	Anonymous 1997

WHO has considered leishmaniasis to be one of the six priority diseases of its special program for research and training in tropical diseases.[2] Owing to the presence of the kinetoplast mitochondrion and other tryponosomal features, the *Leishmania* are protozoa belonging to the order Kinetoplastida and family Trypanosomatidae (Figure 2-1)

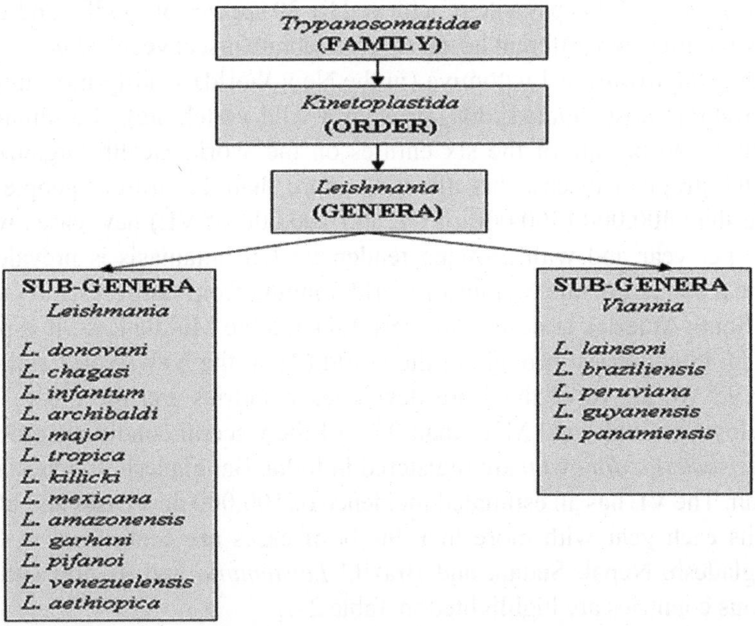

FIGURE 2-1 *Leishmania* parasite classification.[6]

Leishmania spp. essentially requires two different hosts to complete its biological cycle: (1) an invertebrate insect vector, generally females of *Phlebotomus* (in the Old World) or Luztomiya (in the New World) sandfly mosquito and (2) a definitive host, human, dog, or even a wild vertebrate. These sandflies (Diptera: Psychodidae: Phlebotominae) are the main vectors of leishmaniasis, a multi-spectrum disease ranging from self-healing skin lesions to fatal visceral illness. During its life within the sandfly vector, *Leishmania* undergo a complex developmental process, mainly restricted to the midgut, in which the parasites must overcome several documented difficulties. Both parasite and vector achieve a balance that involves significant interplay. In one end, for its survival, *Leishmania* strives to manipulate aspects of the physiology of the sandfly, interfering with digestive proteases,[5] secreting a myoinhibitory peptide that arrests hindgut peristalsis,[5] and causing significant damage to the stomodeal valve (or cardia) of the fly.[5]

Leishmania are the obligate intracellular parasites existing in two morphologic forms: promastigotes and amastigotes. These two forms are morphologically and biochemically different. The insect form, called a promastigote, is a motile parasite closely resembling a hemoflagellate. A promastigote that is found in the digestive tract of sandfly displays one flagellum attached to a mitochondrial-like organelle, called a kinetoplast that contains intertwined circular DNA that are repetitive chains of ring DNA called kinetoplast DNA and DNA (kDNA) molecules known as maxicircles and minicircles. The small, round to oval bodies called amastigotes are the noninfective *Leishmania* parasites that are occurring in monocytes, polymorphonuclear leucocytes, or endothelial cells of vertebrates (hosts) whereas promastigotes represent the infective stage in sandfly (vector). When infected female mosquito bite, promastigotes are rapidly phagocytized by reticular endothelium macrophages, within which the organisms are transformed into the rounded nonmotile form called amastigote. Except for some species of *Leishmania* that have been grown axenically, amastigotes are obligate intramacrophage-phagolysosome microorganisms. Multiplication of amastigotes within the phagolysosomes of macrophages of the skin, mucosa, and viscera gives rise to CL, MCL, and VL, respectively.

2.3 MOLECULAR EPIDEMIOLOGY

Leishmaniasis is caused by protozoan parasites belonging to the genus *Leishmania*, which is further divided into two subgenera, *Leishmania* and *Viannia* and transmitted by female phlebotomine sandflies. Surveillance of the prevalence of *Leishmania* and responsive vector species in endemic and surrounding areas is important for predicting the risk and expansion of the disease. Molecular biological methods are now widely applied to epidemiological studies of infectious diseases including leishmaniasis. These techniques are used to detect the natural infections of sandfly vectors with *Leishmania* protozoa and are becoming powerful tools due to their sensitivity and specificity. Recently, genetic analyses have been performed on sandfly species and genotyping using polymerase chain reaction-restriction fragment length polymorphism has been applied to the sandfly taxonomy. In addition, a molecular mass screening method has been established that enables both sandfly species and natural leishmanial infections to be identified simultaneously in hundreds of sandflies with limited effort. Approximately 20 *Leishmania* species are known to be pathogenic to humans, and the species is the major determinant of clinical outcome (cutaneous, mucocutaneous, and visceral forms).[52]

2.4 TRANSMISSION

The *Leishmania* promastigotes are transmitted by sandfly to vertebrate hosts, for example, canines, marsupials, edentates, and rodents. Once inside the bloodstream of reservoirs for the disease, promastigotes are phagocytosed by the mononuclear phagocytic cells and are transformed to amastigotes by losing their flagella that multiply by means of binary fission. Entry of promastigotes into host macrophages involves multiple parasite–host interactions such as the recognition of specific ligands on the parasite cell surface by receptors on the macrophage cell surface. A number of studies toward understanding the molecular mechanisms of parasite entry have led to the identification of several candidate receptors facilitating multiple routes of entry there by highlighting the redundancy in the entry process. These include membrane proteins present on the macrophage cell surface such as the mannose-fucose receptor, receptor for advanced glycosylation end products, the fibronectin receptor, the Fc receptor, and complement receptors such as CR1 and CR3. The large number of different receptors responsible for the entry of the parasite into host macrophages makes it difficult to establish a unique therapeutic target for the treatment of leishmaniasis. On lyse of host cell, the free parasites spread to new cells and tissues of different organs including the spleen, liver, and bone marrow. Amastigotes in the blood as well as in the monocytes are ingested during a blood meal by female sandfly. Once ingested, the amastigotes migrate to the midgut of the sandfly and transform into the promastigotes. After a period of 4 to 5 days, promastigotes move forward to the esophagus to reach salivary glands of the sandfly. Infected sandfly during the second blood meal regurgitates the infectious promastigotes from its pharynx into the bloodstream of the host vertebrates and the life cycle is repeated.[1] Entire process of transmission as well as the life cycle of *Leishmania* parasite is illustrated in Figure 2-2.

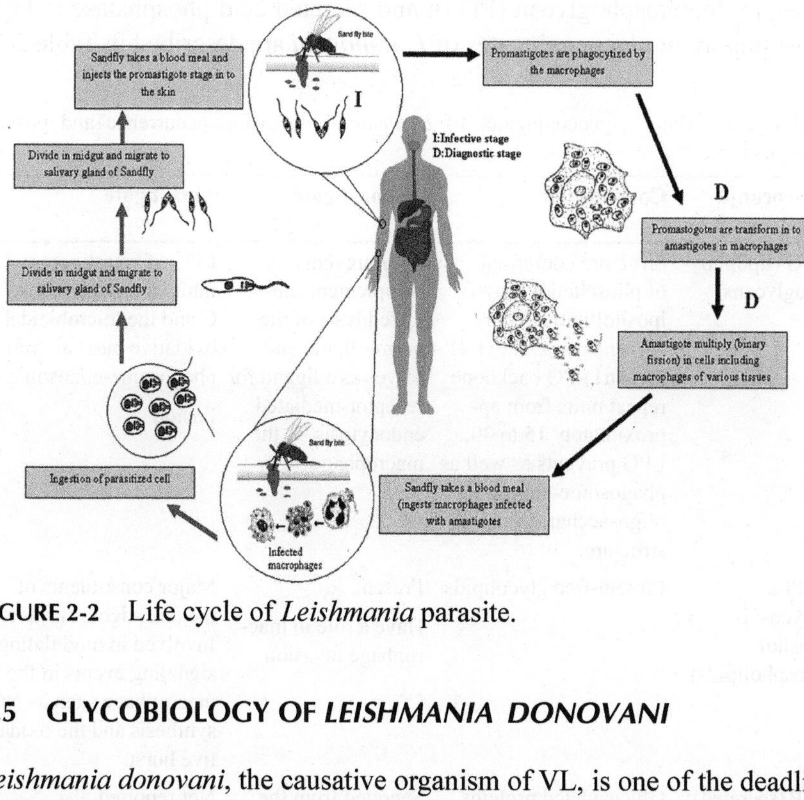

FIGURE 2-2 Life cycle of *Leishmania* parasite.

2.5 GLYCOBIOLOGY OF *LEISHMANIA DONOVANI*

Leishmania donovani, the causative organism of VL, is one of the deadliest of the entire known *Leishmania* species. This protozoan parasite displays immense adaptability to survive under extremely harsh conditions. Cell surface glycoconjugates play a pivotal role in parasite virulence and infectivity. Their survival strategies frequently involve the participation of glycoconjugates that form a protective barrier against hostile environment. In fact, a common feature of parasite cell surface architecture is the presence of an elaborate and highly decorative glycocalyx that allows the parasite to interact with and respond to its external environment.[10] Cell membrane-bound carbohydrates and sugars play a key role in parasite survival and proliferation. Most of these specialized molecules are members of a family of phosphoglycans whereas others are a family of glycoinositol phospholipids. Throughout their life cycle, *Leishmania* survive and proliferate in highly hostile environments and have evolved special mechanisms that enable them to endure these adverse conditions. To protect from such harsh conditions, one of the adaptive mechanisms includes the production of a dense cell surface the glycocalyx which is composed of lipophosphoglycan (LPG) and glycosylinositol phospholipids (GIPLs); secreted glycoconjugates, proteophosphoglycan (PPG); and secreted acid phosphatase (sAP).[10] Most important glycoconjugates of *L. donovani* are described in Table 2-2.

TABLE 2-2 Major glycoconjugates of *Leishmania donovani*: occurrence and possible biological roles[10]

Glycoconjugates	Constitution	Promastigote	Amastigote
LPG (lipophosphoglycans)	Structure composed of phosphatidyl(myo) inositollipid anchor, glycan core, Gal (β1,4) Man(α1)-PO backbone repeat units from approximately 15 to 30. LPG prevents as well as phagosome-endosome oligosaccharide cap structure	LPG prevents complement-mediated lysis of the promastigote and serves as a ligand for receptor-mediated endocytosis by the macrophage	LPG of amastigotes inhibits protein kinase C and the microbicidal oxidative burst as well as phagosome-endosome Fusion
GIPLs (glycosyl-inositol phospholipids)	Protein-free glycolipids	Present. Have a role in macrophage invasion	Major constituents of the amastigote surface. Involved in modulating signaling events in the macrophage such as NO synthesis and the oxidative burst.
sAP (secreted acid phosphatase)	Glycosylated proteins	Secreted from the flagella	Not reported
PPG	Proteophosphoglycans	GPI-anchored cell associated filamentous form termed mPPG The gel-like matrix, formed by these interlocking filaments, traps the parasites in the sandfly anterior gut	Secrete their own nonfilamentous form termed aPPG. aPPG is believed to contribute to the formation of the parasitophorous vacuole, thus participating in the maintenance of infection

TABLE 2-2 *(Continued)*

Glycoconjugates	Constitution	Promastigote	Amastigote
Phosphoglycan	(hydrophilicphosphoglycan consisting of capped oligosaccharide repeat units but minus the GPI anchor and the glycan core	Present function not yet defined.	Not reported
Sialoglycans	Sialic acid derivatives	Sialic acid derivatives present, but Neu 5Gc absent the O acetylated forms activate the classical complement pathway	Sialic acid derivatives present. Neu5Gc present. Role not yet known.

2.6 SANDFLY–*LEISHMANIA* INTERACTIONS

Sandflies (Diptera: Psychodidae: Phlebotominae) are the main vectors of leishmaniasis, a multi-spectrum disease ranging from self-healing skin lesions to fatal visceral illness. Approximately 40 species of *Leishmania* have been described,[8,11] in which different species are associated with distinct disease outcomes. In parallel, over 900 species and subspecies of sandflies have been identified to date (from a recent compilation of all sandfly species, E. Galati personal communication), but only a limited number have been proven or incriminated as vectors of *Leishmania.*[11] A specific relationship exists between sandflies and *Leishmania* such that, in nature, only certain species of sandflies are able to transmit certain species of *Leishmania.*[12] The specificity of this species is driven by several molecular factors that allow the parasite to infect, survive, and multiply within the midgut of the sandfly and be transmitted to a suitable vertebrate host during a blood meal. Some sandfly species are considered permissive (or nonspecific) as they are able to harbor experimental infections of several *Leishmania* species (e.g., *Lutzomyia longipalpis* and *L. infantum chagasi* or *Leishmania mexicana*); other sandfly species are considered restrictive (or specific) as they can only be infected with the *Leishmania* species that they carry in nature (e.g., *Phlebotomus papatasi* and *L. major*). However, the precise interactions that lead to this vectorial capacity in sandflies, whether for permissive or restrictive vectors, remain to be fully elucidated. During its life within the sandfly vector, *Leishmania* undergo a complex developmental process, mainly restricted to the midgut, in which the parasites must overcome several documented difficulties. Both parasite and vector achieve a balance that involves significant interplay. In one end, for its survival, *Leishmania* strives to manipulate aspects of the physiology of the sandfly, interfering with digestive proteases,[13–15] secreting a myoinhibitory peptide that arrests hindgut peristalsis[16] and causing significant damage to the stomodeal valve (or cardia) of the fly.[17,18] In contrast, sandflies probably recognize the presence of *Leishmania* and likely mount an immune response to the infection.[19] In *L. longipalpis*, defensin, glycine-rich proteins (GRP), which are transcripts associated with the innate immunity of insects, are upregulated following a blood meal.[19] Serine protease inhibitors (serpins) also are upregulated following a blood meal and possibly also by *Leishmania*,[19] whereas digestive enzymes may be regulated at the level of transcription and/or activity by the parasite.[20,21] Sandflies also seem to induce programmed cell death (apoptosis) of midgut cells following infection.[19,22] Apoptosis is an innate defense mechanism in insects and known to be used by mosquitoes to eliminate *Plasmodium*-infected midgut cells.[23] Although *Leishmania* do not invade the midgut cells, close contact between the parasites and these cells, that is, adhesion to epithelial cells through the parasite surface, is well documented.[24] Thus, despite their long evolutionary history (fossil records indicate the presence of flagellates), possibly trypanosomatids, within sandflies in the Early Cretaceous[25] the relationship between *Leishmania* and sandflies can be considered an active and intense evolutionary arms race. In this section, we highlight some of the most important events during the development of *Leishmania* in a suitable sandfly vector, and discuss the issues associated with *Leishmania*–sandfly specificity, metacyclogenesis, and sandfly midgut responses to *Leishmania*. Additional themes related to current and future strategies to prevent transmission of *Leishmania* parasites targeting the vector are also discussed.

2.7 *LEISHMANIA*–MACROPHAGE INTERACTIONS

In this section, we have discussed the role of reactive oxygen species (ROS) in parasite survival, macrophage defense, and treatment. Initially the understanding of the different *Leishmania* parasite stages are described with the mechanisms involved in the production and resistance against the various ROS produced by macrophages. This mechanics was described as a function of specific phases in the life cycle. In addition, antioxidant potential of the infective agent is established by reflecting the role of ROS in the treatment of *Leishmania.*

2.7.1 REDOX BIOLOGY

Leishmania–macrophage interactions insight into the redox biology. *Leishmania* organisms have a relatively simple life cycle, characterized by two principal stages, the flagellated mobile promastigotes living in the gut of the sandfly vector and the immobile amastigotes within phagolysosomal vesicles of the vertebrate host macrophages.[26] Infected female sandflies transmit the disease by various life cycle stages have different sensitivities to ROS and provoke different oxidative responses of the macrophage. After recognition of *Leishmania* spp., macrophages are activated and become so-called "effector cells" that can phagocytose and destroy the unwanted guest. Various cellular processes start after macrophage activation, including the production of phagolysosomal degradation enzymes (e.g., proteases, nucleases, phosphatases, lipases, and esterases), oxidative burst generation, and nitric oxide (•NO) production. The production of lysosomal enzymes induces a direct toxic effect and acidification of the environment. The oxidative burst provoked by the enzyme reduced nicotinamide adenine dinucleotide (NADPH) oxidase is a result of the dramatic increase in oxygen consumption that is typical of the phagocytosis process. After macrophage activation, an increased concentrations of various cytokines such as interferon (IFN)-γ and tumor necrosis factor (TNFα) enhance NADPH oxidase activity and subsequently the production of ROS, such as superoxide radical (O_2 •−). The production of O_2 •− leads to the spontaneous or enzymatic formation of hydrogen peroxide (H_2O_2), hydroxyl radical (HO•), hypochlorite (OCl−), and peroxynitrite (ONOO−).[26] The increased •NO and •NO-metabolite levels in activated macrophages are the result of inducible nitric oxide synthase (iNOS or NOS_2) activation. L-arginine acts as a nitrogenous donor of •NO, which spontaneously converts to nitrite and nitrate. Parasite persistence within the macrophages is determined by a balance between the ability of the immune response to sufficiently activate *Leishmania*-infected macrophages and the ability of the parasite to resist cytotoxic mechanisms of macrophage activation.[26] The production of these cytokines, ROS, and •NO derivatives normally leads to destruction of the phagocytosed microorganism, but *Leishmania* spp. are one of the few protozoa that can survive and even replicate in this hostile environment.[26] Understanding this survival process may lead to important information for the research and the development of new antileishmanial drugs. The existing treatment options for *Leishmania* are limited and far from satisfactory, thereby endorsing the need for the development of new drugs or therapies. Although *Leishmania* species are susceptible in vitro to exogenous superoxide radical, hydrogen peroxide, nitric oxide, and peroxynitrite, they manage to survive the endogenous oxidative burst during phagocytosis and the subsequent elevated nitric oxide production in the macrophage. The parasite adopts various defense mechanisms to cope with oxidative stress: the LPG membrane decreases superoxide radical production by inhibiting NADPH oxidase assembly and the parasite also protects itself by expressing antioxidant enzymes and proteins. Some of these enzymes could be considered as potential drug targets because they are not expressed in mammals. In respect to antileishmanial therapy, the effects of current drugs on parasite–macrophage redox biology and its involvement in the development of drug resistance and treatment failure are presented.

2.7.2 LEISHMANIA PARASITES TO EXOGENOUS REACTIVE OXYGEN SPECIES

Leishmania is divided into three major clinical forms: CL, MCL, and VL. *Leishmania* species are transmitted by a phlebotome sandfly vector.[133] Life cycle of *Leishmania* is distinguished by two primary stages:

- Flagellated mobile promastigotes living in the gut of the sandfly vector
- Immobile amastigotes within phagolysosomal vesicles of the vertebrate host macrophages[134]

During their blood meal, infected female sandflies transmit the disease by inoculating the promastigote form into the skin. These parasites are phagocytosed by macrophages and dendritic cells in the dermis of the vertebrate host. Once the promastigotes were uptaken and internalized into a phagosome, eventually the fusion with lysosomes occurs that resulted in to the survival of the parasites in the phagolysosome. In phagolysosome, promastigotes rapidly converted into amastigotes. This transformation process takes 12–24 hours and amastigotes continuously grow and multiply within the phagolysosomal compartment. These amastigotes present in the macrophages and monocytes of an infected vertebrate host are then ingested by sandfly takes its blood meal are released into the sandfly midgut where they develop into flagellated promastigotes. This whole process of transformation of dividing, noninfective procyclic form acquires virulence a capability into a nondividing, infective metacyclic form is called as metacyclogenesis.[6] After the migration of metacyclic promastigotes into the pharynx and buccal cavity of phlebotome sandfly vector, they can be easily transmitted during a next blood meal. Now capability of macrophages toward the production of free radicals (ROS) against this infectious state was varied according to the different life cycle stages of parasite. These various life cycle stages provoke different oxidative responses of the macrophage and have different sensitivities toward various ROS. Macrophages once identify the unwanted guest (*Leishmania* sp.), activated and become effector cells to phagocytose and destroy these parasites. Different types of cellular processes that are initiated after macrophage activation includes the production of phagolysosomal degradation enzymes (e.g., proteases, nucleases, phosphatases, lipases, and esterases), oxidative burst generation, and nitric oxide (•NO) production. Generation of lysosomal enzymes by macrophages furnish the direct toxic effect and acidification of the compartment. During the phagocytosis process, oxygen consumption is increased leading to the production of NADPH oxidase that ultimately triggers oxidative burst. In addition, macrophage activation also enhances the production of different concentrations of cytokines such as IFN-γ and TNFα enhance NADPH oxidase activity and consequently production of ROS, such as superoxide radical ($O_2^{\bullet-}$). Generation of $O_2^{\bullet-}$ radicals lead to the formation of hydrogen peroxide (H_2O_2), hydroxyl radical (HO•), hypochlorite (OCl^-), and peroxynitrite (ONOO−).[135,136] iNOS activation in activated macrophage elevate concentrations of •NO and •NO-metabolites. Amino acid L-arginine is an active nitrogen donor of •NO, which spontaneously converts to nitrite and nitrate. Parasite activation is dependent on the potential of the immune response to activate *Leishmania*-infected macrophages and the strength of the infective agent to resist cytotoxic reactions offered by activated macrophages.[137] Activated macrophage-mediated generation of cytokines, ROS, and •NO derivatives usually leads to the destruction of the phagocytosed microorganism. However, *Leishmania* parasites are well adapted to survive and replicate in this hostile environment. Knowledge of the mechanism and other molecular processes involved in the survival process can furnish the significant information for the future research and the development of new antileishmanial drugs. Limited drugs or therapies for *Leishmania* require more satisfactory research to explore promising novel antileishmanial drug targets.

2.7.3 IMPACT OF REACTIVE OXYGEN SPECIES (ROS) ON THE CONTROL OF PARASITE

Macrophage defense is chiefly controlled by $O^{2\bullet-}$ and • NO. These agents cause toxicity to the parasites and give rise to the production of various metabolites such as H_2O_2 and ONOO.

Superoxide radical ($O^{2\bullet-}$) showed a direct toxic effect on *L. chagasi* promastigotes.[138] Extent of toxicity is dependent on the in vitro and in vivo susceptibility of *Leishmania* to exogenous (which means donated by a donor or exogenously added enzymes and substrates) free radicals. In addition. susceptibility is further dependent on the parasite stage: metacyclic promastigotes were more resistant compared to procyclic promastigotes. By acting as precursor, $O^{2\bullet-}$ further has the capability to generate other toxic oxidants.[139] Since H_20_2 is formed by the dismutation of $O^{2\bullet-}$ [a reaction catalyzed by superoxide dismutase (SOD)] therefore $O^{2\bullet-}$-producing compounds and enzymes are also sources of H_2O_2. It has been discovered that H_2O_2 is more toxic for *Leishmania* spp. than $O^{2\bullet-}$.

In addition to $O^{2\bullet-}$ and H_2O_2, NO is also reported for its potential antileishmanial effects. Potential antileishmanial effects of •NO can be evaluated by the supplementation of •NO donors. It is produced by the tightly regulated enzyme [•NO synthase (NOS)]. Out of its three types (neuronal or nNOS/NOS_1, NOS/NOS_2, and endothelial or eNOS/NOS_3) only iNOS is accountable for the production of •NO in macrophages. iNOS easily solubilize in the biological fluids for conducting the oxidation of L-arginine to •NO and L-citrulline. When compared with eNOS and nNOS, iNOS generated in phagocytes only when suitable stimuli are applied and then produces •NO in large amounts.

Toxicities of peroxynitrite (ONOO) against *Leishmania* are reported at many places. ONOO is formed by the interaction between the free radicals •NO and $O2^{\bullet-}$.[140] It is reported that the occurrence of peroxidoxins (PXNs) in *Leishmania* parasites protect them from $ONOO^-$ toxicity.[141] In contrast to •NO, high in vitro toxic effects of ONOO– are also reported.

2.7.4 PHAGOCYTOSIS OF LEISHMANIA: ROLE OF REACTIVE OXYGEN SPECIES

When infected sandfly bites, promastigotes are released in to blood stream where they are phagocytosed by macrophages. These macrophages when burst for the release of amastigotes are again rapidly phagocytosed by new macrophages. It is well established that generation of $O^{2\bullet-}$ is dependent on the extent of phagocytosis of microbes. More the phagocytosis occurs more the $O^{2\bullet-}$ is produced[142] through the activation of NADPH oxidase.[143] However *Leishmania* parasite can survive after phagocytosis, even after acquiring considerable susceptibility to exogenous ROS and •NO. Now a question raised here that how the parasite escapes from this toxic burst of ROS production. According to various reports *Leishmania* parasite escapes by counteracting the endogenous ROS production through antioxidant systems or by actively decreasing ROS production

2.7.5 LEISHMANIA ANTIOXIDANT DEFENSE SYSTEM

2.7.5.1 TRYPANOTHIONE/TRYPANOTHIONE REDUCTASE

Usually mammalian intracellular thiol redox system is controlled by glutathione (GSH)/glutathione reductase to effectively reduce ROS by GSH forming oxidized glutathione disulfide (GSSG). Glutathione can be restored from oxidized glutathione disulfide by glutathione reductase.[144] *Leishmania* lacks such expression, however. its redox mechanisms is dependent on the glutathione conjugate which is also known as trypanothione ($T(SH)_2$). This glutathione conjugate is produced when $T(SH)_2$ reduces ROS. It has been reported that the antioxidant potential of thiols is due to the generation of γ-glutamylcysteine synthetase (γ-GCS) knockout *L. infantum* mutants. In addition, it was also demonstrated that γ-glutamylcysteine synthetase is the rate-limiting enzyme in the biosynthesis of GSH. Formation of $T(SH)_2$ via the intermediate glutathionyl spermidine by the conjugation of GSH with spermidine[145] is ATP-dependent process. This process is catalyzed by the single enzyme trypanothione synthetase, which has been described in the *Trypanosoma* sp., *Crithidia fasciculata*, and *L. major*.[146] However, heterozygous knockout promastigotes produced lower levels of $T(SH)_2$ and therefore become more vulnerable to oxidative stress in vitro with a decreased survival inside activated macrophages.[147]

2.7.5.2 PEROXIDASES

Leishmania does not produce catalase or classical selenocysteine containing glutathione peroxidase. This might be due to the lack of gene that expresses or responsible for the production of these two major H_2O_2-metabolizing enzymes usually present in eukaryotes. It has been reported that H_2O_2 elimination in parasite is dependent on the $T(SH)_2$.[148] In addition, proteins like tryparedoxin (TXN) and peroxiredoxin (PRX) are essential for $T(SH)_2$ to reduce H_2O_2.[149] These proteins are responsible for the show tryparedoxin peroxidase activity.

2.7.5.3 TRYPANOTHIONE S-TRANSFERASE

These detoxifying enzymes belong to a class of glutathione S-transferases (GSTs) that catalyze the conjugation of GSH to electrophiles through thioether linkages.[150] Moreover these compounds are responsible for the removal of endogenous reactive species formed during oxidative stress, such as lipid hydroperoxides and reactive aldehydes.[151] However no GST activity has been reported in *Leishmania*, whereas trypanothione S-transferase activity was found in *L. major*, *L. infantum*, and *Leishmania tarentolae*.[152]

2.7.5.4 5,6,7,8-TETRAHYDROBIOPTERIN

In addition to these enzymes, a reduced pterin called as 5,6,7,8-tetrahydrobiopterin reported for inducing the antioxidant property to several parasites. 5,6,7,8-tetrahydrobiopterin, acts as a natural cofactor of the aromatic amino acid hydroxylases, as well as of all three forms of NOS.[153] It has been investigated that reduced biopterins (e.g., BH_4) are capable to scavenge free radicals and play an active role in the defense against oxidative stress. 5,6,7,8-tetrahydrobiopterin act as an essential growth factor for *Leishmania*[154] and implicated in the control of metacyclogenesis.[155]

2.7.5.5 SUPEROXIDE DISMUTASE

In eukaryotic organisms, SODs plays an active role in the control of oxidative stress. Mammals cell contains three isoforms of SODs: copper–zinc SOD (encoded by the sod1 gene), manganese SOD (encoded by the sod2 gene), and extracellular SOD (encoded by the sod3 gene).[156] Antioxidant property exhibited by the expression of SODs in *Leishmania* is quite similar, however *Leishmania* SODs contain iron (FeSOD). As reported, SOD is absent in several *Leishmania* sp., which realize its importance in parasite for exhibiting SOD-mediated antioxidant mechanics against toxic ROS.[157]

2.7.5.6 PENTOSE PHOSPHATE METABOLISM

This metabolism is required to sustain intracellular NADPH levels and the cellular redox balance. However, this type of metabolism has been scarcely studied in *Leishmania* redox biology, while enzymes involved in pentose phosphate pathway were found in several *Leishmania* parasite.[158] In addition, it was discovered that supplementation of methylene blue causes depletion of cellular levels of NADPH followed by the considerable increase in the amount of glucose. This makes pathway diverted through the pentose phosphate pathway as reported in *L. mexicana* promastigotes.[159]

2.7.6 ANTILEISHMANIAL DRUGS AFFECTING MACROPHAGE OR LEISHMANIA REDOX SIGNALING

Leishmaniasis treatment is based on the administration of only few drugs that usually causes side effects and increase in resistance. Some drugs are administered orally and some are administered through parenteral route. For leishmaniasis chemotherapy, almost all drugs are administered through parenteral route. Identification of potential targets during chemotherapy is essential to eradicate intracellular amastigote that multiply in macrophages, thereby hinder the task of antileishmanial therapy. Specific experimental conditions are required for potentiating the antileishmania drug research. As it is noteworthy that in vitro drug susceptibility varies differs between log-phase promastigotes, axenic amastigotes, fresh spleen-derived amastigotes, and intracellular amastigotes.[160] However, this is not always reported that the experimental conditions or model can enhance the infectivity of (field isolate) promastigotes.[161] Therefore, it is obligatory for first getting an initial knowledge of in vivo model before finalizing the possible drug targets.

Sb remain the first-line treatment despite its lack of knowledge about exact mechanism of action. It is widely investigated that pentavalent antimonials (SbV) are the prodrug and that they should be converted to trivalent antimonials (SbIII) for antileishmanial activity. While establishing antimonials relation with the antioxidant defense system of the parasite, it was found that SbIII decreases the thiol-reducing capacity of *Leishmania* by inducing an efflux of trypanothione disulfide. In addition, these drugs inhibit the trypanothione reductase that results in the accumulation of trypanothione disulfide. It was further explained that the sensitivity of *Leishmania* spp. is dependent on the tryparedoxin peroxidase activity, that is, increase in *L.*

major SbIII-sensitive promastigotes resulted in a significant decrease in sensitivity to SbIII (Figure 2-3).

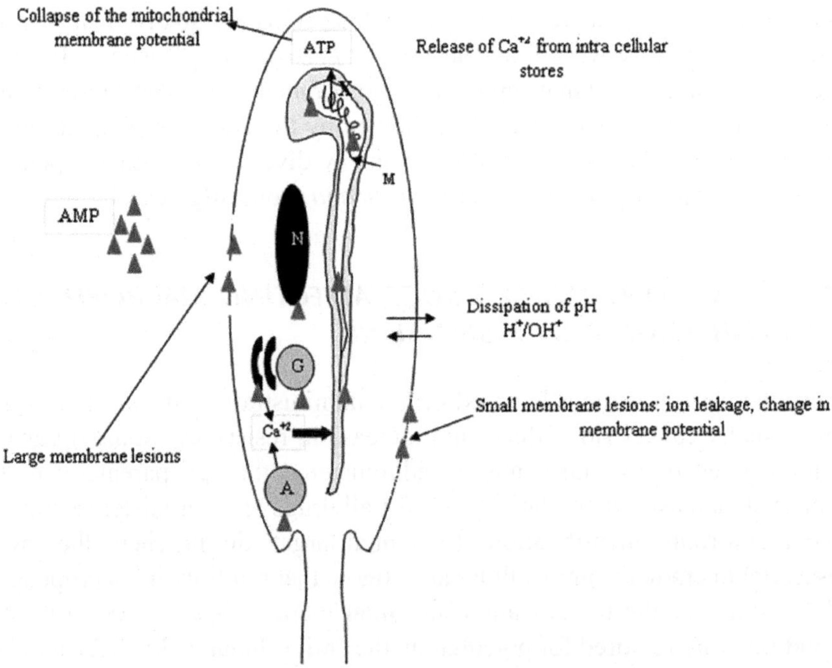

FIGURE 2-3 Redox targets of antileishmanial drugs in macrophage, phagosome, and amastigote. Possible drug targets are (1) increasing oxidative stress in the phagosome (dotted lines), as suggested by in vitro experiments with AmB; (2) decreasing antioxidant defense at the amastigote level (dashed lines), for example, Sb, which showed an induction of $T(SH)_2$ efflux and inhibited TR; and/or (3) interference with amastigote cellular metabolism (solid lines), for example, interference with membranes and membrane-linked enzymes such as PKC and Na/KATPase, which is observed with MILT, and decreasing mitochondrial membrane potential, described as a possible target of PAR. PKCi, inactive PKC; PKCa, active PKC.

2.7.6.1 PAROMOMYCIN

Paromomycin (PAR) is an amino glycoside which is usually administered in combination with Sb to reduce the duration of treatment. Parenteral administration of this drug is found to be not very effective for CL than the topical formulation combined with methylbenzethonium chloride. The possible mechanism of action could be due to respiratory dysfunction and mitochondrial membrane depolarization (Figure 2-3).

2.7.6.2 AMPHOTERICIN B

Amphotericin B (AmB) has been used as a second-line treatment and exhibits an excellent antileishmania activity with higher than 90% cure rates in VL. At present, liposomal formulations of AmB are the first choice in various developed countries. The possible mechanism can be explained on the bases of its chemical structure. AmB bind to ergosterol, the main sterol synthesized in fungal and *Leishmania* membranes by promoting the permeability of the cell membrane followed by the promotion of ion influx into the parasite leading to its death (Figure 2-3).

2.7.6.3 MILTEFOSINE

Miltefosine (MILT) (hexadecylphosphocholine) is the first orally administered drug for *Leishmania* treatment. The use of MILT is now limited because it acquires serious teratogenic potential and its long half-life approximately 150 hours), which may facilitate the emergence of drug resistance. Recent data explore its activity on antioxidant potential of parasite by inhibiting ATPase activity in *Trypanosoma cruzi* and host mammalian cells (Figure 2-3). In addition, MILT is also able to induce IFN-γ production through the host cell, resulting in iNOS activation.

2.8 ANTIMICROBIAL PEPTIDES WITH *LEISHMANIA* AND THEIR FUNCTIONAL ROLE IN HOST PARASITISM

Trypanosomatids of the genera *Leishmania* and Trypanosoma parasites alternately infect blood-feeding insects and mammalian hosts during their complex life cycle. Infection caused by the *Leishmania* and trypanosomes is commenced by the injection of infective metacyclic parasites by insects (sandflies or tsetse flies, respectively) into the skin of the host during feeding. Infective metacyclic forms of *T. cruzi* that are present at the near to the feeding site of hindgut of triatomine bugs are eventually introduced into the wound by contamination. It is not well clear that after having the potential innate immune responses of the insect how the host parasites are adapted to both replicate and differentiate into infective forms.[27] To establish the infection in the mammalian host, parasites overcome innate immune factors and ultimately parasitize phagolysosomes of professional phagocytes whereas intracellular *T. cruzican* reside in any nucleated cell type. The treatment strategies of leishmaniasis and trypanosomiasis are still dependent on outdated drugs, which are becoming ineffective due to the development of parasite resistance and are often poorly tolerated. Exploration of novel therapeutic agents is required to overcome these problems. AMPs are multifunctional components of the innate systems of both insect and mammalian hosts of the pathogenic trypanosomatids *Leishmania* species. The purpose of this chapter is to summarize the work done in the area of AMP–*Leishmania* interactions which have mainly focused on in vitro activity studies as a prerequisite to the development of AMPs as chemotherapeutic agents in leishmaniasis. In addition, effects of these interactions on different parts of the parasite life cycle during natural are also highlighted.

AMPs are gene-encoded, small (10–50 residues long), cationic proteins that are multifunctional components of the innate immune systems of both insect and mammalian hosts of the pathogenic trypanosomatids *Leishmania* and *Trypanosoma* species.[28] In addition to its structural diversity, AMPs contain comparatively high proportion of basic amino acids and form either predominate lya-helical structures, orb-pleated sheets. There are various sources of AMP reported against different *Leishmania* species (Table 2-3). It has been reported that certain subsets of AMPs (defensins and some cathelicidins) are cysteine-rich. These cysteine-rich areas facilitate the extensive intra-disulfide bonding that is crucial for its activity.[29] The amphipathicity property of AMPs allows them to interact with negatively charged microbial membranes. AMPs destabilize surface membranes through a variety of mechanisms and cause the microbial death by inducing autophagic-, necroticor apoptotic-cell death.[30–33] As it is well evidenced that AMPs destabilize cell surface membranes, it has been reported that they also penetrate cells and associate with intracellular organelles. Such association leads to pleiotropic effects on metabolic and bioenergetic pathways.[34,35] It was also proposed that AMPs localize intracellularly to affect calcium levels, mitochondrial function, induce autophagy, necrosis, and apoptosis by disrupting surface membranes and ultimately affects parasite growth and differentiation in their hosts.

The expression of AMPs in various organisms confirms the conservation of AMP functionality as a primitive immune defense response. Several reports confirms the expression of AMPs in mammals through an extensive variety of cell types and dominate at portals of microbial entry such as the gastrointestinal, respiratory, urogenital tracts, and in the skin. The expression of cathelicidin- and defensin-type AMPs in mammals can affect the host inflammatory response. This can be accomplished by behaving as chemokines to directly attract host cells or promoting chemokine secretion by other cells leading to the migration of neutrophils, monocytes, and macrophages into the areas of local inflammation.[36–38] Various classes of parasites such as *Leishmania* and *Trypanosoma* species are successful in their complex life cycles because they can easily flourish in harsh environments within two different hosts. Parasites are exposed to the multitude of different AMPs during their exposure to the immune systems of both insect and mammalian hosts. Owing to their strong adapted mechanisms of parasite to overcome or neutralize deleterious AMPs-mediated effects, they survive and flourish in host cell. Therefore, potential of AMPs need to be strengthen by exposing potential targets of their activity at the cellular level.

TABLE 2-3 Antimicrobial peptides against different leishmania species[12]

Peptide source	Antimicrobial peptides
Frogs	Magainins
	Dermaseptins
	Phylloseptins
	Temporins
	Bombinins
Insects	Cecropins and Melittin
	Gomesin (taranula)
	Sandfly defensin (SD-1)
	Mussel AMPs
	Tachyplesin (horseshoe crab)
	Clavanin A (sea squirt)
	Shrimp AMPs
Plants	Wheat thionin
	Potato defensin (PTH-1)
	Potato snakin1
	Barley lipid-transfer protein
Mammals	Cathelicidins
	Defensins
Other	Seminalplasmin peptides (bovine)
	Histatin 5 (human)

2.8.1 TARGETS AND EFFECTS ON ANTIMICROBIAL PEPTIDE ATTACK ON PARASITES

Whole process of targeting by AMP is illustrated in Figure 2-4. Cationic AMPs (orange circles) are attracted to and insert within the negatively charged parasite membrane. The permeabilization causes small and large lesions in the membrane leading to the equilibration of intracellular and extracellular pH, flow of ions in and out of the cell as well as transit of larger molecules. Some AMPs may penetrate cells and cause an increase in the concentration of intracellular Ca^{2+} from intracellular stores within acidocalcisomes (AC), glycosomes (GLY), and endoplasmic reticulum (purple layered structure). Some AMPs can cause a breakdown in the mitochondrial (M) membrane potential and halt the production of ATP, possibly in whole or in part by the toxic effect of free intracellular Ca^{2+}. ATP can also be lost through the AMP-permeabilized cell membranes. The structure with multiple circles within the mitochondrial represents the specialized mitochondrial DNA (kinetoplast DNA) in this group of parasites. N represents nucleus.

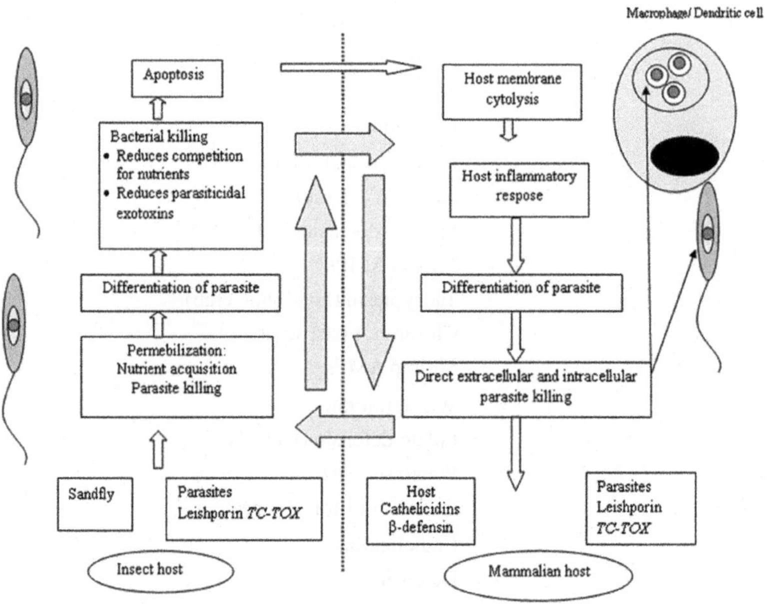

FIGURE 2-4 Targets and effects of antimicrobial peptide attack on parasites.

2.8.2 FUNCTIONAL ROLES OF ANTIMICROBIAL PEPTIDE

Proposed functional roles of AMP interactions in the *Leishmania* life cycle as they circulate within insect to mammalian hosts are illustrated in Figure 2-5. AMPs present within their respective insect vectors (indicated in the boxes at the bottom-left panel) may play a role in limiting the growth of parasites and/or bacteria that coinhabit the insect. AMPs or AMP-like proteins produced by parasites may also be protective and limit competition in a polymicrobic environment. Action of AMPs on parasites may permeabilize cell membranes aiding in nutrient acquisition or lead to intracellular signaling events. AMPs, possibly in conjunction with other stimuli, may lead to parasite differentiation into infective metacyclic forms. Upon infection of mammals, parasites initially encounter several subclasses of AMPs (boxes at the bottom-right panel), which may decrease their numbers. Intracellular parasites *Leishmania* may encounter AMPs within their host cells. For *Leishmania*, AMPs expressed within phagolysosomes may be important for the elimination of parasites. Host cell AMPs may be important for the differentiation of amastigotes into trypomastigotes, which then escape through host cells.

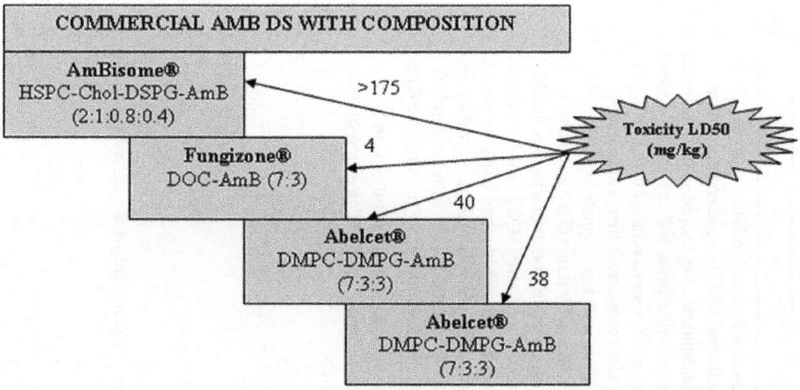

FIGURE 2-5 Functional roles of antimicrobial peptide interactions in the *Leishmania* life cycle.

2.9 BIOCHEMICAL TARGETS FOR THERAPY

Current research on *Leishmania* lead to the exploration of various biochemical targets such as glycolytic enzymes (present in promastigotes and amastigotes), synthesis of sterols, that is, ergosterol (differ from mammalian cholesterol), purine metabolism (enzymatic differences between *Leishmania* and the mammalian host), *de novo* synthesis of pyrimidines (thymidylate synthase in *Leishmania*), polyamines (polyamines putrescine, spermidine, and spermine are short-length cationic molecules), and enzymes responsible for maintaining intracellular reducing environment in parasite.[39] Prominent biochemical targets are highlighted in Table 2-4.

TABLE 2-4 Enzymes as potential drug targets in leishmaniasis[27]

Target	Source	Inhibitors	Role
Sterol biosynthetic pathway (*Squalene synthase & sterol methyl-transferase*)	Membrane, glycosomes, mitochondrial and microsomal vesicles	C14 alpha-demethylase inhibitors such as ketoconazole and D0870, squalene epoxidase inhibitor terbinafine, alkyllsophospho-lipids such as ilmofosine, miltefosine and edelfosine, Ajoene, statins (act on the mevalonate pathway by inhibiting HMG-CoA reductase), bisphosphonates, which interfere with the isoprenoid pathway in the step catalyzed by farnesyl diphosphate synthase, zaragozic acids and quinuclidines, inhibitors of squalene synthase (SQS), which catalyzes the first committed step in sterol biosynthesis, (d) allylamines, inhibitors of squalene epoxidase, (e) azoles, which inhibit C14 -demethylase, and (f) azasterols, which inhibit -sterol methyltransferase	Unlike mammalian cells, which have cholesterol as the major membrane sterol, trypanosomatids synthesize ergosterol and other 24-methyl sterols that are required for their growth and viability. These sterols are absent from the mammalian cells. Therefore, the sterol biosynthetic pathway from *Leishmania* is considered to be an important drug targe
Glycolytic pathway (*Glyceraldehyde-3-phosphate dehydrogenase*)	Glycosomes	Adenosine analogs with substitutions on N-6 of the adenine ring & on the 2' position of the ribose moiety	The energy metabolism of trypanosomatids solely depends on the carbon sources available in the host. African trypanosomes lack a functional Krebs cycle, they use glycolysis as the only source of ATP generation. Seven of the glycolytic enzymes are compartmentalized in peroxisome-like organelles, glycosomes, which is a unique feature of trypanosomatids. The unique compartmentalization of glycolytic enzymes in glycosomes in *Leishmania* and their large phylogenetic distance with the mammalian hosts provides them with unique features.
Purine salvage pathway (*Hypoxanthine-guanine phosphoribosyl transferase*)	Glycosomes	Allopurinol, Phthalic anhydride derivative	The parasitic protozoa, including *Leishmania* lack the enzymes to synthesize purine nucleotides *de novo*, therefore, they have to depend upon the purine salvage system to utilize purine bases from their mammalian hosts (Figure2-3). Purine bases are translocated through the parasite cell surface by nucleoside transporters. Therefore nucleoside transporters and purine salvage enzymes are the key targets for *Leishmania*

TABLE 2-4 *(Continued)*

Target	Source	Inhibitors	Role
GPI biosynthetic pathway (Glycosylphos-phatidylinositol enzymes)	Endoplasmic reticulumn	amino sugars, protease inhibitors and substrate analogues (lipopeptide antibiotic amphomycin that forms a complex with dolichol-P-mannose)	Glycosylphosphatidylinositol glycolipids are major cell surface constituents in the *Leishmania* parasites that act as anchor to various cell surface glycoproteins. The cell surface of the promastigotes is coated by glycocalyx which consists of GPI anchored glycoproteins, GPI-anchored lipophosphoglycan and a family of free GPIs, called as glycoinositolphospholipids, in high densities. They protect the parasite from the alternate complement pathway and external hydrolases.
Protein kinases	Cytosol	Sunitinib, sorafenib, lapatinib	Cyclin dependent kinases are known to play a crucial role in cell division. They have been found to be abnormally regulated in cancer cells and have therefore drawn attention as drug targets. In *Leishmania*, the cdc-2-related kinase (CRK) family has attracted attention as potential drug targets. They are homologs of CDKs and are thought to be essential for cell cycle progression. Two putative CDKs in *L. mexicana*, LmexCRK1 and LmexCRK3 have been found to be essential to the promastigotes form of the parasite.
MAP kinases		Naïve macrophages inactivates the all three MAP kinases ERKI/2, p 38 and JNK, stimulation of leishmania lipopolysaccharide, *phorbol-myristate-acetate*-activated macrophages	Mitogen-activated protein kinases are mediators of signal transduction and important regulators of cell differentiation and cell proliferation in eukaryotic cells. So far, 10 MAP kinases have been identified in *L. mexicana*, of which LmxMKK, LmxMPK and LmxMPK9 have been studied intensely
Folate biosynthesis (Dihydrofolate reductase, Dihydrofolate reductase-thymidylate)	Cytosol	Sulphonamides, trimethoprim, pyrimethamine, 2,4-Diaminoquinazoline analogs Offolate, 4,6-diamino-1,2-dihydro-2,2-dimethyl-1-(3-substituted-phenyl)-s-triazine, methotrexate, 2,4-Diamino-6,7-diisopropylpteridine	Folate pathway has been of interest as a drug target and has been used in anti-cancer and anti-malarial chemotherapy. Folates are important cofactors used in a variety of metabolic pathways like DNA and RNA synthesis and amino acid metabolism.

TABLE 2-4 *(Continued)*

Target	Source	Inhibitors	Role
Glyoxalase system	Kinetoplast	recombinant glyoxalase I (LdGLOI) protein, S-4-bromobenzyl glutathionylspermidi	The Glyoxalase system functions to detoxify the cell by removal of toxic and mutagenic intermediate, methylglyoxal, which is mainly formed as a by-product of glycolysis. It is also formed during threonine catabolism and acetone oxidation (Cooper; Vickers et al.[152]). The glyoxalase system comprises of two enzymes viz. glyoxalase I (lactoyl glutathione lyase) (EC 4.4.1.5) and Glyoxalase II (hydroxyacyl glutathione hydroxylase) (EC 3.1.2.6) and uses glutathione as a cofactor. However, trypanosomatids rely on a trypanothione dependent glyoxalase system
Trypanothione pathway (trypanothione reductase)	Cytosol and mitochondria	Auranofin, Ag(I), Sb(III) Melarsen oxide, Nifurtimox	As discussed above, trypanothione (bis-(glutathionyl) spermidine) is a key molecule against oxidative stress in Trypanosoma and *Leishmania*. It is not only unique to the parasite but is also crucial in maintaining the cellular redox potential and thus is essential for parasite survival. Trypanothione synthesis is catalyzed by two enzymes, namely, trypanothione synthetase (TS) (EC 6.3.1.9) and trypanothione reductase (TR) (EC 1.8.1.12).
Topoisomerases	Kinetoplast and mitochondria	8-prenylmucronulatol, lyasperin H and smiranicin, 9-anilinoacridine, Dihydrobetulinic acid, Camptothecin, stibogluconate and urea stibamine,	DNA topoisomerases are ubiquitous enzymes that play an important role in many essential processes like DNA replication, transcription, recombination and repair. They are broadly classified as type I and type II topoisomerases that cleave single stranded and double stranded DNA, respectively. DNA topoisomerases have been used as chemotherapeutic targets for anti-bacterial and anti-parasitic diseases. Type I topoisomerase (EC 5.99.1.2) have been characterized from *L. donovani* and *T. cruzi*. The enzyme was found to be independent of ATP. *L. donovani* topoisomerase I was found to be present in both kinetoplast and nucleus.

TABLE 2-4 *(Continued)*

Target		Source	Inhibitors	Role
Metacaspases		Cytosol	Trypsin inhibitors, such as leupeptin, antipain, and N^{α}-tosyl-l-lysine-chloromethyl ketone, Peptidomimetic metalloproteases inhibitors	Essential for proper segregation of nucleus and kinetoplast of the parasite.
Proteases	*Aspartic proteases*	Flagellar pocket, membrane, megasomes, and endocytic/ exocytic vescicles	HIV protease inhibitors (Indinavir, Saquinavir, Nelfi navir, Saquinavir Ritonavir, Lopinavir, and Atanazavir)	Proteinases are of four main types- cysteine, serine, aspartate and metallo-enzymes. The name is given on the basis of the residue present in the active site. In case of parasitic protozoa, the most identified and characterized are the cysteine proteinases (CPs), which are homologous to mammalian cathepsins. CPs have attracted attention as potential drug targets because of their role in host cell–parasite interaction, as putative virulence factor, and being structurally different from the mammalian homolog.
	Metallo-proteases		Peptide inhibitors, Peptidomimetic metalloproteases inhibitors	
	Serine proteases		N-tosyl-L:-phenylalanine chloromethyl ketone, Benzamidine, Aprotinin, Kunitz-type protease inhibitor, Ecotin-like inhibitors of serine peptidases	Play crucial roles in *Leishmania* parasite physiology and in host-parasite interaction such as migration through tissue barrier, cleavage of host proteins for nutrition acquisition, immune evasion, and activation of inflammation and subversion of host cell signaling system.
	Cysteine protease		Cystatin, biflavonoids orelloflavone fukugiside and morelloflavone, organic tellurium compound, palladacycle complex, tetromycin derivatives, cathepsin b inhibitor (CA074, CLIK-60) MDL 28170 (a potent calpain inhibitor) K11777, aziridine-2,3-dicarboxylates, Leupeptin, E-64, crystal structures of papain, cruzain, and human liver cathepsin B (molecular modeling), Brugia malayi cysteine protease inhibitor-2 in which the amino acid Asn66 was mutated to Lys66 (Bm-CPI-2M), *N*-methylpiperazine-phenylalanyl-homophenylalanyl-vinylsulfonephenyl	.
Protein disulfide isomerase		Cytosol	Bacitracin, hexachlorophene and a mixture of the aflavin monogallates	Essential for intracellular survival of the parasites

2.10 DRUG DELIVERY SYSTEMS

From their earliest days, delivery system (DS) found application for VL mainly due to the fact that *Leishmania* parasites colonize macrophages in liver and spleen, which are also responsible for clearance of DS.[40] The first use of liposomal drugs in the treatment of infectious diseases was made in the case of *Leishmania*. Liposome-encapsulated antimonials were found to be 700 times more effective than unencapsulated drug in hamsters.[40] After this seminal work, extensive literature reported that the activity of the most currently antileishmanial drugs was improved by encapsulation in DS. Actually there are three lipidic DS of AmB licensed for clinical use (Ambisome, Amphocil, and Albecet),[40] although only one of them, Ambisome, is recommended for treating patients with leishmaniasis who are unresponsive to antimonial. The three were found more effective than antimonials even with a single dose treatment. However, Ambisome was better tolerated.[40] Ambisome was effective when intravenously administered but not given by subcutaneous or intraperitoneal route, although in general the treatment of CL required higher doses than for VL. The efficacy of Ambisome and Amphocil, but not Albecet, to treat CL was ascribed to the smaller size (100 nm) of the former that prolongs their circulation before to extravasate toward the skin lesions where the inflammation generated. The composition and toxicity profile of these formulations are illustrated in Figure 2-6.

Current treatment is based on chemotherapy, which relies on a handful of drugs with serious limitations such as high cost, toxicity, difficult route of administration, and lack of efficacy in endemic areas. Pentavalent antimonials have been the mainstay of antileishmanial therapy for over 70 years with second-line drugs, AmB and Pentamidine, used in case of antimonial failure. Since the introduction of MILT at the beginning of this century, no new antileishmanial compounds have been approved for human treatment.[40] Conceptually, many of the unlikely properties of conventional antileishmanial drugs or the poor immunogenicity of subcellular compounds of *Leishmania* could be improved through the use of DSs and nanodevices provided by the pharmaceutical technology. DS could improve the solubility of poorly water-soluble drugs (e.g., AmB or atovaquone) or protect antigenic proteins, DNA, or RNA from rapid degradation. Needle-free administration of antileishmanial drugs or vaccines (e.g., by oral or topical routes) would be also feasible. Because of their particulate nature, DS should provide more selective targeting of drugs or antigens (Ags) toward monocyte phagocyte system (MPS). As *Leishmania* parasites are also mainly confined in macrophages, DS could improve the therapeutic index of antileishmanial drugs, decreasing the effective dose and the off-target toxic effects produced by an inadequate biodistribution. As Ag presenting cells belong to MPS, DS should enhance the Ag uptake and contribute to increase the immunogenicity of subcellular vaccines.

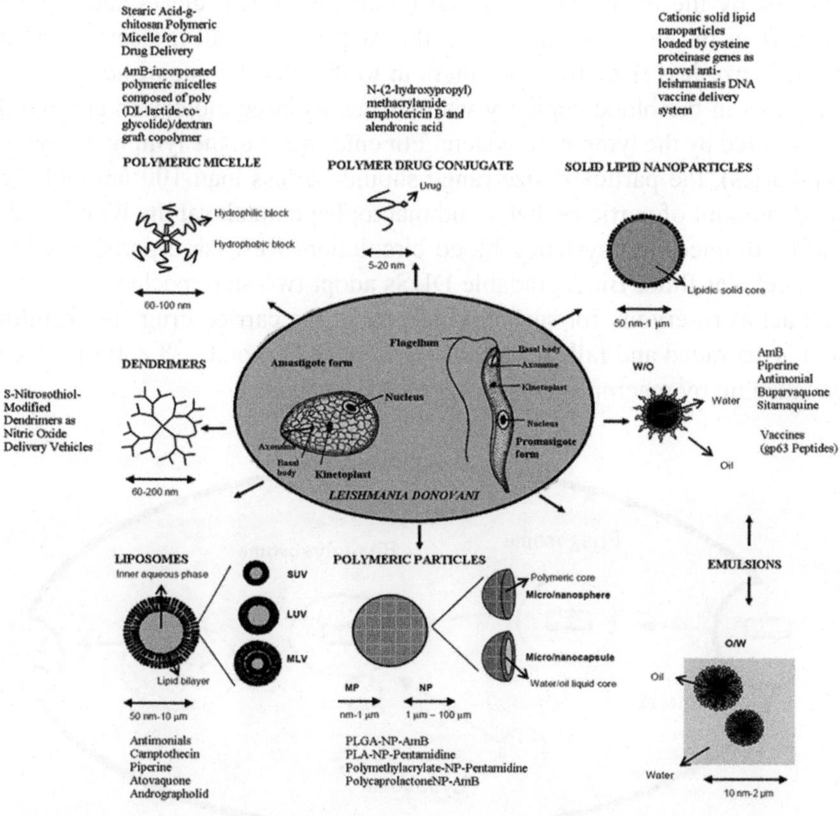

FIGURE 2-6 The composition and toxicity profile of these formulations are mentioned.

Leishmania amastigotes live inside resident macrophages in different anatomic sites. Their hidden location is responsible for impairing the accession of therapeutic drugs. DDSs should allow the adverse effects caused by problematic routes of administration to be avoided as well as enhancing the antileishmanial activity and reducing the toxicity of the medication (Figure 2-7). There are various types of DDS that are reported for antileishmanian drugs (Figure 2-7). However, after 30 years of research in the field, and since leishmaniasis is mostly a disease affecting the poorest populations, currently Ambisome is the only DDS used against the visceral form, and most experimental development only relates to parenteral administration. Because of blockage of lung capillary bed, rigid or solid drug particles smaller than 3 × 10^4 nm administered through parenteral route. Particles those are targeted or desired to site into the interstitial/extracellular space can deliver by subcutaneous, intramuscular, and intraperitoneal route. Once retained by the interstitial fluid, the lymphatic system clears and separate them from the interstitial tissue. In this step, only small molecules having particle size less than 16 KDa enters in to the blood compartment through the pores in the blood capillary walls, whereas large molecules are mainly transported by the lymphatic system. For entering in to the lymphatic (lymph capillaries), the particles' size range should be less than 100 nm and only small amount of particles that avoid macrophage uptake at the lymph nodes can be drained into systemic blood circulation. Rest large particle remain extracellular fluid. Biodegradable DDSs adopt two step mechanisms. They first act as reservoirs for sustained release of the carried drug and formulation is degraded and falls in suitable size range (beyond 7–8 × 10^3 nm), can be taken up by macrophages to start phagocytosis.[40]

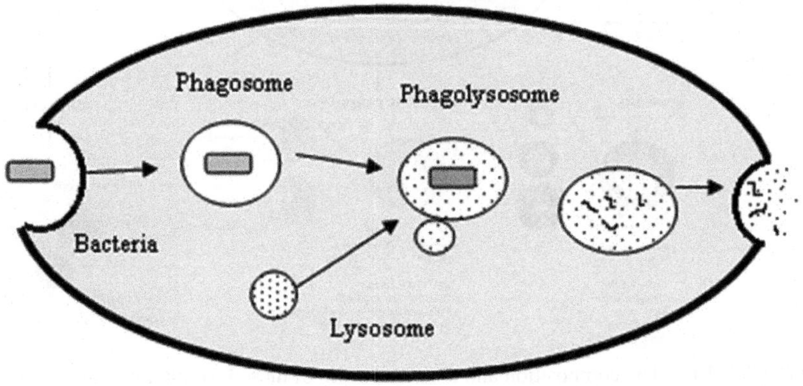

FIGURE 2-7 Various types of DDS that are reported for antileishmanian drugs.

For designing oral DS, particles should be stable at low pH and resist the degradation against lipases, proteases, and bile salts. DS preferably mucoadhesive usually taken up by enterocytes followed by M cells from the Peyer's patch and delivered to the lymphatic circulation. Topical route allows particles below 5 nm to cross the dry surface of the stratum corneum cell layers; however, delivery is independent of structure and shape of the drug. One of the major constrain if the stratum corneum is absent, the diffusion barrier is decreased that may certainly affects the whole delivery procedure. In the CL epithelial membrane get ruptured and more often changes in the skin physiology occurs, which allows particles in blood circulation can cross the permeability barrier to get close to the infected cell.[40]

Particles from any DDSs when reached to blood circulation faces continuous endothelium, which contains pores that allow the passage of small molecules (2–3 nm) outside the circulation, for example, fenestrated endothelium present in in kidneys allow urinary elimination of small particles those are less than 5 nm. However, transport of particles also dependent on their charge and hydrophilic/hydrophobic nature. Most of particles higher than 5 nm are retained by the blood vessels and their leakage to peripheral tissues is impaired. Here the nature of coating decides the fate of the particles, for example, particles coated with protein (lipoproteins) promotes particle recognition and further removal from blood by the accessible cells from the mononuclear phagocyte system. Coated proteins are called as opsonins and the process is called as opsonization. According to the designed DS, protein-coated particles or opsonized particles are generally removed in organs compartment with fenestrate endothelium, chiefly by the Kupffer cells from liver vasculature followed by macrophages in spleen, and rarely by macrophages in lung and bone marrow. Particles that are designed without protein coat, that is, nonopsonized particles are less rapidly cleared from circulation. These particles remain in blood circulation and are easily allowed to extravagate to peripheral tissues where local destruction of the basal membrane and the permeability were increased by inflammation. For designing suitable DDS, it is very important to study the cell uptake modalities for particles such as endocytosis and phagocytosis.[40] There are various novel nano-DDSs that are currently experimented and utilized against leishmaniasis such as dendrimers (monodisperse polymers), solid and nanostructured lipid nanoparticles (SLNs and NLPs), ultradeformable lipid matrices, and various nano-structured polyelectrolyte complexes. Dendrimers are their highly stable water soluble unimolecular micelles that forms complexes with hydrophobic drugs in their inner hydrophobic pockets and can be administered by the oral route. SLNs and NLPs are having solid hydrophobic core of variable crystallinity, stabilized by amphipathic surface. Drugs loaded in particles are retained and released in a controlled manner, as a function of core phase transitions in response to external stimuli such as changes in humidity, heat, light, or mechanical stress. They can be administered by the oral and topical route. Ultradeformable lipid matrices are those vesicles that are capable of experiencing spontaneous locomotion and penetration to deeper layers across water nanochannels in the stratum corneum. Ultradeformable liposomes do not fuse on the surface of the stratum corneum, and penetrate without being destroyed. Ultradeformable liposomes could efficiently transport low- or high-molecular weight hydrophilic drugs across thickened lesions that represent an additional barrier to absorption in the CL.[40]

2.10.1 PHAGOCYTOSIS AND POTENTIAL DRUG DELIVERY SYSTEM

This section demonstrates various nonbiological and biological DSs used to improve the uptake of antibiotics by phagocytic cells, as well as the in vitro and in vivo studies performed with these types of carrier and their efficacy against different types of pathogens. In addition, this chapter also describes nanoparticulate DDS as the most reliable method utilized for the treatment of *Leishmania*

Defense-controlling phagocytic cells are an essential component of the immune system. The main function of these cells is to ingest and destroy microorganisms.[41] These phagocytes are further classified in to various types of cells such as blood polymorphonuclear leucocytes, neutrophils, or granulocytes. When required, these cells migrate to sites of infection. One of the subtype of phagocytes are called as monocytes, also found in the blood stream has the tendency to leave the circulation and penetrate tissues. After penetration, they change shape and become macrophages. Some infectious agents usually parasites are survived and flourish after they have been ingested by phagocytic cells, chiefly macrophages. This type of adaptation exhibited by the pathogen hinders the treatment of this type of infection. The strong adaptation quality of the pathogen at specified intracellular locations allows their internalization in microorganisms. This can protect them from the host defense mechanisms and from the action of various therapeutic agents especially antibiotics. Thus parasite may successfully encounter difficulties in penetrating phagocytic cells.[42,43] Intracellular microorganisms are mainly responsible for various severe pathologic conditions such as leishmaniasis, tuberculosis, or histoplasmosis. Such pathologic conditions are mainly found in immunodepressed patients especially among acquired immunodeficiency syndrome (AIDS) patients.[44] To cure such type of infectious diseases, currently various antibiotics of different groups (aminoglycosides, the fluoroquinolones, the beta-lactams, the macrolides, etc.) are utilized. Penetration ability of these antibiotics in phagocytic cells varies which may limit their potential in the treatment of intracellular infections.

The use of these antibiotics with suitable DSs may enhance their penetration and selective distribution and activate the antibiotic therapy against intracellular infections.

The use of nonviral nanoparticulate systems for the delivery of anti-leishmania drugs is gaining significant focus for medical and pharmaceutical applications. DDS can be designed to meet specific physicochemical requirements, and should be low toxic and produce minimal antigenic reaction. Macrophages are considered as the most potential cellular targets by drug-loaded nanoparticles as they play a central role in inflammation and they act as reservoirs for microorganisms that are involved with deadly infectious diseases such as *Leishmania*. Effective drugs in the treatment of macrophage-mediated diseases usually induce serious adverse effects, when administered as a free form, owing to the requirement of satisfactory concentration to induce a desirable effect. Thus administration of free form of drug could give rise to many problems such as their systemic spreading, a lack of bioavailability at the desired sites, and a short half-life. Employment of drug-loaded nanoparticles for macrophage-mediated diseases represents a better alternative to avoid such problems face by effective drug in free form. This system decreases the side effects and increases efficacy of the therapeutic drug selected for the treatment.

2.10.1.1 MECHANISM OF THE UPTAKE OF ANTIBIOTICS BY PHAGOCYTIC CELLS

Phagocytic cells cause phagocytosis consisting of the ingestion of microorganisms by the cell and their later destruction and elimination. Phagocytosis is also adopted by macrophages and neutrophils (Figure 2-8). It is very essential to explore the exact mechanism involved during this whole process. Uptake of pathogen in phagocyte is dependent on the stimulation of specific surface receptors. Stimulation of selective receptors leads to internalization followed by the formation of a vesicle or phagosome that eventually fuses with lysosomes to give rise to a phagolysosome. This process is sometimes mediated by antibodies. Entry of pathogen in phagocyte also leads to the activation of redox mechanism that may give rise to derivatives of oxygen, halogen ions in the case of neutrophils, and cationic proteins and nitric oxide in the case of macrophages[45,46] (Figure 2-8). The strong adaptive mechanisms followed by intracellular parasites often handicap the phagocytic potential to destroy the germs responsible for an infection. This may give rise to the population or pathogenicity of parasite to further strengthen their survival rate in one cellular compartment or another, or in the cytoplasm if they are able to break down or cross the membrane.[45,47] As mentioned earlier, internalization of these parasites at specified location in phagocytic cells provide them protection from the host defense mechanisms (antibodies or complement) and from the action of antibiotics that are unable to penetrate the cell.[42,43] These infectious agents present in intracellular reservoirs can prevent the action of the antibiotic by penetrating in cells. They leave the host compartment during the entry of antibodies or antibiotics making the cell more susceptible for further relapses and increase the chances of chronic disease.[43,48] Because of their high phagocytic capacity, reduced microbiocidal properties and their long half-lives, monocytes and macrophages are the usual reservoirs for these infective agents.[49] Antibiotics play an important role in destroying intraphagocytic accumulation of parasites. These antibiotics are transported by the phagocytic cells from the blood or a tissue to the site of infection by chemotactic mechanisms. After reaching at desirable site of infection, these phagocytic cells release the drug to kill the pathogen. One of the characters of antibiotic to retain its high concentration in phagocytic cells makes the process easier to exhibit its action against extracellular microorganisms located at the site of infection or inflammation.[50–52] Different types of *Leishmania* pathogen that can cause intracellular infections are highlighted in Table 2-5.

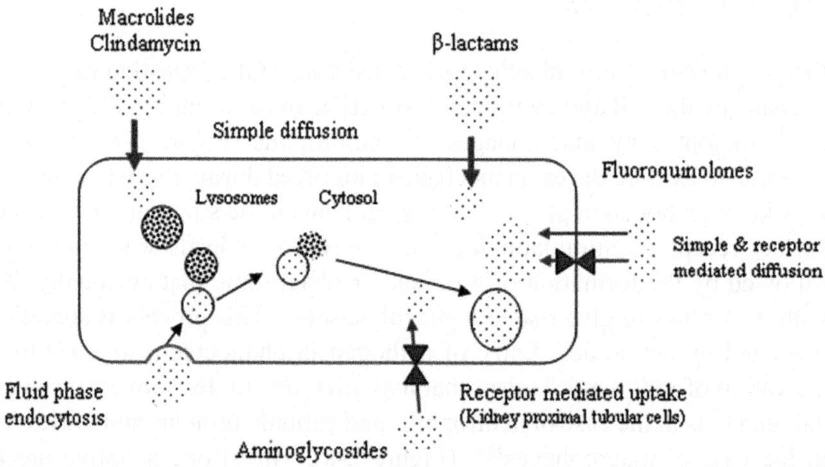

FIGURE 2-8 Phagocytosis of microorganisms by phagocytic cells.

TABLE 2-5 Intracellular microorganisms mediated infections and various antibiotics usually employed for their treatment

Type of infection	Microorganism	Disease	Antibiotic
Protozoarian	*Leishmania donovani*	Visceral leishmaniasis	Pentavalent antimonials, polyene antibiotics, pentamidine, sulphamides, pyrimethamine, suramine, melarsoprol, nifurtimox, tryparsamide
	Leishmania infantum	Visceral leishmaniasis	
	Leishmania major	Cutaneous leishmaniasis	
	Toxoplasma gondii	Toxoplasmosis	
	Trypanosoma cruzi	Chagas disease	

2.10.1.2 ANTIBIOTICS PENETRATION IN PHAGOCYTIC CELLS

Incapability of some antibiotics to penetrate in phagocytic cell and tend to remain in the extracellular space limits its applications in the treatment of various infectious diseases. Therapeutic antibiotic concentrations are required inside the cells to kill all pathogens before their escape. It has been proven that due to the low intracellular concentration retained by most of the antibiotics in vitro shows little or no antibacterial activity in vivo. Therefore the antibiotic must be present at a sufficiently high concentration to be able to destroy the microorganism directly or to increase the antibacterial function of phagocytic cells.[53] The majority of the antibiotics are incapable to penetrate cells (beta-lactams and aminoglycosides) and only some (quinolones, macrolides, and clindamycin) are efficiently taken up by phagocytic cells.[54] The antibiotics that are efficient in infiltrating phagocytes usually adopt several mechanisms, such as diffusion or by receptor-mediated uptake, as shown in Figure 2-9. Fluoroquinolones, beta-lactams, and macrolides infiltrate the cell by diffusion whereas aminoglycosides penetrate by receptor-mediated uptake.[43] The phagocytic concentration of antibiotic is dependent on drug metabolism, elimination, absorption, and binding or accumulation in different intracellular structures such as phagolysosomes. Activity of antibiotics is also dependent on factors like state of bacterial responsiveness, physicochemical environment at the site of infection, and the degree of cooperation with the host defenses.[43,55,56] In addition, metabolic state (sensitive toward the antibiotics) of pathogen and phagocytic capacity also determines the action of the antibiotic[43,56–58] (Figure 2-9). It is more important to look after pharmacodynamic parameters for maintaining the intracellular concentration of certain antibiotic such as macrolides, fluoroquinolones, and aminoglycosides. In addition, the time of exposure is important in beta-lactams and glycopeptides. Physiological intracellular conditions such as acid pH of lysosomes and related vacuoles may decrease the activity of aminoglycosides or macrolides.[43,59,60] It was studied that the intracellular activities of several antibiotics are lower than that observed extracellularly through an in vitro model of infected THP-1 human macrophages with *Staphylococcus*. This was dependent on the extracellular concentration and the time lasting duration of cell exposure to antibiotics.[56] Therefore for exerting intracellular action penetration of antibiotics in phagocytic cells is obligatory (Figure 2-9).[53] This was particularly observed in the case of clindamycin, which is highly concentrated in phagocytic cells however acquired low or no activity against sensitive microorganisms. Perhaps this was due to the inhibitory effects of drug on the antimicrobial action of phagocytic cells.[52,61–65]

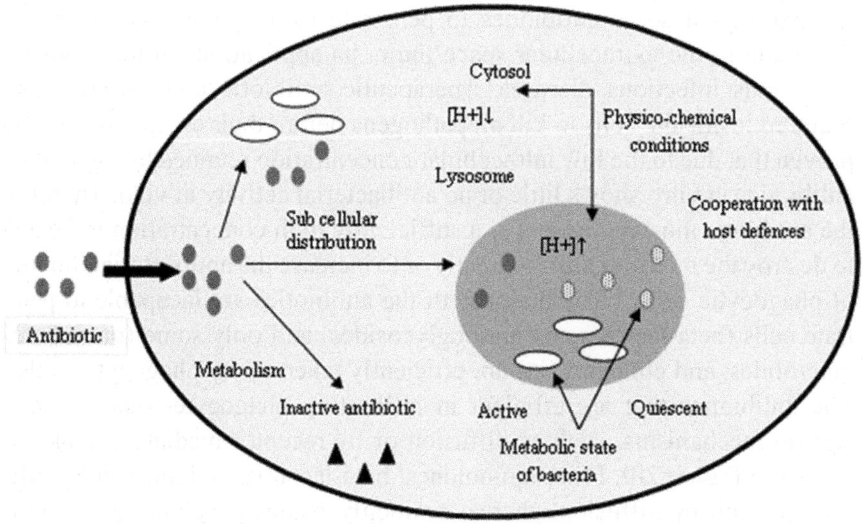

FIGURE 2-9 Mechanism of penetration of antibiotics in phagocytic cells.

2.10.3 DELIVERY SYSTEMS IN ANTIBIOTIC THERAPY FOR PHAGOCYTIC CELLS

DS in the form of suitable carrier systems is required to increase their cellular penetration of antibiotics in order to treat intracellular infections. Such DS is applicable for those antibiotics which are effective against intracellular microorganisms but have a low intracellular penetration capacity. These carrier systems should be having some obligatory characteristics for their application or utilization against intracellular infections such as biodegradable, biocompatible, and they must remain stable under their in vivo conditions,[70,71] must be rapidly recognized and withdrawn from the circulation by the phagocytic cells of the reticuloendothelial system (RES), must achieve elevated drug concentrations in the target cells, should allow sustained release of the drug for prolonged period at the site of infection, prevent premature degradation of the drug, enhance drug retention in tissues, reduce the appearance of resistances due to low drug permeation, increase the therapeutic index, and decrease the toxicity of drug.[44,66–69,72–78] For designing the more specific intracellular DDS, the carrier system must be vectored by using passive or active vectoring process. In passive vectoring, carrier systems are prepared in such a way that they can be easily recognized and ingested by the phagocytic cells as foreign substances. This process is achieved by the opsonization of carriers by serum proteins when they arrive in the bloodstream, hence stimulates the inherent capacity of phagocytic cells to ingest carrier systems. On contrary, active vectoring is done by using surface modifications in the carriers to enhance the affinity for recognizing and specifically interacting with target cells. Surface of the carrier systems are modified by the binding of ligands. These ligands are easily recognized by specific receptors of phagocytic cells. Such recognition promotes the ligand–receptor binding with great affinity and allows their internalization via receptor-mediated endocytosis. Most of the ligands are prepared according to the structure of some selected receptors found on macrophages such as mannosyl/fucosyl receptors and macrophage scavenger receptors. Most of the current research focused on the utilization of glycoproteins or polysaccharides ending in mannose or fucose radicals, and polyanionic macromolecules such as acetylated low density lipoproteins (LDLs), with affinity for scavenger receptors.[79,80] Surface modification of carrier system by fixation of specific antibodies is another alternative to increase selectivity for infected cells. Drug release from these carrier system is chiefly dependent on the nature of the DS. During liposomal delivery, drug is released into the biophase by passive diffusion of the drug through the bilayer and when the liposome is degraded in the lysosome.[72] Carrier systems are made up of synthetic polymers release the drug by several mechanisms such as polymer degradation or chemical cleavage of the drug from the polymer, swelling of the polymers and releasing the drug entrapped within them, osmotic pressure effects creating pores, and by simple diffusion.[77,81] There are various types of carrier system reported for the intracellular delivery of antibiotics such as liposomes, micro- and nanoparticles, nanosuspensions and conjugates with water-soluble polymers and with lipoproteins. Nowadays, biological carrier systems such as cell ghosts are also utilized for treating such type of infection. Factors affecting the intracellular activity of antibiotics are illustrated in Figure 2-10.

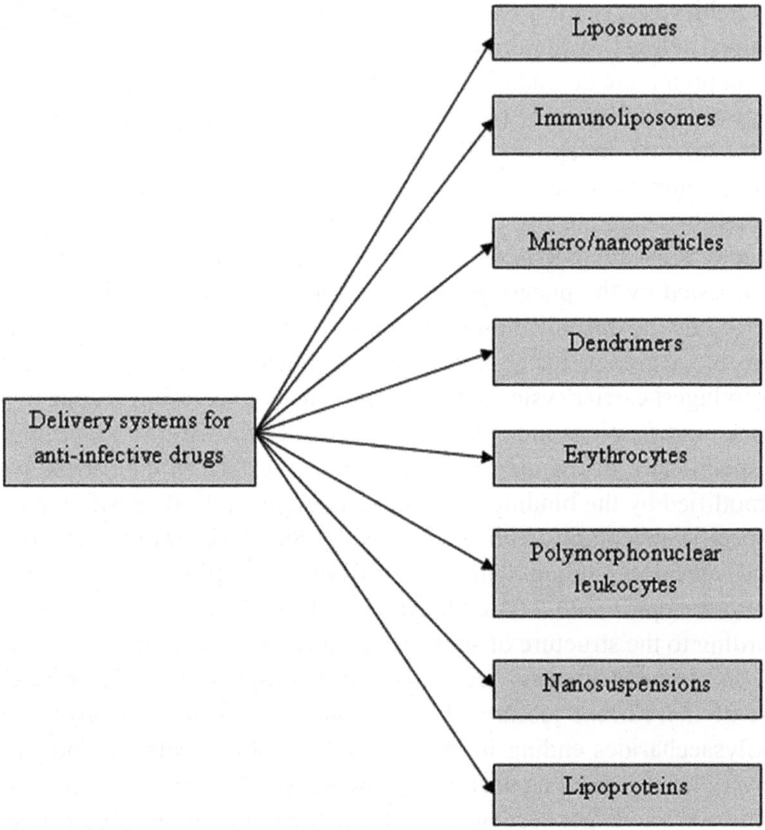

FIGURE 2-10 Factors affecting the intracellular activity of antibiotics.

2.10.4 NANOPARTICULATE SYSTEMS FOR MACROPHAGE TARGETING

Owing to low toxicity and selective nature for targeting tissue and cells, nonviral nanoparticulate systems are promoted nowadays in DDS.[82] To prepare the suitable nanoparticulate systems drugs, peptides, and nucleic acids of poor stability are combined with polymers and lipids to obtain very fine, sub-micron particulate systems. Such prepared forms acquire the ability to interact with the cells and be internalized by them. There are enormous therapeutic applications of these systems such as DDSs, cancer therapy and diagnosis, gene therapy, and immunomodulating activities have been reported.[83] Nanoparticulate system is advantageous in conjugating them to specific ligands so that they can be easily targeted at desired cell type, tissue, or organ; whereas optimization and physicochemical characterization could facilitate a desired therapeutic level to be reached. One of the main disadvantage of nanoparticulate system is that they can be easily recognized by the RES, hence eliminated from the bloodstream within short period after intravenous injection, depending on their size and surface characteristics. In addition, the rapid uptake of nanoparticles is problematic when the long-term circulation of nanoparticle-loaded drug systems is needed. This problem limits most of the applications of nanoparticles. To combat with such problem nanoparticles are modified at their surface. This surface modification is achieved by using polyethylene glycol (PEG) in case of polymeric drug carriers and liposomes. Moreover utilization of amphiphilic diblock copolymer monomethoxypoly(ethylene oxide)–poly(lactic acid) (MPEO–PLA) in the preparation of nanoparticles was also promoted for extending their phagocytosis. However, surface modification or coating protocol to delay opsonization process depends on the chain length and the density of these moieties at the surface of the particles. Recent reports confirms the promising effects of polyalkylcyanoacrylate (PACA) nanoparticles that can be prepared either by polymerization of alkylcyanoacrylate monomers or directly from the polymers. Nanospheres obtained from PACA have the potential to bind a wide array of drugs in a nonspecific manner, thus expanding their significance for several treatments. Various methods have been used to derive nanospheres, oil- and water-containing nanocapsules and core-shell nanospheres. Couvreur et al. demonstrated role of PACA nanoparticles in drug targeting to specific sites in the body, with a particular emphasis on cancer chemotherapy. Their potential use of PACA nanoparticles as carriers for antisense oligonucleotides (ODN) has also been reported.[84] Combining together PACA nanoparticles are considered for their dual and synergistic action by combining different drugs during the synthesis and loading process. Nanoparticles are proven as best candidate for functional small interfering RNA (siRNA). These siRNA are composed of 21–23 nucleotides and are designed to degrade a specifically targeted mRNA. Among the recent applications, targeting the lung in mice in order to modulate respiratory syncytial virus (RSV) infection and potential inhibition of vascular endothelial growth factor (VEGF) expression followed by the inhibition of tumor are the prominent one.[85]

2.10.5 NANOPARTICLE-MEDIATED THERAPY FOR LEISHMANIAL PATHOGEN

Nowadays phagocyte-mediated therapies constitute various promising approaches to treat diseases. For the effective targeting a profound knowledge of surface receptors and nanoparticulate surface modification or conjugation strategies are required for their efficient interaction with cell systems. Various strategies used against infective agents are demonstrated in Figure 2-11. Our main purpose is to address significance of nanoparticulate systems for macrophage therapies of bacterial infections especially *Leishmania*. Parasites that are responsible for *Leishmania* causes several infectious diseases which can spread to the visceral organs, such as liver and spleen, resulting in VL, or to mucous membranes of the mouth and nose. Progression will occurs if disease is not diagnosed or untreated at initial stages. It may also diseases provoke high rates of mortality. As mentioned earlier, the adaptation and internalization of these parasites at specific location (organelles or cytoplasm e.g., the lysosomal vacuoles of reticuloendothelial macrophages) hinder the accessibility of antileishmanial drugs. This issue attracts several researchers to design nanocarriers for targeting antileishmanial drugs to macrophages so as to increase their penetration across the macrophage and to increase the retention time period of the drug inside the compartment. In addition, the encapsulation of antileishmanial drugs overcomes their side effects. Natural polymers are also proved to be effective in encapsulation of AmB as recently investigated by Bhatia et al. (in significance of algal polymer in designing AmB nanoparticles).[86] AmB-mediated nanoparticles are responsible for the stimulation of inflammatory mediators, such as IL-1 and TNF-α, in human and murine mononuclear cells,[47–49] acting as secondary defense mechanism against the parasitic infection.[47–49] It has been studied that this drug showed an improvement in its efficacy when encapsulated in poly (e-caprolactone) nanospheres stabilized with poloxamer 188. Furthermore drug also acquired inhibitory effect on the IL-1 and TNF-acytokines production in mouse peritoneal macrophages.[90] Quercetin-encapsulated nano forms was found to reduce the parasite burden in the spleen and reduces hepatotoxicity and renaltoxicity.[91] Nano forms of gentamycin with polybutylcyanoacrylate as coating polymer improve the side effects of this drug during its administration for intracellular delivery to mouse intraperitoneal macrophages.[92] Poly (D,L-lactide) nanoparticles were also used against *L. donovani* activity after loading them with primaquine. This type of association improves the efficacy of the drug than the free form and resulted in a reduced toxicity. Similarly no systemic toxicity was observed with PLA nanoparticles-loaded primaquine after intravenous injection in BALB/c mice; however, administration of same dose of free drug resulted in weight loss of the animals.[93] polyisohexylcyanoacrylate (PIHCA) nanoparticles were also found to improve the efficacy of primaquine.[94] In addition, phagocytosis of PACA nanoparticles by J-744 macrophages induced the activation of a respiratory burst, which led to augmented antileishmanial action. Methacrylate-mediated pentamidine nanospheres were found to be 25 times more active than in the case of the free form.[95] Therefore the treatment of infected macrophages with nanoforms-mediated DDSs is proved to be an effective therapy for increasing the infiltration, retention bioavailability, and concentration inside the infected monocyte/macrophagic system.

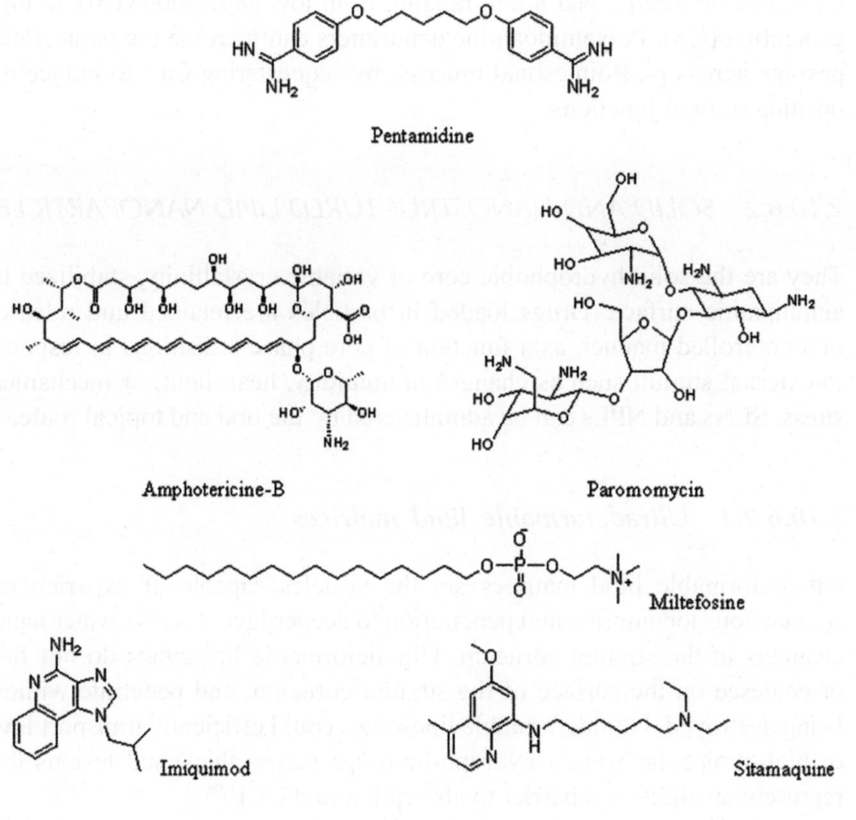

FIGURE 2-11 Strategies used against infective agents.

2.10.6 POTENTIAL NANO DRUG DELIVERY SYSTEMS AGAINST LEISHMANIASIS

2.10.6.1 DENDRIMERS

Dendrimers are water soluble and act as unimolecular micelles to form complexes with hydrophobic drugs in their inner hydrophobic pockets. Because of their high structural stability dendrimers can be administered by the oral route.[96] Different to conventional polymeric particles, the issues associated with scaling up, presence of by-products and reproducible size are resolved for dendrimers. On the basis of polymers dispersion, there are two types of dendrimers (monodisperse and polyamidoamine). Monodisperse dendrimers are made up of monodisperse polymers with high area/volume ratio, size between 2 and 8 nm, ranging from low generation (G0), to high generation (G8). Polyamidoamine dendrimers can increase the paracellular passage across gastrointestinal mucosa, by sequestering Ca^{2+} to induce the opening of tight junctions.

2.10.6.2 SOLID AND NANOSTRUCTURED LIPID NANOPARTICLES

They are the solid hydrophobic core of variable crystallinity, stabilized by amphipathic surface. Drugs loaded in particles are retained and released in a controlled manner, as a function of core phase transitions in response to external stimuli such as changes in humidity, heat, light, or mechanical stress. SLNs and NPLs can be administered by the oral and topical route.[97]

2.10.6.2.1 Ultradeformable lipid matrices

Ultradeformable lipid matrices are the vesicles capable of experiencing spontaneous locomotion and penetration to deeper layers across water nano-channels in the stratum corneum. Ultradeformable liposomes do not fuse or coalesce on the surface of the stratum corneum, and penetrate without being destroyed. Ultradeformable liposomes could efficiently transport low- or high-molecular weight hydrophilic drugs across thickened lesions that represent an additional barrier to absorption in the CL.[98]

2.11 CURRENT THERAPIES

Current treatment of leishmaniasis is primarily based on chemotherapy with some attempts at immunotherapy.[99] Despite substantial research, there is currently no vaccine against *Leishmania* infection.[100] Treatment of the disease is predominantly based on the pentavalent antimonials, a group of drugs introduced in the first half of the 20th century.[101,102] Although this is the classic treatment in most endemic areas, its usefulness has been compromised by the emergence of resistance and its variable efficacy against different forms of disease. Second line treatment includes drugs such as AmB and pentamidine. These are characterized by high efficacy, but are also relatively expensive and have severe side effects.[102–104] These factors affect all currently available antileishmanial drugs, prompting a search for novel drug targets and new approaches to drug development. Structures of various antileishmanial drugs published in the past few years are demonstrated in Figure 2-12.

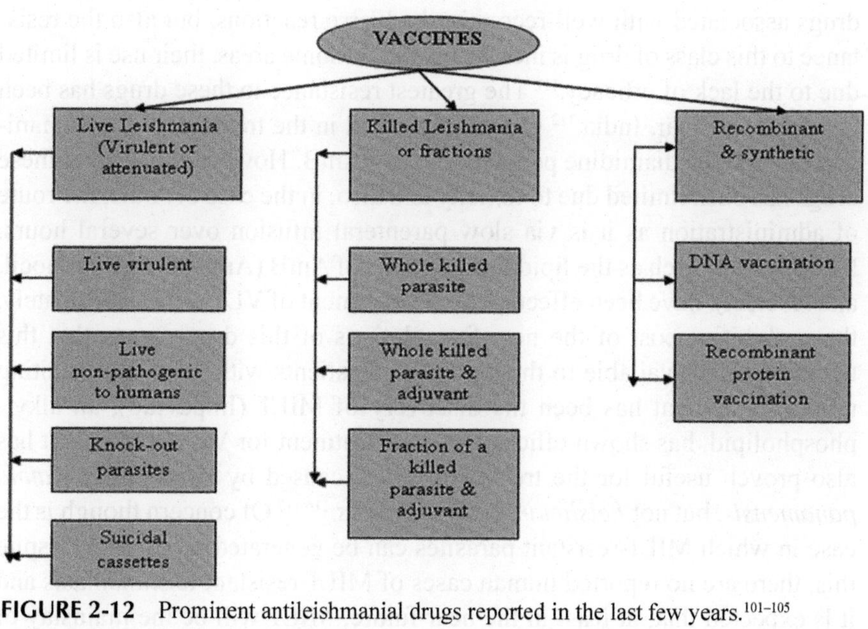

FIGURE 2-12 Prominent antileishmanial drugs reported in the last few years.[101–105]

Pentamidine and other aromatic diamidines (Figure 2-12) were synthesized as hypoglycemic drugs, where their chemotherapeutic profile against antiprotozoal therapy was early discovered. Diamidines have been used against *Leishmania* infections since 1939, with pentamidine being the one that has displayed higher chemical stability, as it eases administration and contains less toxicity. The chemical delivery of pentamidine is in the form of isehionate salts, whereas the pharmaceutic presentation is an intravenous or intramuscular injection (Pentam 300) or nebulizer (Nebupent). Pentamidine and other diamidines have developed good therapeutic indexes against Indian and African leishmaniasis in humans, although their toxicity rates have precluded this group of drugs as second-line chemotherapeutic compounds against *Leishmania.* However, pentamidine is the drug of choice in arsenic- or antimony-relapsed *Leishmania* strains and especially in *Pneumocystis carinii* pneumonia patients affected with human immunodeficiency virus (HIV). The pentamidine mode of action is controversial and not completely understood. The cationic structure of this molecule is due to its strong cationic nature at physiological pH, thus being responsible for its strong cationic nature at physiological pH, thus being responsible for the host.[105–109]

The pentavalent antimonials have been recommended for the treatment of leishmaniasis for over 50 years.[110] Not only is the treatment with these drugs associated with well-recognized adverse reactions, but also the resistance to this class of drug is increasing and, in some areas, their use is limited due to the lack of efficacy.[111] The greatest resistance to these drugs has been observed in Bihar, India.[112] Other drugs used in the treatment of leishmaniasis include the diamidine pentamidine and AmB. However, the use of these drugs has been limited due to toxicity and also, in the case of AmB, the route of administration as it is via slow parenteral infusion over several hours. Newer drugs, such as the lipid formulations of AmB (Ambisome, Amphocil, and Abelcet), have been effective in the treatment of VL.[113,114] Unfortunately, the prohibitive cost of the new formulations of this drug means that this treatment is unavailable to the majority of patients with VL.[113] An exciting new development has been the discovery of MILT (Impavido), an alkylphospholipid, has shown efficacy as oral treatment for VL in India.[115] It has also proven useful for the treatment of CL caused by *Leishmania vianna panamensis*, but not *Leishmania v braziliensis.*[116,117] Of concern though is the ease in which MILT-resistant parasites can be generated in vitro.[118] Despite this, there are no reported human cases of MILT-resistant leishmaniasis and it is expected that, at least in the near future, MILT will be the mainstay of treatment in India and surrounding regions. Various antileishmanial drugs and their mode of action, toxicity, route of administration, regimen, efficacy, resistance, and price are mentioned in Table 2-6.

TABLE 2-6 Antileishmanial drugs and their mode of action

Antileishmanial drugs	Mechanism of action	Toxicity	Visceral leishmaniasis	Cutaneous leishmaniasis	Administration regimen, efficacy, resistance, price
Pentavalent antimonials (sodium stibogluconate) (Pentostam) OSbOHO	Action on the macrophage, Activated within the amastigote form	Limited information regarding chemistry and mode of action: cardio toxicity, renal insufficiency, pancreatitis, anemia, leucopenia headache, nausea, vomiting, abdominal pain on long-term administration.	First-line drugs Sodium stibogluconate (Pentostam, SSG)	First-line drugs Sodium stibogluconate (Pentostam)	*Administration:* IV, IM, and IL, *Regimen:* 30 days 20 mg/kg/day *Efficacy:* 35–95% (depending on area) *Resistance:* Common (>60% in Bihar, India) *Price:* $50–70
Pentamidines [Dimedene analogs such as mepacrine, pentamidine isethionate (Pentam-300)]	Binds to tRNA and inhibits aminoacylation and translation of the replicating parasite.	Emergence of drug resistance especially in HIV coinfections. Adverse reactions of injectable form of pentamidine: hypotension, hypoglycemia, leucopenia, thrombocytopenia, cardiac arrhythmia, acute renal failure, elevated serum creatinine level, nausea, fever.	First-line drugs	First-line drugs	

TABLE 2-6 *(Continued)*

Antileishmanial drugs	Mechanism of action	Toxicity	Visceral leishmaniasis	Cutaneous leishmaniasis	Administration regimen, efficacy, resistance, price
Amphotericin B (Polyene antibiotics) Ambisome, Amphocil,Acelcet	Binds with the ergosterols of the parasitic cell membranes thus forming a binary complex with the membrane sterols resulting in pores which causes changes in membrane permeability and ionic balance leading to parasitic cell death	Nephrotoxicity Poor gastro-intestinal absorption and negligible bioavailability. Also may react with mammalian cell membrane causing cellular dysfunction. ± Rigors and chills during infusion	First line drugs Amphotericin B (Fungizone) Liposomal amphotericin B (AmBisome)	First line drugs Amphotericin B (Fungizone)	*Administration:* IV, Lip AmB: *Regimen:* 30 days 1 mg/kg (15 mg/kg total dose), Lip AmB: 5–20 mg/kg total dose 4–10 doses over 10– 20 days *Efficacy* >90%, Lip AmB: >97% *Resistance:* Laboratory strains, Lip AmB: Not documented *Price :* $100, Lip AmB: $280

TABLE 2-6 *(Continued)*

Antileishmanial drugs	Mechanism of action	Toxicity	Visceral leishmaniasis	Cutaneous leishmaniasis	Administration regimen, efficacy, resistance, price
Paromomycin (an aminocyclitol-aminoglycoside antibiotic)	Impairs the macromolecular synthesis and alters the membrane properties of leishmania	Mainly used in the cutaneous form of the disease Has limited use in the treatment of visceral leishmaniasis. + Nephrotoxicity, ototoxicity, hepatotoxicity	Clinical trials (Paromomycin (Phase III))	First line drugs Paromomycin (topical formulations with methylbenzethonium chloride or urea) Clinical trials Paromomycin (topical formulation with gentamicin and surfactants, Phase II)	*Administration:* IM *Regimen:* 21 days 15 mg/kg/day *Efficacy:* 94% (India) 46–85% (Africa, depending on dose) *Resistance:* Laboratory strains <u>Price</u> :$10
5. Miltefosine	Mechanism of action uncertain, possible inhibition by phosphatidylcholine biosynthesis, signal transduction and regulation of calcium homeostasis	Development of quick drug resistance + Gastrointestinal, nephrotoxicity, hepatotoxicity, teratogenicity	Clinical trials Miltefosine (oral, Phase IV; registered in India)	Clinical trials Miltefosine (oral, Phase III, registered in Colombia)	*Administration:* IM *Regimen:* 28 days 1.5–2.5 mg/day *Efficacy:* 94–97% *Resistance:* Laboratory strains *Price:* $70

2.11.1 DRUGS IN CLINICAL DEVELOPMENT

2.11.1.1 MILTEFOSINE

MILT, initially developed as an anticancer drug, is the first effective oral treatment of VL and the latest antileishmanial drug to enter the market. Its antileishmanial activity was initially discovered in the mid-1980s and efficacy demonstrated in a number of experimental models in vitro and in vivo. These findings led to clinical trials and registration in India in March 2002 for oral treatment of VL and in Colombia for CL in 2005. There are concerns about teratogenicity and the long half-life of the drug, and that the latter might encourage the emergence of resistance.[119]

2.11.1.2 PAROMOMYCIN

PAR, an aminoglycoside antibiotic, was originally identified as an antileishmanial in the 1960s and has been used in clinical trials for both VL and CL. Development of the parenteral formulation of PAR, a drug with poor oral bioavailability, for VL has been slow, but phase III trials are currently ongoing in India under the aegis of the Institute of One World Health (*www.iowh.org*) and in East Africa managed by DNDi and partner institutes (*www.dndi.org*). As with MILT, resistance to PAR could be induced in *L. donovani* promastigotes experimentally in vitro. The resistance was specific to PAR and stable and its mechanism seems to be due to decreased drug uptake.[119] PAR might also be a drug suitable for the topical treatment of CL.

2.11.1.3 AMPHOTERICIN B FORMULATIONS

AmB in the form of AmB deoxycholate (Fungizone) is the second-line treatment for VL when antimonial therapy fails. Originally developed as a systemic antifungal, it is also an efficient antileishmanial, but has the major drawback of being acutely toxic and thus must be carefully administered. To ameliorate this, reformulations of AmB have been developed to alter its pharmacokinetics. By changing the serum-binding properties, its high affinity for LDLs being the major cause of toxicity, lipid-associated AmB preparations have been made with varying degrees of success. The liposomal AmB formulation, Ambisome, is registered treatment for VL, but use in VL endemic regions is limited by cost.[119]

2.11.1.4 SITAMAQUINE

Sitamaquine (WR6026) is an 8-aminoquinoline currently in clinical development by Glaxo Smith Kline for oral treatment of VL.[119] Discovery of sitamaquine as antileishmanial agent was based on extensive efforts in synthetic chemistry at the Walter Reed Army Institute for Research (WRAIR). Recently, results were reported from phase II dose ranging studies in India and Kenya. The overall cure rate at day 180 in the intention-to-treat-population was 83% in Kenyan patients[119] and 87% in Indian patients.[119] Abdominal pain and headache were reported in the Kenyan study and vomiting, dyspepsia, and cyanosis by the Indian investigators. Methemoglobinemia is associated with 8-aminoquinolines, but was only reported in Indian patients.[119] Sitamaquine is rapidly metabolized, forming desethyl and 4-CH_2OH derivatives, which might be responsible for its activity.

2.11.1.5 IMIQUIMOD

Imiquimod (Aldara, 3M Pharmaceuticals) is an antiviral compound [1-(2-methylropyl)-1*H*-imidazo(4,5-c)quinolin-4-amine] used extensively for the topical treatment of genital warts caused by the human papillomavirus. It is an immunomodulator, stimulating a local immune response at the site of application, which in turn resolves the infection. Imiqimod induces the production of cytokines and nitric oxide in macrophages and has been shown to have an effect in experimental infections of CL,[119] and in conjunction with standard antimonial chemotherapy, has been used to successfully treat patients with cutaneous lesions, which did not respond to antimonial therapy alone.[119] It is suggested that the topical treatment activates localized macrophages to kill the parasite, whereas the antimonial eliminates systemic amastigotes that are responsible for persistence of infection.[119]

2.11.2 LEISHMANIA VACCINES

Leishmania are obligate intracellular vector-borne parasites that cause significant morbidity and mortality in many countries worldwide. There are several species of the parasite that vary according to geographical location and cause a variety of clinical syndromes ranging from self-limiting cutaneous lesions to potentially fatal infection of the viscera. The disease manifested is dependent on both the species of the parasite and the immune response of the host. Depending on the species of the parasite, resistance to infection is generally associated with a T-helper-1 immune response that activates macrophages to kill intracellular *Leishmania* in a nitric oxide-dependent manner. Conversely, disease progression is generally associated with a T-helper-2 response that activates humoral immunity.[50] Chemotherapeutic treatments for leishmaniasis exist but are expensive, toxic, and ineffective against resistant strains. A vaccine against leishmaniasis is feasible since most individuals that were once infected become resistant to clinical infection when later exposed. However, despite the wealth of information regarding the genetics of the parasite and the experimental immunology of the disease, there is currently no vaccine against *Leishmania.* A multitude of vaccine strategies have been pursued including the use of killed and genetically modified parasites. Immunization with naked plasmid DNA encoding *Leishmania* Ags represents a new approach to a *Leishmania* vaccine and confers several advantages over the more traditional vaccination methods.[120] In order to develop an effective vaccine against leishmaniasis, it is important to understand the mechanisms of the immune response to *Leishmania* infection. Classification of *Leishmania* vaccine is demonstrated in Figure 2-13.

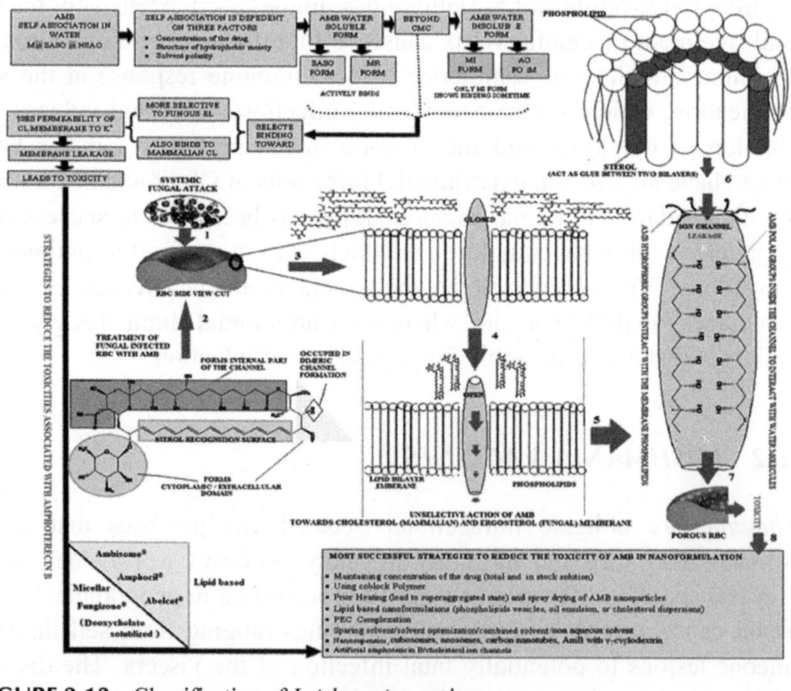

FIGURE 2-13 Classification of *Leishmania* vaccines.

Live virulent vaccination with live, virulent *L. major* called as leishmanization that resulted in a lifelong protection against *L. major* after cure. Live vaccines that are carrying the live species (*L. tarentolae*), which is nonpathogenic to humans and induced a protective immune response against *L. donovani*. Knock-out parasites vaccines are those vaccines in which removal/blocking/replacement of parasite genes is made for survival. It was reported that administration of DHFR-TS (enzyme gene) *L. major* knock-out gene resulted in a survival of knock-out in mice for about 2 months without producing a lesion. Such type of vaccines provides short-term protection against wild-type strain. Suicidal cassettes-type vaccines are those vaccines that contain genetically modified Ag. Parasites are genetically modified to induce suicide in response to external signals or to produce biological substances that activate immune attack against them.[120] Administration of *L. major* strains producing biologically active granulocyte-macrophage colony-stimulating factor–enhanced parasite killing and delayed lesion development in susceptible BALB/c mice. Whole-killed parasite vaccines are a single species of killed promastigotes or more than one species of killed strains. Recent report related with killed parasite vaccines suggested that a delivery of such killed single strain of *Leishmania amazonensis* significantly increases protection from natural infection and Th1 responses. Whole-killed parasite and adjuvant are those vaccines that are made up of whole dead promastigotes and an adjuvant to stimulate immune response, for example, killed *L. mexicana/L. braziliensis* promastigotes and BCG. Such types of vaccines are used in severe cases to develop Th1 immune response. Fraction of a killed parasite and adjuvant vaccines are made up of *Leishmania* Ags and an adjuvant to stimulate an immune response, for example, fructose mannose ligand (FML) Ag from surface of parasite and saponin adjuvant (Leishmunew). The first vaccines against canine VL are called as potential transmission-blocking vaccine. DNA vaccination are those that are made by introduction of bacterial plasmid DNA encoding Ags into host cells in vivo, for example, multi-antigenic DNA vaccine encoding KMPII, TRYP, LACK, and CP636 DNA vaccine against parasite enzyme *gamma-glutamylcysteine synthetase* (g-GCS). These vaccines increases the production of IgG1 and IgG2 and provides cell-mediated immunity but are unable to induce protection in dogs against *L. infantum*. Recombinant protein vaccination are such vaccination that are provided with recombinant proteins, for example, recombinant hydrophilic acylated surface protein B1 (HASPB1) that provides protection against experimental challenge with *L. donovani*.[120]

2.11.3 ADJUVANTS FOR LEISHMANIA VACCINE

The term adjuvant has been used for any material that can increase the humoral or cellular immune response to an Ag. In the conventional vaccines, adjuvants are used to elicit an early, high, and long-lasting immune response. The mode of action of adjuvants was described[121–122] as the formation of a depot of Ag at the site of inoculation, with slow release; the presentation of Ag to immunocompetent cells; and the production of various and different lymphokines. Over the past decade, there has been a flurry of research on adjuvants for vaccines, and several novel adjuvants are now licensed products or in late stage clinical development. The success of adjuvants in enhancing the immune response to Ags has led many researchers to refocus their vaccine development programs. Although several vaccine candidates have been tested against leishmaniasis, there is yet no effective vaccine against this parasitic disease. Recent research has documented that efforts to develop effective *Leishmania* vaccine have been limited due to the lack of an appropriate adjuvant. It seems likely that adjuvants will be increasingly important as the science of *Leishmania* vaccine advances. First generation (killed) vaccines, which are relatively safe, have been made and they could be improved by the addition of appropriate adjuvants to provide longer lasting protection with fewer inoculations.[121] Criteria involved in selecting the formulation for a given vaccine include the nature of the antigenic components, type of immune response desired, preferred route of delivery, avoidance of considerable adverse effects, and stability of the vaccine. The optimally formulated adjuvant will be safe, stable before administration, readily biodegraded and eliminated, able to promote an Ag-specific immune response, and inexpensive to produce. New vaccines are urgently needed for many infections caused by intracellular infections including HIV, leishmaniasis, malaria, and tuberculosis.[121] They will require a more sophisticated approach. These intracellular pathogens are well-adapted parasites with sophisticated mechanisms for evading immune responses. In developing vaccines for leishmaniasis, it will be necessary to consider adjuvants as sophisticated agents which can critically influence many parameters of immune responses including specificity, type, intensity, duration, and genetic variability. The study of adjuvants is, in reality, the study of factors that control the expression of different types of immune responses. It would be exciting to discover an adjuvant that, when combined with a suitable Ag, will be able to induce an early, potent and long-lasting *Leishmania*-specific cellular immune response. Adjuvants used for *Leishmania* vaccine are listed in Table 2-7.

TABLE 2-7 List of adjuvants used for *Leishmania* vaccine[51]

Adjuvants	Composition of whole vaccine	Mechanism of action	Limitation
Interleukin-12 (IL-12)	*Leishmania* antigen (SLA)+IL-12	CD4 differentiation of +Th 1 cells in the lymph node and spleen Production of IFN-γ from T-cell and natural killer cells	High cost, difficult to manufacture, its efficacy and safety as an adjuvant for human use is questionable
Granolucyte macrophage-colony stimulating factor (GM-CSF)	Antigens, TSA, LmSTII, rLb-hsp83 and 10 mg of LeIF in combination with 50 mg of GM-CSF (Leukine)	Dominant Th 1 type response	Erythema, induration at the injection site, high doses injection with pentavalent antimony shortens the healingtime
Bacille Calmette Guérin (BCG)	*Mycobacterium bovis*, (*Mycobacterium tuberculosis*) e.g., BCG vectors carrying gp63 against *L. major*	Induction of a Th 1 immune response And production of IFN-γ	Inflammatory arthritis and autoimmune reactions
Montanide ISA 720	*Montanide ISA 720* (ICC-1132/ ISA 720: malaria vaccine) *Montanide ISA 720-TAB9* (HIV vaccine) *Montanide ISA 720-L. major* (*Leishmania* vaccine)	Alternative adjuvant to aluminium hydroxide inducing both Th 1-type cellular and humoral immune responses in humans	Transient injection site pain, Montanide ISA 720-TAB9 showed reactogenicity
Aluminium salts	Noncrystalline gels based on aluminium oxyhydroxide, aluminium hydroxyphosphate or various e.g., *L. amazonensis* promastigotes + rhIL-12 + Alum; Alum-precipitated; ALM vaccine + BCG against *L. donovani*	Approved for use in humans and enhances the primary immunization series, reducing the amount of antigen needed per dose	Salts have little effect on peptide and polysaccharide antigens; general local reactions (sterile abscesses, erythema, subcutaneous nodules, granulomatous inflammation and contact hypersensitivity

TABLE 2-7 *(Continued)*

Adjuvants	Composition of whole vaccine	Mechanism of action	Limitation
Monophosphoryl lipid A (MPL)	LeIF, LmSTI-1 and TSA + MPL+ squalene (MPL-SE) in squalene oil as adjuvant; Leish-111f-MPL-SE vaccine (most effective formulation); *L. major* SEAgs	Leish-111f-MPL-SE vaccine first defined vaccine for leishmaniasis (increases CD4, T cells producing IFN-γ, IL- 2, and tumor necrosis factor, cytokines, indicating a Th 1-type immune response)	In human clinical trials and has completed phases I and II safety and immunogenicity testing in normal, healthy human subjects with no adverse effects being observed
CPG Oligodeoxynucleotide (CpG ODN)	Unmethylated CpG dinucleotide motifs present in bacterial genomes or synthetic oligodeoxynucleotides (ODNs)	Strong immunostimulatory agents in mice boosting the humoral and cellular response (promote Th 1 responses)	CpG ODN has very rare limitations and provide stable, cost effective adjuvant for use in vaccination
Liposomes	Dehydration-rehydration vesicle (DRV)- *L. major;* positively charged liposomes- *L. donovani* promastigotes (PLLD)	PLLD: With BCG could be used to induce a Th 1 response in resistant C57 BL/6 mice; DRV: significant T-cell activation	DRV liposomesnot suitable for I.V. route immunization with the leishmanial antigen preparation; DRV was not protective when the subcutaneous route
Glucan	Glucan is a β 1,3 polyglucose derivative of baker's Yeast+ formalin-killed *L. donovani*	Variable protection and immune response against visceral infection with the parasite was seen in groups vaccinated with glucan and soluble antigens	Injections of glucan alone induced a lesser degree of resistance against infection
Corynabacterium parvum	*Bordetella pertussis* components + cholera toxin + Mycobacteria + Corynabacteria (commonly used micro-organisms, whole or their parts) *C. parvum* + low infection dose (*L. amazonensis*; *C. parvum* + *L. major* promastigote surface antigen-2 complex)	C. parvum + 46-kilodalton glycoprotein (M-2) of *L. amazonensis* appeared to be the Th1 immune response as CD4 + T cells and produce large amounts of IFN-γ	

TABLE 2-7 *(Continued)*

Adjuvants	Composition of whole vaccine	Mechanism of action	Limitation
Saponins (Quil-A, ISCOM and QS-21)	Quil-A and its derivatives, extracted from the bark of the *Quillaja saponaria* tree (*L. braziliensis* promastigote protein + Quil-A, ISCOM and QS-21)	Saponins have been widely used as an adjuvant in veterinary vaccines, increases anti-*Leishmania* IgG isotypes, together with higher levels of lymphocytes, particularly of circulating CD8 and T lymphocytes	
Freund's adjuvants (FCA)	FCA is a mixture of non-metabolizable oil (mineral oil), a surfactant (Arlacel A), and mycobacteria (*M. tuberculosis or M. butyricum*); Freund's adjuvants + killed *L. infantum* promastigotes	Antibody production is increased by FCA primarily because of the depot effect and nonspecific immunopotentiation of macrophages by surfactant and the mycobacteria	Pathologic reaction to the Freund's adjuvants starts at the injection site with mild erythema and swelling followed by tissue necrosis, and intense inflammation

2.11.4 CLINICAL MANIFESTATIONS

Clinical manifestations of a disease mean those that can be determined by history (talking to the patient) and examination (observing the patient, including with some simple tools such as a stethoscope or thermometer). The clinical manifestations of *Leishmania* vary with geography, epidemiology, immunity, and age.

2.11.4.1 CUTANEOUS LEISHMANIASIS

The clinical manifestation of CL is often compared with that of leprosy. There can be two types of clinical manifestations found in CL: simple or diffuse (disseminated). In CL, various types of parasitic species cause the "wet" ulcers and "dry" ulcers. The primary indication of this infectious disease is skin lesions, which can spontaneously cure before 10 months. When wound is infected against sandfly bites the inoculation occurs. This may usually occur on legs, arms, neck, or face. Incubative period of parasite extends from weeks to months, followed by the appearance of an erythematous papule. This erythematous stage can transform in to painless lesion stage or plaque or ulcer. These lesions are usually painless.[39] There are no systemic symptoms reported for CL. The key feature of CL after recovery or successful treatment is that it induces immunity to reinfection by the species of *Leishmania* that caused the disease. Clinical features of CL according to their types are highlighted in Table 2-8.

2.11.4.2 MUCOCUTANEOUS LEISHMANIASIS

In South America, it is also referred as *espundia*. It is generally characterized by metastasis stage from disseminated protozoa rather than by local spread. MCL is usually caused by New World species. However Old World *Leishmania aethiopica* has also been reported to cause this syndrome.

Secondary infection plays a prominent role in the size and persistence of ulcers. Infection by *L. (Viannia) braziliensis* may lead to mucosal involvement in up to 10% of infections, depending on the region in which it was acquired. The incubation period is from 1 to 3 months. The initial infection is characterized by a persistent cutaneous lesion that eventually heals, although as many as 30% of patients report no prior evidence of leishmaniasis. Ulcer progression is slow and steady. Several years later, oral and respiratory

TABLE 2-8 Types of cutaneous leishmaniasis

Types of CL	Clinical manifestation	General remarks
Localized cutaneous disease	• Lesions are without pain or pruritus • Scarring and changes in pigmentation • Exhibit localized lymphangitic spread.	• Both New World and Old World species cause localized cutaneous leishmaniasis. • New World disease usually presents with a solitary nodule, whereas Old World disease is associated with multiple lesions.
Diffuse cutaneous leishmaniasis	• Diffuse cutaneous disease develops in an anergic host with poor immune response. • Individual with a deficient cell-mediated immunity is most vunerable for this type of disease (human immunodeficiency virus (HIV) infection) • Characterized by a primary lesion, which may spread to multiple areas of the skin (face, ears, extremities, buttocks) until the whole body is affected. • Plaques, ulcers, and nodules may form over the entire body, resembling lepromatous leprosy (see the image below). • No neurologic or systemic invasion is involved • Lesions are neither destructive nor erosive, they are disfiguring. • Infections are chronic and may recur after treatment	• Diffuse disease is more common with New World species • Old World *L. aethiopica* may progress to diffuse disease in East Africa
Leishmaniasis recidivans	• Leishmaniasis recidivans may occur years after a localized cutaneous • lesion has healed, commonly presenting on the face • New ulcers and papules form over the edge of the old scar and proceed inward to form a psoriasiform lesion. • Infection may be from reactivation of dormant parasites or new infection from a different species. • Skin trauma can result in activation of seemingly latent cutaneous infection long after the initial bite.	The infections tend to be resistant to treatment.

TABLE 2-8 *(Continued)*

Types of CL	Clinical manifestation	General remarks
Post-kala-azar dermal leishmaniasis	• Characterized by multiple, hypopigmented, erythematous macules. • Over time, these macules can transform into large nontender plaques and nodules that involve the face and trunk • Disease resembles lepromatous leprosy	• Post-kala-azar dermal leishmaniasis follows the treatment of visceral leishmaniasis • In Africa (about 2% of cases) and India (about 10% of cases)
The African variant	• This may occurs shortly after treatment of visceral leishmaniasis • Characterized by an erythematous papular rash on the face, buttocks, and extremities. • Lesions spontaneously resolve over the course of several months.	

mucosal involvement occurs, causing inflammation and mutilation of the nose, mouth, oropharynx, and trachea (see the following image), resulting in symptoms of nasal obstruction and bleeding. These can become sites of infection, sometimes leading to sepsis. Cases in which the time between the primary lesion and the appearance of mucosal involvement is up to 2 decades have been reported. Progressive mucocutaneous disease is difficult to treat and often recurs. With prolonged infection, death occurs from respiratory compromise and malnutrition. MCL may arise after inadequate treatment of certain *Leishmania* species. Children are rarely affected.[39]

2.11.4.3 VISCERAL LEISHMANIASIS

Among the most destructive and fatal form of leishmaniasis is VL which is traditionally known as kala-azar or the Indian name for "black fever/disease." Black fever or kala-azar named because of its characteristic darkening of the skin that is seen in patients with this condition. In Indian, it is called by several names such as Dumdum fever, Assam fever. Its termed as infantile splenomegaly in various parts of the world. In contrast with other *Leishmania*, it is characterized by systemic infection of the liver, spleen, and bone marrow. This disease occurs with both New and Old World species. Intensity of illness ranges from asymptomatic infection or self-resolving disease to fulminant, severe, life-threatening infection. Various subclinical cases occur and remain unrecognized, so proper diagnosis is required. VL can be well characterized by fever (continuous or remittent and becomes intermittent at a later stage), weight loss, hepatosplenomegaly, pancytopenia, and hypergammaglobulinemia. Patients of VL can also suffer from night sweats, weakness, diarrhea, malaise, and anorexia. Skin hyperpigmentation caused due to the melanocyte stimulation and xerosis. Beginning of VL can be insidious or sudden. Young malnourished children are most susceptible and present with edema caused by hypoalbuminemia, hemorrhage caused by thrombocytopenia, or growth failure caused by features of chronic infection. The incubation period varies after infection (usually 3–6 months, but can be months or years) and may depend on the patient's age and immune status as well as the species of *Leishmania*. VL if remain untreated, chances of death frequently occurs within 2 years which may be due to hemorrhage (secondary to infiltration of the hematopoietic system), severe anemia, immunosuppression, and/or secondary infections.

2.11.4.4 VISCEROTROPIC LEISHMANIASIS

Viscerotropic leishmaniasis has an indolent but distinct clinical presentation. It does not appear to progress to full VL. Patients suffering from viscerotropic leishmaniasis have gone through an array of symptoms. Period of infection or progression may be from months to years after infection. This infective period can be presented by fever, rigors, fatigue, malaise, nonproductive cough, intermittent diarrhea, headache, arthralgias, myalgias, nausea, adenopathy, transient hepatosplenomegaly, and abdominal pain.

2.11.5 VISCERAL LEISHMANIASIS AND AMPHOTERECIN B

The leishmaniases are protozoan diseases caused by *Leishmania* parasites. The standard and first-line treatment of VLs is pentavalent antimony (meglumine antimoniate or sodium stibogluconate), but toxicity is frequent with this drug. Moreover antimony unresponsiveness is increasing in *L. infantum* and *L. donovani* foci, both in immunocompetent and in immunosuppressed patients. AmB is a polyene macrolide antibiotic that binds to sterols in cell membranes. It is the most active antileishmanial agent in use. Its infusion-related and renal toxicity may be reduced by lipid-based delivery. Liposomal AmB (Ambisome) seems to be less toxic than other AmB lipid formulations (Amphocil); Liposome Technology Inc., Menlo Park, CA, USA, Amphotec); Ben Venue Laboratories Inc., Bedford, OH, USA). Optimal drug regimens of Ambisome vary from one geographical area to another. Shortening the duration of treatment without decreasing the total dose (i.e., 10 mg/kg/day for 2 days) seems promising to reduce the global cost of the therapy. AmB lipid complex is a lipid formulation of AmB, an antifungal drug with activity against *Leishmania* spp. AmB lipid complex appears to enhance uptake of AmB by infected macrophages in patients with VL. In Bihar, India, where VL is hyperendemic, AmB deoxycholate is now first-line parenteral treatment.

A protozoal disease *Leishmania* is responsible for considerable health problems in public domain especially in tropical and subtropical regions. Among the various types of *Leishmania*, a vector-borne systemic disease called as VL caused by obligate intramacrophage protozoan parasites such as *L. donovani*, becomes fatal in the absence of treatment.[123] It is predicted that 88 countries are leishmaniasis-endemic and there are approximately 500,000 new cases of VL and more than 50,000 deaths from the disease every year. According to data, VL is reported in those patients where their whole immune system is compromised, for example, AIDS patients are more susceptible against VL than others.[124] This has created a necessity to present treatment for this disease. As we have already discussed, the sandfly life cycle including the developmental stages of *L. donovani* and its two distinct forms (an extracellular promastigote flagellar form found in the midgut of sandflies and an intracellular amastigote form that resides in phagolysosomes of mammalian (host) macrophages), we are directly moving toward host–parasite interaction. Once the female sandflies transmit the disease by flagellar promastigotes during a blood meal, parasites are internalized by dendritic cells and macrophages. This transformation leads to the loss of flagella by amastigotes[123] and allows the multiplication of amastigotes into host macrophages. Infection caused by promastigotes into host macrophages involves various parasite–host interactions such as recognition of specific ligands on the parasite cell surface by receptors on the macrophage cell surface. Various studies have been reported to understand the molecular mechanisms of parasite entry. This facilitates the recognition of specified receptors that promotes or allows the infiltration of parasite or led to the identification of multiple routes in the entry process.[123] Such receptors includes membrane proteins that are present on the macrophage cell surface such as receptor for advanced glycosylation end products, the mannose–fucose receptor, the fibronectin receptor, the Fc receptor, and complement receptors such as CR1 and CR3. However, occurrence of diverse receptors that are accountable for the entry of the parasite into host macrophages makes it difficult to establish a unique or ideal therapeutic target for the treatment of leishmaniasis. Initial barrier of host cell that initially interacts with *L. donovani* is plasma membrane of host cells. Plasma membrane of host cell is made up of cholesterol, which is an essential component of higher eukaryotic cellular membranes and is crucial in membrane organization, dynamics, function, and sorting.[124] Cholesterol also known as "lipid rafts" is usually nonrandomly distributed in biological membranes[125] and important for the maintenance of membrane structure and function. These specialized membrane domains or lipid rafts made of cholesterol facilitates the infiltration of pathogens[126] and hence plays a vital role in the function and organization of membrane proteins and receptors.[127] Earlier reports have proven the requirement of host membrane cholesterol in the binding and internalization of *Leishmania* promastigotes into macrophage cells.[128] AmB a polyene antibiotic and its leishmanicidal-based formulations are considered as the best existing drugs against VL and have a 97% cure rate without any resistance.[129] AmB potentially binds to ergosterol, major sterol in *Leishmania*, leads to the formation of transmembrane AmB channels followed by the alteration of permeability to cations, water, glucose, and affect membrane-bound enzymes. The most interesting about AmB is that it binds with ergosterol with the same affinity as with cholesterol.[130] It has been reported that in vivo treatment of AmB affects the integrity of both host and parasite membranes. During in vivo both host and parasite membranes are exposed to AmB, consequently effect on both sterols (ergosterol of *Leishmania* and cholesterol of host macrophages) is reported. It was also demonstrated that AmB interacts with host membrane cholesterol to sequester it in the membrane, thereby effectively reducing the ability of cholesterol to interact with and exert its effects on other membrane components such as receptors responsible for leishmanial entry.

2.11.5.1 AMPHOTERECIN B NANOPARTICULATE DRUG DELIVERY

Increasing prevalence of serious systemic infections such as aspergillosis, candidiasis, and cryptococcosis demands a potent fungicidal agent that effectively destroys the fungal growth without the development of any resistance and toxicity. AmB is a broad-spectrum polyene macrolide antifungal agent that does not induce resistance, widely known for the treatment of life-threatening systemic fungal infections and act as second-line drug of choice for VL.[131] However its poor water solubility, poor stability (in acidic pH), low intestinal permeability, and various dose-related serious side effects, for example, nephro and hemolytic toxicity limits its therapeutic efficacy in oral DDS. All these problems are associated with different states of AmB in aqueous media that determines the overall activity of drug. That is why it is conventionally administrated parenterally. Nanoparticulate DS is the most suitable mode for delivering AmB. Most of the currently available AmB nano formulations are lipid based (Ambisome, Amphocil, and Abelcet) though some are also available in micellar (Fungizone) and nanosuspension form. These all formulations have their serious concerns such as rapid release, surfactant-related toxicities, low drug-loading capacity, difficult route of administration, limited in vivo efficacy, and high price. Thus, there is an urgent need for effective oral antifungal DDS that not only reduces the side effects but also increases the absorption of AmB in a controlled manner.

Polyelectrolyte complexation (PEC) technique for nanoparticles involves the controlled mixing of diluted polycation and polyanion solutions that gives the size range of 20 to 500 nm with various shapes such as spherical, toroid, rod-like shapes, or have a loose gel-like up to compact internal structure. They are easily prepared (usually does not require any stabilizer or surfactant), economic, and are nontoxic in nature. PEC particles can serve as carrier for low- (drug) to high-molecular weight (protein) compounds. They are efficient in binding or internalization at various types of human cells. One of the major problems associated with PEC is their strong aggregation tendencies. Usually this type of aggregation has sufficient colloidal stability which can be modulated by polyelectrolyte concentration, ionic strength, pH, polyelectrolyte structure, and molecular weight.[7]

Biodegradable polymeric nanocarriers have attracted a lot of attention toward drug delivery for hydrophobic drugs. They are reported as the best candidates for delivering optimum drug with increased absorption at targeted site. Loading of these drugs in form of polyelectrolyte complex was proved to be a good strategy to control the drug release rate and to improve their bioavailability. Therefore due to established advantages and suitable features of two biopolymers, chitosan (CS) and porphyram (POR) are selected for present study for the formulation and development of AmB.

Due to various appealing properties such as biodegradability, biocompatibility, low toxicity, and relatively low production cost, hydrophilic nature, chitosan is widely used as a polymeric drug carrier material in several dosage forms. Fast dissolution at low pH and insolubility above pH 6 hinders some of its applications in pharmaceutical field. Chemical modification such as copolymerization or derivatization helps in improving its properties but they may also lead to the formation of new chemical entities with unknown toxicological profiles. Thus physical modification of the polymer is preferred than chemical modifications. Formation of stoichiometric polyelectrolyte complexes by addition of polyanion is an excellent strategy to overcome these problems. Currently most of the researchers are focusing toward discovery/selection/exploration of natural polyanion which could be not only safe, biodregerable, biocompatible but also form stable complex without or with least amount of cross-linking agent.[132]

2.11.5.2 MECHANISM OF ACTION OF AMPHOTERECIN B

Hypothetical illustration of how the association of AmB affects antifungal activity of the whole dug is shown in Figure 2-14. AmB, oldest drug that does not induce resistance, possess poor solubility in water (soluble in some organic solvent e.g., DMSO/DMF) but beyond critical micellar concentration (CMC) AmB starts self-association in aqueous media. This type of association in aqueous media creates the equilibrium stage [between monomers (M), self-associated soluble oligomers (SASO), and nonsoluble aggregation of oligomers (NSAO)] which is dependent on several factors as illustrated in Figure 2-14. Beyond CMC, the solubilized form [monomeric (MR) and self-associated oligomer] is converted into insoluble form aggregated [(AG)/ micellar (MI) form]. Therefore due to availability of several forms of single drug, it attains different types of activity. The soluble form can be an active form since it actively binds to the membrane either at once or after reconstitution in micelles within the lipid bilayer but it is only possible beyond CMC. Among insoluble, the micellar form can be active in some cases. As a result the overall activity of AmB is dependent on the equilibrium stage between the different forms present in the aqueous medium. Factors influencing this stage can change the whole activity of the drug. Among these two forms, soluble form (self-associated oligomer) effectively/unselectively binds with the fungal ergosterol membrane and cholesterol membrane by increasing permeability to K^+ but proved to be more toxic than aggregated form as it causes leakage to mammalian cholesterol also. This leakage is governed by the formation of AmB-sterol complex in a fashion where polar groups head toward the inside of the channel and hydrophobic groups interact with the outside phospholipid membrane. This may lead to various toxicity problems. At the present time, various strategies has been adopted to reduce these toxicities while formulating AmB in nano form.[86–89]

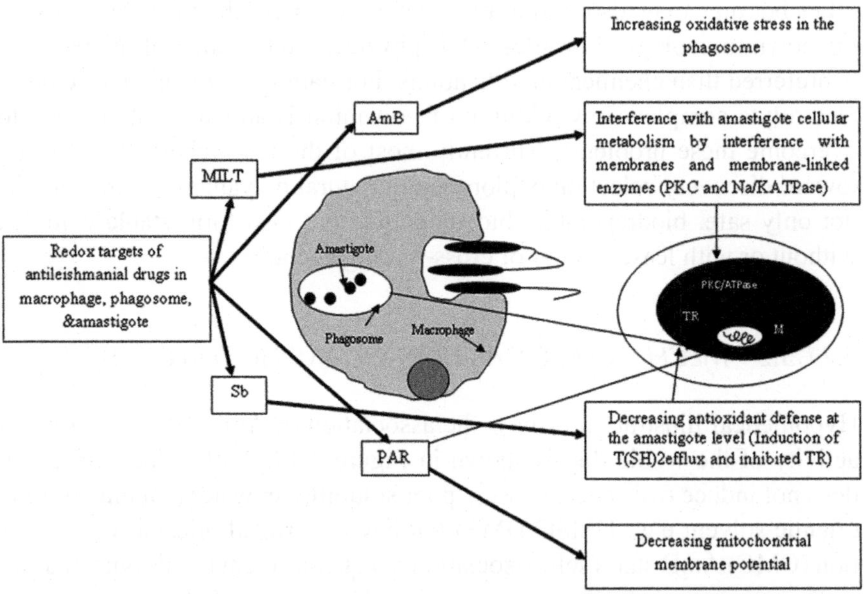

FIGURE 2-14 Mechanism of antifungal action of Amphoterecin B representing it's relation with the nature of arrangement (form) in aqueous state with its associated toxicities and cures.[13]

2.11.6 RECENT ADVANCES IN THE DEVELOPMENT OF NOVEL CHEMOTHERAPIES AGAINST LEISHMANIASIS

According to the WHO, leishmaniasis is a major tropical disease. Effective treatment against leishmaniasis (vaccine) is not available. Treatment with chemotherapeutic agents is the better way to treat various disease conditions. Nevertheless, currently available therapeutic agents are toxic and expensive. In addition, the resistant strains emerged against these therapeutic agents is still acknowledged as a serious problem, which has compelled the search for new antileishmanial agents. Here in this chapter, we have described the overview of current antileishmanian agents clinically used with new compounds that are under development. As discussed in earlier chapters, pentavalent antimonials are still the first choice among drugs used for the treatment of leishmaniasis. Alternatively, AmB, pentamidine, MILT, and PAR can be used. For the discovery of potential leishmanicidal agents with least side effects, various other synthetic products and compounds isolated from natural sources were explored.

Leishmaniasis is a highly communicable disease caused by parasites of the genus *Leishmania*. The disease manifests as three types: CL, MCL, and VL, which is also known as kala-azar. Among these the most common form is CL. It is a group of diseases with a varied range of clinical manifestations. This may vary from small cutaneous nodules to gross mucosal tissue destruction. The most severe form and debilitating disease is VL, in which the parasites migrated to vital organs and characterized by prolonged fever, splenomegaly, hypergammaglobulinemia, and pancytopenia. During this infection, patients gradually become ill over a period of few months. There are chances of death if remain untreated.[162]

In leishmaniasis, the transmission of parasite occurs through the bite of female phlebotomine sandflies infected with the protozoan, followed by the internalization of these parasites via macrophages in the liver, spleen, and bone marrow.[163]

Progression of the disease is dependent on the life cycle of parasite and its dimorphic forms (amastigotes and promastigotes). During the infection to mammalian host, amastigotes forms of parasites are present in the mononuclear phagocytic system and promastigotes in the digestive organs of the vector.[164]

Recent report suggested the 1.5 million new cases of cutaneous leishmaniasis and over 500,000 new cases of visceral leishmaniasis occur each year around the worldwide and 90% of cases occur in Afghanistan, Algeria,

Brazil, Pakistan, Peru, Saudi Arabia, and Syria.[164] The most severe form of *Leishmania* is VL that occurs in 65 countries; the majority (90%) of cases occur in agricultural areas and among the suburban, poor five countries: Bangladesh, India, Nepal, Sudan, and Brazil.[165] Propensity of *Leishmania* is increasing globally at an alarming rate. Various efforts have been applied to prevent the expansion of leishmaniases beyond their natural ecotopes.[166] Susceptibility of *Leishmania* in immune composed of patients especially in immunodeficiency virus (HIV), where *Leishmania* is present as coinfection.[167]

Wide acceptance of the classical treatment of disease with pentavalent antimonial compounds is reported. This classical treatment involved the administration of toxic and poorly tolerated drugs. The most old drugs introduced in earlier times are pentavalent antimonials. These antimonials compounds include meglumine antimoniate (Glucantime) and sodium stibogluconate (Pentostam). They are known to be the first-line compounds used to treat leishmaniasis. Many other drugs that may be used against leishmaniasis are pentamidine and AmB.[168] Lack of knowledge regarding the adverse effects of conventional medications and their misapplication enabled the development of generalized resistance to these agents.[168] Unavailability of effective vaccines and[9] serious adverse effects of conventional medications open the scope for new antileishmanian drugs from various other synthetic and natural resources.[169] These drugs require suitable DDSs for the development as novel chemotherapeutics. Various researches have been implicated in developing biopharmaceutical technologies for the design of the delivery strategy, such as nanoparticles, liposomes, cochleates, and nonspecific lipid transfer proteins.

2.11.6.1 CURRENT TREATMENT AND RECENT ADVANCES

In 1945, pentavalent antimonials become the first-choice treatment for both VL and CL. AmB and pentamidine are known to be the second-line antileishmanial drugs. However, both these drugs require extensive courses of parenteral administration. Selection of treatment is dependent on the type of the causative agents in leishmaniasis.[170] As mentioned earlier, the most common syndrome is localized CL, which is most frequently caused by *L. major* and *Leishmania tropica* in the Old World (Mediterranean basin, Middle East, and Africa), and by *L. braziliensis*, *L. mexicana*, and related species in the New World (Mexico, Central America, and South America).

It has been studied that several CL patients from Peru did not respond to pentavalent antimonial compounds. After analysis, it was found that these patients are infected with different types of *Leishmania* parasitic strains. Therefore the exact identification of parasite assists in selecting appropriate choice of a treatment against leishmaniasis. One dominating rule to treat the *Leishmania* is its spontaneous cure. Though depending on the *Leishmania* species, the chances of recovery fluctuates. This variation affects the time period consumed during the treatment, which may extend from months to years for proving the complete cure. Toxicity of the current drugs and inefficiency in eliminating the parasite from infected individuals makes the patient more susceptible against chemoresistance potential of the parasite.[171] Therefore the research on new antileishmania treatment attracts the development of new medicines that can replace or complement the presently available therapeutic alternatives. Encouraging the various chemotherapeutics agents for testing against Leishmanais is essential nowadays. Potential treatments for VL and their characteristics are highlighted in Table 2-9.

Potential of chemotherapeutic agents was more improved after the development of antileishmanial chemotherapy in form of lipid formulations of AmB. This lipid-based formulation was found to be less toxic for the treatment for fungal infections, and has been exploited for the treatment of leishmaniasis.[172] These unilamellar lipid-based vesicles (Ambisome 1), lipid complex (Abelcet 1), and colloidal dispersion (Amphocil) have all been evaluated in clinical trials for VL and/or MCL. It was found in 2000, Ambisome and Amphocil are more effective than against *L. donovani* in a mouse model. Ambisome (25 mg/kg) potentially reduces the size of lesions caused by *L. major*, and Amphocil (12.5 mg/kg) also showed activity, Abelcet was inactive against this species.[173] Nevertheless, the high price of these AmB-based preparations prevent their extensive utilization in developing countries. Several new economic formulations such as microcapsules made up of albumin (an effective carrier system) provides efficient protection to drug against phagocytic cells. Micospheric encapsulation of AmB in three different forms (monomeric, dimeric, and multiaggregate) and a multiaggregate form encapsulated with two commercial polymers were evaluated against *L. infantum* (both extracellular promastigote and intracellular amastigote forms). It was found that albumin-encapsulated forms exhibit no toxicity to murine cells. In addition, it was also observed that albumin-encapsulated forms showed lower EC50 values (0.003 mg/mL) for amastigotes than the free formulations (0.03 mg/mL). Recently Bhatia et al. have successfully prepared the AmB nanoparticles by using polyelectrolyte

TABLE 2-9 Current VL treatments and their main characteristics

Drugs	Administration	Regimen	Efficacy (*)	Resistance	Toxicity	Price
Pentavalent antimonials	IV, IM and IL	30 days 20 mg/kg/day	35–95%(depending on area)	Common (>60% in Bihar, India)	+++ Cardiotoxicity, pancreatitis, nephrotoxicity, hepatotoxicity	$50–70
Amphotericin B	IV	30 days 1 mg/kg (15 mg/kg total dose)	>90%	Laboratory strains	Nephrotoxicity	$100
Liposomal amphotericin B	IV	5–20 mg/kg total dose 4–10 doses over 10–20 days	>97%	Not documented	Rigors and chills during infusion	$280
Miltefosine	PO	28 days 1.5–2.5 mg/day	94–97%	Laboratory strains	Gastrointestinal, nephrotoxicity, hepatotoxicity, teratogenicity	$70
Paromomycin sulfate	IM	21 days 15 mg/kg/day 94% (India)	46–85% (Africa, depending on dose)	Laboratory strains	Nephrotoxicity, ototoxicity, hepatotoxicity	$10

IV = intravenous administration; IM = intramuscular administration; IL = intralymphatic administration; PO = oral administration. * Definitive cure at 6 months.

complexation technique.[86] During this study, they have explored the significance of using algal-based polymer with chitosan to encapsulate AmB against fungal infection. In vivo toxicity of this AmB was also evaluated. This and many other similar reports increased interest in AmB encapsulated in microspheres, and in exploring new chemotherapeutic approaches.[174]

An alkylphospholipid and oral antineoplastic agent known as MILT was developed for cutaneous cancers. This drug is currently applied to treat leishmaniasis. Exploration of potential antileishmanian effects of this drug led to the detection of new antiprotozoal medicines. MILT was approved as Impavido treatment for visceral and cutaneous leishmaniasis, including for antimony-resistant infections.[175] MILT has become the first oral treatment for leishmaniasis in some countries. However, this drug may not necessarily be superior to parenteral therapies for all forms of leishmaniasis. Longer (28 days) treatment in *Leishmania* is obligatory sometime. Such longer treatment strategies with antibiotic formulations must be more rational and prevents the patients from developing resistance to the drug. Several examinations were performed to understand the resistance mechanisms are mentioned in Table 2-10. The resistance mechanisms include a decrease in drug uptake, differential plasma membrane permeability, more rapid drug metabolism, and efflux of the drug. In 2002, MILT was approved in India for the treatment of visceral leishmaniasis.[176] Since this drug acquires the teratogenic potential, therefore it should not be administered to pregnant women.[177] After MILT, various other drugs belonging to the same category of alkylphospholipids such as edelfosine and ilmofosine, perifosine, were evaluated and have proved to possess potent in vitro antiparasitic activity. Oral administration of edelfosine and perifosine were recently tested against BALB/c mice infected with *L. amazonensis.* Preclinical treatment has been proven that perifosine possess higher activity in the in vivo assay. In addition, it was also discovered that it may be used as possible alternative treatment against CL.[178]

For oral treatment of VL, sitamaquine known to be a promising drug in Africa. It has been proven that 28-day course of oral administration of sitamaquine at 2.0 mg/kg/day provides well cure and tolerance in patients infected by *L. donovani.* Some adverse effects such as abdominal pain, headache, and especially renal event and optimal dose selection need further investigation.[179]

An aminoglycoside known as PAR is widely accepted for clinically important antileishmanial activity. Oral administration of PAR is efficient in the treatment of both VL and CL, however poor absorption has led to the development of parenteral and topical formulations for the visceral and cutaneous forms, respectively. Recent research put more light over the significance of using PAR as a potent antileishmania drug. It was studied that deep gluteal intramuscular injection (11 mg/kg/day) for 21 days was proved to be equally effective as infusion of AmB (1 mg/kg/day) for 30 days.[180] In contrast, it was also proven that treatment of CL with PAR ointment has not shown any difference with control groups. Nevertheless, the new topical formulations of PAR have given good results. Therefore topical PAR can also be a therapeutic alternative for cutaneous leishmaniasis, whereas longer treatment is required for clinical healing.[182] Moreover hydrophilic gel containing 10% PAR topical formulation was found to be effective against *L. amazonensis* than antimony treatment, whereas these two medications were equally effective against *L. braziliensis*. Therefore the gel formulation may represent an alternative topical treatment for CL. Currently, various antileishmanial drugs are available: their mechanism of action on parasites, dosage, advantages, and limitations are mentioned in Table 2-10.

KEYWORDS

- ***Leishmania***
- **pharmacology**
- **drug**
- **target**
- **delivery**
- **vaccine**
- **etiology**
- **epidemiology**
- **transmission**
- **amphoterecin B**
- **macrophage targeting**
- **Antibiotic therapy**
- **antimicrobial peptide (AMP)**
- **ROS**
- **reactive oxygen species**

TABLE 2-10 Currently available anti-leishmanial drugs: their mechanism of action on parasites, dosage, advantages and limitations[184,185]

Drug	Mode(s) of action	Dosage (for VL)	advantages	Limitations
Pentavalent antimonials: Meglumine antimoniate (Glucantime) or sodium stibogluconate (Pentostam)	Activated within the amastigote/macrophage after conversion to the trivalent form. Shows direct parasiticidal activity by generation of ROS, depletion of thiols, modulation of bioenergetic pathways (glycolysis, fatty acid beta oxidation, inhibition of ADP phosphorylation, blocking of SH groups of amastigote proteins) and inhibition of topoisomerase I	20 mg/kg b.w., i.m., daily (600 mg total) for 30 days in India	Easily availability and low cost	Myalgia, pancreatitis, cardiac arrhythmias, hepatitis Acquired resistance
Amphotericin B (polyene antibiotic	Complexes with 24-substituted sterols, such as ergosterol in the cell membrane, causing pores that alter ion balance, increase membrane permeability resulting in cell death; also acts as an inhibitor of ergosterol biosynthesis	0.75–1.0 mg/kg for 15–20 infusions either daily on alternate days in India	Primary resistance is unknown	Need for prolonged hospitalization High cost, high fever with rigor, chills, hypokalemia, renal dysfunction
Lipid formulation of amphotericin B Ambisome/Abelcet/ Amphotec		Ambisome: 2.0 mg/kg × 5 days, i.v. in	Highly effective, low toxicity	High cost
Paromomycin (aminoglycoside antibiotic), also known as aminosidine or monomyc	In bacteria, inhibits protein synthesis, but in *Leishmania*, the exact mechanism is not yet known. It is proposed to induce respiratory dysfunction in *L. donovani* promastigotes. It also promoted ribosomalsubunit association of both cytoplasmic and mitochondrial forms, low Mg + 2 which induced dissociation	16 mg/kg × 21 days, i.m.: 20 mg/kg × 17 days, i.m.	Effective, well tolerated and relatively cheap, acts synergistically with antimonials	Lack of efficacy in East Africa

TABLE 2-10 *(Continued)*

Drug	Mode(s) of action	Dosage (for VL)	advantages	Limitations
Miltefosine (hexadecy-lphosph-ocholine)	It interacts with the cell membrane of *Leishmania* by modulation of cell surface receptors, inositol metabolism and phospholipase activation, cell death being mediated by apoptosis	100–150 mg for four weeks, p.o. in India	Effective and safe	Vomiting and diarrhoea. nephrotoxic, teratogenic
Sitamaquine (8-aminoquinoline, originally WR6026)	Unknown, possibly affects mitochondrial electron transport chain	1.75–2 mg/kg/day for 28 days in India.	Little is known about its efficacy and toxicity	

REFERENCES

1. Mishra, B. B.; Kale, R. R.; Prasad, V.; Tiwari V. K.; Singh, R. K. Scope of natural products in fighting against leishmaniasis. In *Opportunity, Challenge and Scope of Natural Products in Medicinal Chemistry*; Research Signpost: Varanasi, India, 2011; pp 121–154.
2. WHO. Control of the Leishmaniases. Report of a WHO Expert Committee. *World Health Organ. Tech. Rep. Ser.* **1990,** *793*, 1–1583.
3. Desjeux, P.; Meert, J.; Piot, B.;, Alvar, J.; Medrano, F.; Portus, M.; Munoz, C.; Laguna, F.; Velez, R. L.; Salas, A.; Sirera, G.; Cisterna, R.; Montalban, C.; Quero, H.; Gradoni, L.; Gramiccia, M.; Russo, R.; Dedet, J.; Pratlong, F.; Dereure, J.; Deniau, M.; Izri, A.; Matheron, S.; Farault, F.; Marty, P.; Rosenthal, E.; Antunes, F.; Abranches, P.; Pradinaud, R. *Leishmania*/HIV Co-infection in South-western Europe 1990–1998: Retrospective Analysis of 965 Cases. *Wkly Epidemiol. Rec.* **1999,** *74* (44), :365–375. http://whqlibdoc.who.int/hq/2000/WHO_LEISH_2000.42.pdf
4. Murray, H. W. Kala-azar—Progress Against a Neglected Disease. N. Engl. J. Med. **2002,** *347*, 1793–1794.
5. Ramalho-Ortigao, M.; Saraiva, E. M.; Traub-Csekö, Y. M.. Sand Fly–*Leishmania* Interactions: Long Relationships Are Not Necessarily Easy. *Open Parasitol. J.* **2010,** *4*, 195–204.
6. Grimaldi, G. J.; Momen, H.; Naiff R. D.; McMahon-Pratt, D.; Barrett, T. V. Characterization and Classification of Leishmanial Parasites from Humans, Wild Mammals, and Sand Flies in the Amazon Region of Brazil. *Am. J. Trop. Med. Hyg.* **1991,** *44* (6), 645–661.
7. Desjeux, P. The Increase of Risk Factors for Leishmaniasis Worldwide. *Trans. R. Soc. Trop. Med. Hyg.* **2001,** *95*, 239–243.
8. Desjeux, P. Leishmaniasis: Current Situation and New Perspectives. *Comp. Immunol. Microbiol. Infect. Dis.* **2004,** *27*, 305–318.
9. Choi, C. M.; Lerner, E. A. Leishmaniasis as an Emerging Infection. *J. Invest. Dermatol. Symp. Proc.* **2001,** *6*, 175–182.
10. Mukhopadhyay, S.; Mandal, C. Glycobiology of *Leishmania donovani*. *Indian J. Med. Res.* **2006,** 123, 203–220.
11. Killick-Kendrick, R. Phlebotomine Vectors of the Leishmaniases: A Review. *Med. Vet. Entomol.* **1990,** *4*, 1–24.
12. Sacks, D.; Kamhawi, S. Molecular Aspects of Parasite-Vector and Vector–Host Interactions in Leishmaniasis. *Annu. Rev. Microbiol.* **2001,** *55*, 453–483.
13. Schlein, Y.; Jacobson, R. L. Resistance of *Phlebotomus papatasito* Infection with *Leishmania donovaniis* Modulated by Components of the Infective Blood Meal. *Parasitology* **1998,** *117*, 467–473.
14. Schlein, Y.; Warburg, A.; Schnur, L. F.; Shlomai, J. Vector Compatibility of *Phlebotomus papatasi* Dependent on Differentially Induced Digestion. *Acta. Trop.* **1983,** *40*, 65–70.
15. Borovsky, D.; Schlein, Y. Trypsin and Chymotrypsin-like Enzymes of the Sandfly *Phlebotomus papatasi* Infected with *Leishmania* and their Possible Role in Vector Competence. *Med. Vet. Entomol.* **1987,** *1*, 235–242.
16. Vaidyanathan, R. Isolation of a Myoinhibitory Peptide from *Leishmania major* (Kinetoplastida: Trypanosomatidae) and its Function in the Vector Sand Fly *Phlebotomus papatasi* (Diptera: Psychodidae). *J. Med. Entomol.* **2005,** *42*, 142–152.

17. Schlein, Y.; Jacobson, R. L.; Messer, G. *Leishmania* Infections Damage the Feeding Mechanism of the Sandfly Vector and Implement Parasite Transmission by Bite. *Proc. Natl. Acad. Sci. USA.* **1992,** *89*, 9944–9948.
18. Volf, P.; Hajmova, M.; Sadlova, J.; Votypka, J. Blocked Stomodeal Valve of the Insect Vector: Similar Mechanism of Transmission in Two Trypanosomatid Models. *Int. J. Parasitol.* **2004,** *34*, 1221–1227.
19. Pitaluga, A. N.; Beteille, V.; Lobo, A. R.; Ortigão-Farias, J. R.; Dávila, A. M.; Souza, A. A.; Ramalho-Ortigão, J. M.; Traub-Cseko, Y. M. EST Sequencing of Blood Fed and *Leishmania*-infected Midgut of *Lutzomyia longipalpis*, the Principal Visceral Leishmaniasis Vector in the Americas. *Mol. Genet. Genomics* **2009,** *282*, 307–317.
20. Ramalho-Ortigao, M.; Jochim, R. C.; Anderson, J. M.; Anderson, J. M.; Lawyer, P. G.; Pham, V. M.; Kamhawi, S.; Valenzuela, J. G. Exploring the Midgut Transcriptome of *Phlebotomus papatasi*: Comparative Analysis of Expression Profiles of Sugar-fed, Blood-fed and *Leishmania major*-infected Sandflies. *BMC. Genomics* **2007,** *8*, 300.
21. Dillon, R .J.; Lane, R. P. Influence of *Leishmania* Infection on Bloodmeal Digestion in the Sandflies *Phlebotomus papatasi* and *P. langeroni*. *Parasitol. Res.* **1993,** *79*, 492–496.
22. Boulanger, N.; Lowenberger C.; Volf, P.; Ursic, R.; Sigutova, L.; Sabatier, L.; Svobodova, M.; Beverley, S. M.; Späth, G.; Brun, R.; Pesson, B.; Bulet, P. Characterization of a Defensin from the Sand Fly *Phlebotomus duboscqi* Induced by Challenge with Bacteria or the Protozoan Parasite *Leishmania major*. *Infect. Immun.* **2004**, *72*, 7140–7146.
23. Hurd, H.; Carter, V. The Role of Programmed Cell Death in Plasmodium-mosquito Interactions. *Int. J. Parasitol.* **2004,** *34*, 1459–1472.
24. Killick-Kendrick, R.; Rioux, J. A. Intravectorial Cycle of *Leishmania* in Sandflies. *Ann. Parasitol. Hum. Comp.* **1991,** *66* (Suppl. 1), 71–74.
25. Poinar, G. J. Early Cretaceous Trypanosomatids Associated with Fossil Sand Fly Larvae in *Burmese amber*. *Mem. Inst. Oswaldo. Cruz.* **2007,** *102*, 635–637.
26. Assche, T. V.; Deschacht, M.; Inocêncio da, L. R. A.; Maes, L.; Cos, P. *Leishmania*–macrophage Interactions: Insights into the Redox Biology. *Free Radic. Biol. Med.* **2011,** *51*, 337–351.
27. Boulanger, N.; Bulet, P.; Lowenberger, C. Antimicrobial Peptides in the Interactions between Insects and Flagellate Parasites. *Trends Parasitol.* **2006**, *22*, 262–268.
28. Hancock, R. E.; Diamond, G. The Role of Cationic Antimicrobial Peptides in Innate Host Defences. *Trends Microbiol.* **2000,** *8*, 402–410.
29. Ganz, T.; Lehrer, R. I. Defensins. *Current Opin. Immunol.* **1994,** *6*, 584–589.
30. Kulkarni, M. M.; McMaster, W. R.; Kamysz, E.; Kamysz, W.; Engman, D. M.; McGwire, B. S. The Major Surface-metalloprotease of the Parasitic Protozoan, *Leishmania*, Protects against Antimicrobial Peptide-induced Apoptotic Killing. *Mol. Microbiol.* **2006,** *62*, 1484–1497.
31. Kulkarni, M. M.; McMaster, W. R.; Kamysz, W.; McGwire, B. S. Antimicrobial Peptide-induced Apoptotic Death of *Leishmania* Results from Calcium-dependent, Caspase-independent Mitochondrial Toxicity. *J. Biol. Chem.* **2009,** *284*, 15496–15504.
32. Brogden, K. A. Antimicrobial Peptides: Pore Formers or Metabolic Inhibitors in Bacteria? *Nature Rev. Microbiol.* **2005,** *3*, 238–250.
33. Bera, A.; Singh, S.; Nagaraj, R.; Vaidya, T. Induction of Autophagic Cell Death in *Leishmania donovani* by Antimicrobial Peptides. *Molecul. Biochem. Parasitol.* **2003,** *127*, 23–35.

34. Luque-Ortega, J. R.; Rivero-Lezcano, O. M.; Croft, S. L.; Rivas, L. *In vivo* Monitoring of Intracellular ATP Levels in *Leishmania donovani* Promastigotes as a Rapid Method to Screen Drugs Targeting Bioenergetic Metabolism. *Antimicrob. Agents Chemother.* **2001,** *45,* 1121–1125.
35. Luque-Ortega, J. R.; van't Hof, W.; Veerman, E. C.; Saugar, J. M.; Rivas, L. Human Antimicrobial Peptide Histatin 5 is a Cell-penetrating Peptide Targeting Mitochondrial ATP Synthesis in *Leishmania. FASEB. J.* **2008,** *22,* 1817–1828.
36. Izadpanah, A.; Gallo, R. L. Antimicrobial Peptides. *J. American Acad. Dermatol.* **2005,** *52,* 381–390.
37. Braff, M. H.; Hawkins, M. A.; Di Nardo, A.; Lopez-Garcia, B.; Howell, M. D.; Wong, C.; Lin, K.; Streib, J. E.; Dorschner, R.; Leung, D. Y.; Gallo, R. L. Structure–function Relationships among Human Cathelicidin Peptides: Dissociation of Antimicrobial Properties from Host Immunostimulatory Activities. *J. Immunol.* **2005,** *174,* 4271–4278.
38. McGwire, B. S.; Kulkarni, M. M. Interactions of Antimicrobial Peptides with *Leishmania* and Trypanosomes and their Functional Role in Host Parasitism. *Exp. Parasitol.* **2010,** *126,* 397–405.
39. Balan˜a-Fouce, R.; Reguera, R. M.; Cubrıa, J. C.; Ordonez, D. The Pharmacology of Leishmaniasis. *Gen. Pharmac.* **1998,** *30* (4), 435–443.
40. Espuelas, S. Delivery Systems for the Treatment and Prevention of Leishmaniasis. *Gaz. méd. Bahia* **2009,** *79,* 134–146.
41. Luo, D.; Saltzman, W. M. Synthetic DNA Delivery Systems. *Nat. Biotechnol.* **2000,** *18,* 33–37.
42. Mainardes, R. M.; Silva, L. P. Drug Delivery Systems: Past, Present, and Future. *Curr. Drug Targets* **2004,** *5,* 449–455.
43. Brannon-Peppas, L.; Blanchette, J. O. Nanoparticle and Targeted Systems for Cancer Therapy. *Adv. Drug Del. Rev.* **2004,** *56,* 1649–1659.
44. Brigger, I.; Dubernet, C.; Couvreur, P. Nanoparticles in Cancer Therapy and Diagnosis. *Adv. Drug Del. Rev.* **2002,** *54,* 631–651.
45. Ravi Kumar, M.; Hellermann, G.; Lockey, R. F.; Mohapatra, S. S. Nanoparticle-mediated Gene Delivery: State of the Art. *Expert Opin. Biol. Ther.* **2004,** *4,* 1213–1224.
46. Rihova, B. Immunomodulating Activities of Soluble Synthetic Polymer-bound Drugs. *Adv. Drug Del. Rev.* **2002,** *54,* 653–674.
47. Moghimi, S. M.; Hunter, A. C.; Murray, J. C. Long-circulating and Target Specific Nanoparticles: Theory to Practice. *Pharmacol. Rev.* **2001,** *53,* 283–318.
48. Sakuma, S.; Suzuki, N.; Sudo, R.; Hiwatari, K.; Kishida, A.; Akashi, M. Optimized Chemical Structure of Nanoparticles as Carriers for Oral Delivery of Salmon Calcitonin. *Int. J. Pharm.* **2002,** *239,* 185–195.
49. Kreuter, J. Influence of the Surface Properties on Nanoparticle Mediated Transport of Drugs to the Brain. *J. Nanosci. Nanotechnol.* **2004,** *4,* 484-488.
50. Verdun, C.; Brasseur, F.; Vranckx, H.; Couvreur, P.; Roland, M. Tissue Distribution of Doxorubicin Associated with Polyisohexylcyanoacrylate Nanoparticles. *Cancer Chemother. Pharmacol.* **1990,** *26,* 13–18.
51. Moghimi, S. M.; Szebeni, J. Stealth Liposomes and Long Circulating Nanoparticles: Critical Issues in Pharmacokinetics, Opsonization and Protein-binding Properties. *Prog. Lipid Res.* **2003,** *42,* 463–478.
52. Illum, L.; Davis, S. S.; Muller, R. H.; Mak, E.; West, P. The Organ Distribution and Circulation Time of Intravenously Injected Colloidal Carriers Sterically Stabilized with a Block Copolymer-poloxamine 908. *Life Sci.* **1987,** *40,* 367–374.

53. Allen, T. M. Long-circulating (Sterically Stabilized) Liposomes for Targeted Drug Delivery. *Trends Pharmacol. Sci.* **1994,** *15*, 215–220.
54. Bazile, D.; Michalon, J. P.; Prud'homme, C.; Spenlehauer, G.; Veillard, M. Nanoparticles Having a Prolonged Reticulo-endothelial System Capture Rate. *French Patent No.* 08041, 1991.
55. Bazile, D.; Prud'homme, C.; Bassoullet, M. T.; Marlard, M.; Spenlehauer, G.; Veillard, M. Stealth Me.PEG-PLA Nanoparticles Avoid Uptake by the Mononuclear Phagocytes System. *J. Pharm. Sci.* **1995,** *84*, 493–498.
56. Vauthier, C.; Dubernet, C.; Fattal, E.; Pinto-Alphandary, H.; Couvreur, P. Poly(alkylcyanoacrylates) as Biodegradable Materials for Biomedical Applications. *Adv. Drug Del Rev.* **2003,** *55*, 519–548.
57. Couvreur, P.; Kante, B.; Roland, M.; Speiser, P. Adsorption of Antineoplastic Drugs to Polyalkylcyanoacrylate Nanoparticles and their Release in Calf Serum. *J. Pharm. Sci.* **1979**, *68*, 1521–1524.
58. Douglas, S. J.; Davis, S. S.; Illum, L. Nanoparticles in Drug Delivery. *Crit. Rev. Ther. Drug Carrier Syst.* **1987,** *3*, 233–261.
59. Couvreur, P. Polyalkylcyanoacrylates as Colloidal Drug Carriers. *Crit. Rev. Ther. Drug Carrier Syst.* **1988,** *5*, 1–20.
60. Gibaud, S.; Andreux, J. P.; Weingarten, C.; Renard, M.; Couvreur, P. Increased Bone Marrow Toxicity of Doxorubicin Bound to Nanoparticles. *Eur. J. Cancer* **1994,** *30A*, 820–826.
61. Damge, C.; Michel, C.; Aprahamian, M.; Couvreur, P. New Approach for Oral Administration of Insulin with Polyalkylcyanoacrylate Nanocapsules as Drug Carrier. *Diabetes* **1988,** *37*, 246–251.
62. Chavany, C.; Le Doan, T.; Couvreur, P.; Puisieux, F.; Helene, C. Polyalkylcyanoacrylate Nanoparticles as Polymeric Carriers for Antisense Oligonucleotides. *Pharm. Res.* **1992,** *9*, 441–449.
63. Schwab, G.; Chavany, C.; Duroux, I.; Goubin, G.; Lebeau, J.; Helene, C., Saison-Behmoaras, T. Antisense Oligonucleotides Adsorbed to Polyalkylcyanoacrylate Nanoparticles Specifically Inhibit Mutated Ha-ras-mediated Cell Proliferation and Tumorigenicity in Nude Mice. *Proc. Natl. Acad. Sci. USA* **1994,** *91*, 10460–10464.
64. Soma, C. E., Dubernet, C., Bentolila, D., Benita, S., Couvreur, P. Reversion of Multidrug Resistance by Co-encapsulation of Doxorubicin and Cyclosporin A in Polyalkylcyanoacrylate Nanoparticles. *Biomaterials* **2000,** *21*, 1–7.
65. Chiu, Y. L.; Ali, A.; Chu, C. Y.; Cao, H.; Rana, T. M. Visualizing a Correlation between siRNA Localization, Cellular Uptake, and RNAi in Living Cells. *Chem. Biol.* **2004,** *11*, 1165–1175.
66. Kakizawa, Y.; Furukawa, S.; Kataoka, K. Block Copolymer-coated Calcium Phosphate Nanoparticles Sensing Intracellular Environment for Oligodeoxynucleotide and siRNA Delivery. *J. Control. Release* **2004,** *97*, 345–356.
67. Elbashir, S. M.; Harborth, J.; Lendeckel, W.; Yalcin, A.; Weber, K.; Tuschl, T. Duplexes of 21-Nucleotide RNAs Mediate RNA Interference in Cultured Mammalian Cells. *Nature* **2001,** *411*, 494–498.
68. Hammond, S. M.; Caudy, A. A.; Hannon, G. J. Post-transcriptional Gene Silencing by Double-Stranded RNA. *Nat. Rev. Genet.* **2001,** *2*, 110–119.
69. McManus, M. T.; Sharp, P. A. Gene Silencing in Mammals by Small Interfering RNAs. *Nat. Rev. Genet.* **2002,** *3*, 737–747.

70. Zhang, W.; Yang, H.; Kong, X.; Mohapatra, S.; Juan-Vergara, H. S.; Hellermann, G.; Behera S.; Singam, R.; Lockey, R. F.; Mohapatra, S. S. Inhibition of Respiratory Syncytial Virus Infection with Intranasal siRNA Nanoparticles Targeting the Viral NS1 Gene. *Nat. Med.* **2005,** *11*, 56–62.
71. Schiffelers, R. M.; Ansari, A.; Xu, J., Zhou, Q.; Tang, Q.; Storm, G.; Molema, G.; Lu, P. Y.; Scaria P. V.; Woodle, M. C. Cancer siRNA Therapy by Tumor Selective Delivery with Ligand-targeted Sterically Stabilized Nanoparticle. *Nucleic Acids Res.* **2004,** *32*, e149.
72. Leu, D., Manthey, B.; Kreuter, J.; Speiser, P.; De Luca, P. Distribution and Elimination of Coated Polymethyl [2-14C]methacrylate Nanoparticles after Intravenous Injection in Rats. *J. Pharm. Sci.* **1984,** *73*, 1433–1437.
73. Leroux, J. C.; De Jaeghere, F.; Anner, B.; Doelker, E.; Gurny, R. An Investigation on the Role of Plasma and Serum Opsonins on the Internalization of Biodegradable Poly(D,L-lactic acid) Nanoparticles by Human Monocytes. *Life Sci.* **1995,** *57*, 695–703.
74. Peracchia, M. T.; Harnisch, S.; Pinto-Alphandary, H.; Gulik, A.; Dedieu, J. C.; Desmaele, D.; d'Angelo, J.; Muller, R. H.; Couvreur, P. Visualization of in vitro Protein-rejecting Properties of PEGylated Stealth Polycyanoacrylate Nanoparticles. *Biomaterials* **1999,** *20*, 1269–1275.
75. Wagner, E.; Plank, C.; Zatloukal, K.; Cotton, M.; Birnstiel, M. L. Influenza Virus Hemagglutinin HA-2 N-terminal Fusogenic Peptides Augment Gene Transfer by Transferrin-polylysine-DNA Complexes: Toward a Synthetic Virus-like Gene-transfer Vehicle. *Proc. Natl. Acad. Sci. USA* **1992,** *89*, 7934–7938.
76. Plank, C.; Oberhauser, B.; Mechtler, K.; Koch, C.; Wagner, E. The Influence of Endosome-Disruptive Peptides on Gene Transfer Using Synthetic Virus-like Gene Transfer Systems. *J. Biol. Chem.* **1994,** *269*, 12918–12924.
77. Panyam, J.; Zhou, W. Z.; Prabha, S.; Sahoo, S. K.; Labhasetwar, V. Rapid Endo-lysosomal Escape of Poly(DL-lactide-co-glycolide) Nanoparticles: Implications for Drug and Gene Delivery. *FASEB. J.* **2002,** *16*, 1217–1226.
78. Boussif, O.; Lezoualc'h, F.; Zanta, M. A.; Mergny, M. D.; Scherman, D.; Demeneix, B.; Behr, J. P. A Versatile Vector for Gene and Oligonucleotide Transfer into Cells in Culture and in vivo: Polyethylenimine. *Proc. Natl. Acad. Sci. USA* **1995,** *92*, 7297–7301.
79. Pack, D. W.; Putnam, D.; Langer, R. Design of Imidazole-containing Endosomolytic Biopolymers for Gene Delivery. *Biotechnol. Bioeng.* **2000,** *67*, 217–223.
80. East, L.; Isacke, C. M. The Mannose Receptor Family. *Biochem. Biophys. Acta.* **2002,** *1572*, 364–386.
81. Warr G. A. A Macrophage Receptor for (Mannose/glucosamine)-glycoproteins of Potential Importance in Phagocytic Activity. *Biochem. Biophys. Res. Commun.* **1980,** *93*,737–745.
82. Luo, D.; Saltzman, W. M. Synthetic DNA Delivery Systems. *Nat. Biotechnol.* **2000,** *18*, 33–37.
83. Bazile, D.; Michalon, J. P.; Prud'homme, C.; Spenlehauer, G.; Veillard, M. Nanoparticles Having a Prolonged Reticulo-endothelial System Capture Rate. *French Patent No.* 08041, 1991.
84. Chavany, C.; Le Doan, T.; Couvreur, P.; Puisieux, F.; Helene, C. Polyalkylcyanoacrylate Nanoparticles as Polymeric Carriers for Antisense Oligonucleotides. *Pharm. Res.* **1992,** *9*, 441–449.
85. Schiffelers, R. M.; Ansari, A.; Xu, J.; Zhou, Q.; Tang, Q.; Storm, G.; Molema, G.; Lu, P. Y.; Scaria, P. V.; Woodle, M. C. Cancer siRNA Therapy by Tumor Selective Delivery

with Ligand-targeted Sterically Stabilized Nanoparticle. *Nucleic Acids Res.* **2004,** *32*, e149.

86. Bhatia, S.; Kumar, V.; Sharma, K.; Nagpal, K.; Bera, T. Significance of Algal Polymer in Designing Amphotericin B Nanoparticles. *ScientificWorldJournal.* **2014,** *2014*, 564573.
87. Chia, J. K.; Pollack, M. Amphotericin B Induces Tumor Necrosis Factor Production by Murine Macrophages. *J. Infect. Dis.* **1989,** *159*, 113–116.
88. Cleary, J. D.; Chapman, S. W.; Nolan, R. L. Pharmacologic Modulation of Interleukin-1 Expression by Amphotericin B-stimulated Human Mononuclear Cells. *Antimicrob. Agents Chemother.* **1992,** *36*, 977–981.
89. Gelfand, J. A.; Kimball, K.; Burke, J. K.; Dinarello, C. A. Amphotericin B Treatment of Human Mononuclear Cells in vitro Results in Secretion of Tumor Necrosis Factor and Interleukin-1. *Clin. Res.* **1988,** *36*, 456A.
90. Espuelas, M. S.; Legrand, P.; Loiseau, P. M, Bories C.; Barratt, G.; Irache, J. M. *In vitro* Antileishmanial Activity of Amphotericin B Loaded in Poly(epsilon-caprolactone) Nanospheres. *J. Drug Target* **2002,** *10*, 593–599.
91. Sarkar, S.; Mandal, S.; Sinha, J.; Mukhopadhyay, S.; Das, N.; Basu, M. K. Quercetin: Critical Evaluation as an Antileishmanial Agent in vivo in Hamsters Using Different Vesicular Delivery Modes. *J. Drug Target* **2002,** *10*, 573–578.
92. Zhang, Q.; Liao, G. T.; Wei, D. P.; Zhang, C. J. Increase of Gentamicin Uptake in Cultured Mouse Peritoneal Macrophage and Rat Hepatocytes When Used in the Form of Nanoparticles. *Yao. Xue. Xue. Bao.* **1996,** *31*, 375–380.
93. Rodrigues, J. J. M.; Croft, S. L.; Fessi, H.; Bories, C.; Devissaguet, J. P. The Activity and Ultrastructural Localization of Primaquineloaded Poly(D,L-lactide) Nanoparticles in *Leishmania donovani* Infected Mice. *Trop. Med. Parasitol.* **1994,** *45*, 223–228.
94. Gaspar, R.; Opperdoes, F. R.; Preat, V.; Roland, M. Drug Targeting with Polyalkylcyanoacrylate Nanoparticles: in vitro Activity of Primaquine-loaded Nanoparticles against Intracellular *Leishmania donovani. Ann. Trop. Med. Parasitol.* **1992,** *86*, 41–49.
95. Deniau, M.; Durand, R.; Bories, C.; Paul M.; Astier, A.; Couvreur, P.; Houin, R. *In vitro* Study of Leishmanicidal Agents with Drug Carriers. *Ann. Parasitol. Hum. Comp.* **1993,** *68*, 34–37.
96. Gillies, E. R.; Fréchet, J. M. J. Dendrimers and Dendritic Polymers in Drug Delivery. *Drug Discov. Today* **2005,** *10*, 35–43.
97. Muller, R. H.; Mader, K.; Gohla, S. Solid Lipid Nanoparticles (SLN) for Controlled Drug Delivery—a Review of the State of the Art. *Eur. J. Pharm. Biopharm.* **2000,** *50*, 161–177.
98. Cevc, G. Lipid Vesicles and Other Colloids as Drug Carriers on the Skin. *Adv. Drug Del. Rev.* **2004,** *56*, 675.
99. Convit, J.; Ulrich, M.; Zerpa, O.; Borges, R.; Aranzazu, N.; Valera, M.; Villarroel, H.; Zapata, Z.; Tomedes, I. Immunotherapy of American Cutaneous Leishmaniasis in Venezuela during the Period 1990–99. *Trans. R. Soc. Trop. Med. Hyg.* **2003,** *97* (4), 469–472.
100. Handman, E. Leishmaniasis: Current Status of Vaccine Development. *Clin. Microbiol. Rev.* **2001,** *14* (2), 229–243.
101. Murray, H. W. Progress in the Treatment of a Neglected Infectious Disease: Visceral Leishmaniasis. *Expert. Rev. Anti. Infect. Ther.* **2004,** *2* (2), 279–292.

102. Davis, A. J.; Murray, H. W.; Handman, E. Drugs against Leishmaniasis: A Synergy of Technology and Partnerships. *Trends Parasitol.* **2004,** *20* (2), 73–76.
102. Croft, S. L.; Coombs, G. H. Leishmaniasis - Current Chemotherapy and Recent Advances in the Search for Novel Drugs. *Trends Parasitol.* **2003,** *19* (11), 502–508.
103. Berman, J. Current Treatment Approaches to Leishmaniasis. *Curr. Opin. Infect. Dis.* **2003,** *16* (5), 397–401.
104. Sundar, S.; Rai, M. Advances in the Treatment of Leishmaniasis. *Curr. Opin. Infect. Dis.* **2002,** *15* (6), 593–598.
104. Croft, S. L.; Coombs, G. H. Leishmaniasis–Current Chemotherapy and Recent Advances in the Search for Novel Drugs. *Trends Parasitol.* **2003,** *19*, 502–508.
105. Antimony sodium gluconate, CSID: 20017501, in: http://www.chemspider.com/ChemicalStructure.20017501.html, Royal Society of Chemistry, 2013.
106. A. B, CSID:10237579, in: http://www.chemspider.com/Chemical-Structure.10237579.html Royal Society of Chemistry, 2013.
107. Miltefosine, CSID:3473, in: http://www.chemspider.com/Chemical-Structure.3473.html Royal Society of Chemistry, 2013.
108. Pentamidine, CSID:4573, in: http://www.chemspider.com/Chemical-Structure.4573.html Royal Society of Chemistry, 2013.
109. Paromomycin, CSID:145115, in: http://www.chemspider.com/Chemical-Structure.145115.html Royal Society of Chemistry, 2013.
110. Croft, S. L.; Coombs, G. H. Leishmaniasis - Current chemotherapy and Recent Advances in the Search for Novel Drugs. *Trends Parasitol.* **2003,** *19* (11), 502–508.
111. Sundar, S.; More, D. K.; Singh, M. K.; Singh, V. P.; Sharma, S.; Makharia, A.; Kumar, P. C.; Murray, H. W. Failure of Pentavalent Antimony in Visceral Leishmaniasis in India: Report from the Center of the Indian Epidemic. *Clin. Infect. Dis.* **2000,** *31* (4), 1104–1107.
112. Sundar, S. Drug Resistance in Indian Visceral Leishmaniasis. *Trop. Med. Int. Health* **2001,** *6* (11), 849–854.
113. Murray, H. W. Progress in the Treatment of a Neglected Infectious Disease: Visceral Leishmaniasis. *Expert. Rev. Anti. Infect. Ther.* **2004,** *2* (2), 279–292.
114. Berman, J. D.; Badaro, R.; Thakur, C. P.; Wasunna, K. M.; Behbehani, K.; Davidson, R.; Kuzoe, F.; Pang, L.; Weerasuriya, K.; Bryceson, A. D. Efficacy and Safety of Liposomal Amphotericin B (AmBisome) for Visceral Leishmaniasis in Endemic Developing Countries. *Bull. World Health Organ.* **1998,** *76* (1), 25–32.
115. Sundar, S.; Jha, T. K.; Thakur, C. P.; Engel, J.; Sindermann, H.; Fischer, C.; Junge, K.; Bryceson, A.; Berman, J. Oral Miltefosine for Indian Visceral Leishmaniasis. *N. Engl. J. Med.* **2002,** *347* (22), 1739–1746.
116. Soto, J.; Toledo, J.; Gutierrez, P.; Nicholls, R. S.; Padilla, J.; Engel, J.; Fischer, C.; Voss, A.; Berman, J. Treatment of American Cutaneous Leishmaniasis with Miltefosine, an Oral Agent. *Clin. Infect. Dis.* **2001,** *33* (7), E57–E61.
117. Soto J.; Arana B. A.; Toledo, J.; Rizzo, N.; Vega, J. C.; Diaz, A.; Luz, M.; Gutierrez, P.; Arboleda, M.; Berman, J. D.; Junge, K.; Engel, J.; Sindermann, H. Miltefosine for New World Cutaneous Leishmaniasis. *Clin. Infect. Dis.* **2004,** *38* (9), 1266–1272.
118. Perez-Victoria F. J.; Castanys, S.; Gamarro, F. *Leishmania donovani* Resistance to Miltefosine Involves a Defective Inward Translocation of the Drug. *Antimicrob. Agents Chemother*. **2003,** *47* (8), 2397–2403.
119. Seifert, K. Structures, Targets and Recent Approaches in Anti-leishmanial Drug Discovery and Development. *Open Med. Chem. J.* **2011,** *5*, 31–39.

120. Palatnik-de-Sousa, C. B. Vaccines for Leishmaniasis in the Fore Coming 25 Years. *Vaccine* **2008,** *26*, 1709–1724.
121. Mutiso, J. M.; Macharia, J. C.; Gicheru, M. M. A Review of Adjuvants for Vaccine Candidates. *J. Biomed. Res.* **2010,** *24* (1), 16–25.
122. Kato, H.; Gomez, E. A.; Cáceres, A. G.; Uezato, H.; Mimori, T.; Hashiguchi, Y. Molecular Epidemiology for Vector Research on Leishmaniasis. *Int. J. Environ. Res. Public Health* **2010,** *7*, 814–826.
123. Chappuis, F.; Sundar, S.; Hailu, A.; Ghalib, H.; Rijal, S.; Peeling, R.W.; Alvar, J.; Boelaert, M. Visceral Leishmaniasis: What Are the Needs for Diagnosis, Treatment and Control? *Nat. Rev. Microbiol.* **2007,** *5*, 873–882.
122. Wolday, D.; Berhe, N.; Akuffo, H.; Britton, S. *Leishmania*–HIV Interaction: Immunopathogenic Mechanisms. *Parasitol. Today* **1999,** *15*, 182–187.
123. Alexander, J.; Satoskar, A. R.; Russell, D. G. *Leishmania* Species: Models of Intracellular Parasitism. *J. Cell Sci.* **1999,** *112*, 2993–3002.
124. Mouritsen, O. G.; Zuckermann, M. J. What's So Special About Cholesterol? *Lipids* **2004,** *39*, 1101–1113.
125. Mukherjee, S.; Maxfield, F. R. Membrane Domains. *Annu. Rev. Cell Dev. Biol.* **2004,** *20*, 839–866.
126. Riethmüller, J.; Riehle, A.; Grassmé, H.; Gulbins, E. Membrane Rafts in Host–pathogen Interactions, *Biochem. Biophys. Acta.* **2006,** *1758*, 2139–2147.
127. Paila, Y. D.; Chattopadhyay, A. Membrane Cholesterol in the Function and Organization of G-protein Coupled Receptors. *Subcell. Biochem.* **2010,** *51*, 439–466.
128. Rodríguez, N. E.; Gaur, U.; Wilson, M. E. Role of Caveolae in *Leishmania chagasi* Phagocytosis and Intracellular Survival in Macrophages. *Cell. Microbiol.* **2006,** *8*, 1106–1120.
129. Cohen, B. E.; Ramos, H.; Gamargo, M.; Urbina, J. The Water and Ionic Permeability Induced by Polyene Antibiotics Across Plasma Membrane Vesicles from *Leishmania* sp. *Biochem. Biophys. Acta.* **1986,** *860*, 57–65.
130. Readio, J. D.; Bittman R. Equilibrium Binding of Amphotericin B and its Methyl Ester and Borate Complex to Sterols. *Biochem. Biophys. Acta.* **1982,** *685*, 219–224.
131. Datta, G.; Bera, T. The Effects of Clofazimine, Niclosamide and Amphotericin B, on Electron Transport of *Leishmania donovani* Promastigotes. *Indian J.* Med. Res. **2000,** *112*, 15–20.
132. Nagpal, K.; Singh, S. K.; Mishra, D. N. Chitosan Nanoparticles: A Promising System in Novel Drug Delivery. *Chem. Pharm. Bull.* 2010, *58*, 1423–1430.
133. Sharma, U.; Singh, S. Insect Vectors of *Leishmania*: Distribution, Physiology and Their Control. *J. Vector Borne Dis.* **2008,** *45*, 255–272.
134. Dedet, J. P.; Pratlong, F. Protozoa infection. In *Manson's Tropical Diseases*; Cook, G., Zumla, A., Eds. Saunders: Philadelphia, 2009; pp 1341–1367.
135. da Silva, R.; Sacks, D. L. Metacyclogenesis is a Major Determinant of *Leishmania* Promastigote Virulence and Attenuation. *Infect. Immun.* **1987,** *55*, 2802–2806.
136. Babior, B. M. Phagocytes and Oxidative Stress. *Am. J. Med.* **2000,** *109*, 33–44.
137. Mukbel, R. M.; Patten Jr., C.; Gibson, K.; Ghosh, M.; Petersen, C.; Jones, D. E. Macrophage Killing of *Leishmania amazonensis* Amastigotes Requires Both Nitric Oxide and Superoxide. *Am. J. Trop. Med. Hyg.* **2007,** *76*, 669–675.
138. Wilson, M. E.; Andersen, K. A.; Britigan, B. E. Response of *Leishmania chagasi* Promastigotes to Oxidant Stress. *Infect. Immun.* **1994,** *62*, 5133–5141.

139. Haidaris, C. G.; Bonventre, P. F. A Role for Oxygen-dependent Mechanisms in Killing of *Leishmania donovani* Tissue Forms by Activated Macrophages. *J. Immunol.* **1982,** *129*, 850–855.
140. Blough, N. V.; Zafiriou, O. C. Reaction of Superoxide with Nitric Oxide to form Peroxynitrite in Alkaline Aqueous Solution. *Inorg. Chem.* **1985,** *24*, 3502–3504.
141. Barr, S. D.; Gedamu, L. Role of Peroxidoxins in *Leishmania chagasi* Survival: Evidence of an Enzymatic Defense against Nitrosative Stress. *J. Biol. Chem.* **2003,** *278*, 10816–10823.
142. Babior, B. M.; Kipnes, R. S.; Curnutte, J. T. Biological Defense Mechanisms: The Production by Leukocytes of Superoxide, a Potential Bactericidal Agent. *J. Clin. Invest.* **1973,** *52*,741–744.
143. Minakami, R.; Sumimotoa, H. Phagocytosis-coupled Activation of the Superoxide-producing Phagocyte Oxidase, a Member of the NADPH Oxidase (Nox) Family. *Int. J. Hematol.* **2006,** *84*,193–198.
144. Monostori, P.; Wittmann, G.; Karg, E.; Turi, S. Determination of Glutathione and Glutathione Disulfide in Biological Samples: an In-depth Review. *J. Chromatogr. B Analyt. Technol. Biomed. Life Sci.* **2009,** *877*, 3331–3346.
145. Krauth-Siegel, R. L.; Comini, M. A. Redox Control in Trypanosomatids, Parasitic Protozoa with Trypanothione-based Thiol Metabolism. *Biochem. Biophys. Acta.* **2008,** *1780*, 1236–1248.
146. Comini, M.; Menge, U.; Wissing, J.; Flohe, L. Trypanothione Synthesis in Crithidia Revisited. *J. Biol. Chem.* **2005,** *280*, 6850–6860.
147. Oza, S. L.; Tetaud, E.; Ariyanayagam, M. R.; Warnon, S. S.; Fairlamb, A. H. A Single Enzyme Catalyses Formation of Trypanothione from Glutathione and Spermidine in *Trypanosoma cruzi. J. Biol. Chem.* **2002,** *277*, 35853–35861.
148. Penketh, P. G.; Kennedy, W. P.; Patton, C. L.; Sartorelli, A. C. Trypanosomatid Hydrogen Peroxide [corrected] Metabolism. *FEBS Lett.* **1987,** *221*, 427–431.
149. Rhee, S. G.; Chae, H. Z.; Kim, K. Peroxiredoxins: A Historical Overview and Speculative Preview of Novel Mechanisms and Emerging Concepts in Cell Signaling. *Free Radic. Biol. Med.* **2005,** *38*, 1543–1552.
150. Townsend, D. M. S-glutathionylation: Indicator of Cell Stress and Regulator of the Unfolded Protein Response. *Mol. Interv.* **2007,** *7*, 313–324.
151. Berhane, K.; Widersten, M.; Engstrom, A.; Kozarich, J. W.; Mannervik, B. Detoxification of Base Propenals and Other Alpha, Beta-unsaturated Aldehyde Products of Radical Reactions and Lipid Peroxidation by Human Glutathione Transferases. *Proc. Natl Acad. Sci. USA* **1994,** *91*, 1480–1484.
152. Vickers, T. J.; Fairlamb, A. H. Trypanothione S-transferase Activity in a Trypanosomatid Ribosomal Elongation Factor 1B. *J. Biol. Chem.* **2004,** *279*, 27246–27256.
153. Thony, B.; Auerbach, G.; Blau, N. Tetrahydrobiopterin Biosynthesis, Regeneration and Functions. *Biochem. J.* **2000,** *347* (Pt 1), 1–16.
154. Trager, W. Pteridine Requirement of the Hemoflagellate *Leishmania tarentolae. J. Protozool.* **1969,** *16*, 372–375.
155. Cunningham, M. L.; Titus, R. G.; Turco, S. J.; Beverley, S. M. Regulation of Differentiation to the Infective Stage of the Protozoan Parasite *Leishmania major* by Tetrahydrobiopterin. *Science* **2001,** *292*, 285–287.
156. Miao, L.; St Clair, D. K. Regulation of Superoxide Dismutase Genes: Implications in Disease. *Free Radic. Biol. Med.* **2009,** *47*,344–356.

157. Ghosh, S.; Goswami, S.; Adhya, S. Role of Superoxide Dismutase in Survive *Leishmania* within the Macrophage. *Biochem. J.* **2003,** *369*, 447–452.
158. Ghosh, D. K.; Datta, A. G. *Leishmania donovani*: Assay for a Functional Pentose Phosphate Pathway. *Exp. Parasitol.* **1971,** *29*, 103–109.
159. Maugeri, D. A.; Cazzulo, J. J.; Burchmore, R. J.; Barrett, M. P.; Ogbunude, P. O. Pentose Phosphate Metabolism in *Leishmania mexicana. Mol. Biochem. Parasitol.* **2003,** *130*, 117–125.
160 Callahan, H. L.; Portal, A. C.; Devereaux, R.; Grogl, M. An Axenic Amastigote System for Drug Screening. *Antimicrob. Agents Chemother.* **1997,** *41*, 818–822.
161. da Luz, R. I.; Vermeersch, M.; Dujardin, J. C.; Cos, P.; Maes, L. *In vitro* Sensitivity Testing of *Leishmania* Clinical Field Isolates: Preconditioning of Promastigotes Enhances Infectivity for Macrophage Host Cells. *Antimicrob. Agents Chemother.* **2009,** *53*, 5197–5203.
162. Boelaert, M.; Criel, B.; Leeuwenburg, J.; Van Damme, W.; Le Ray, D.; Van der Stuyft, P. Visceral Leishmaniasis Control: A Public Health Perspective. *Trans. R. Soc. Trop. Med. Hyg.* **2000,** *94*, 465–471.
163. Kamhawi, S. Phlebotomine Sand Flies and *Leishmania* Parasites: Friends or Foes? *Trends Parasitol.* **2006,** *22*, 439–445.
164. Hepburn, N. C. Cutaneous Leishmaniasis. *Clin. Exp. Dermatol.* **2000,** *25*, 363–370.
165. Maltezou, H. C. Drug Resistance in Visceral Leishmaniasis. *J. Biomed. Biotechnol.* **2010,** *2010*, 617521.
166. Shaw, J. The Leishmaniases—Survival and Expansion in a Changing World. *Mem. Inst. Oswaldo. Cruz.* **2007,** *102*, 541–547.
167. Carnau´ba, J. D.; Konishi, C. T.; Petri. V., Martinez, I. C. P., Shimizu, L., Pereira-Chioccola, V. L. Atypical Disseminated Leishmaniasis Similar to Post-kala-azar Dermal Leishmaniasis in a Brazilian AIDS Patient Infected with *Leishmania (Leishmania) infantum chagasi*: A Case Report. *Int. J. Infect. Dis.* **2009,** *13*, 504–507.
168. Croft, S. L.; Barret, M. P.; Urbina, J. A. Chemotherapy of Trypanosomiases and Leishmaniasis. *Trends Parasitol.* **2005,** *21*, 508–512.
169. Croft, S. L.; Sundar, S.; Fairlamb, A. H. Drug Resistance in Leishmaniasis. *Clin. Microbiol. Rev.* **2006,** *19*, 111–126.
170. Arevalo, J.; Ramirez, L.; Adaui, V.; Zimic, M.; Tulliano, G.; Miranda-Vera´stegui, C.; Lazo, M.; Loayza-Muro, R.; De Doncker, S.; Maurer, A.; Chappuis, F.; Dujardin, J. C.; Llanos-Cuentas, A. Influence of *Leishmania* (Viannia) Species on the Response to Antimonial Treatment in Patients with American Tegumentary Leishmaniasis. *J. Infect. Dis.* **2007,** *195*, 1846–1851.
171. Ouellette, M.; Drummelsmith, J.; Papadopoulou, B. Leishmaniasis: Drugs in the Clinic, Resistance and New Developments. *Drug Resist. Updat.* **2004,** *7*, 257–266.
172. Croft, S. L.; Coombs, G. H. Leishmaniasis-current Chemotherapy and Recent Advances in the Search for Novel Drugs. *Trends Parasitol.* **2003,** *19*, 502–508.
173. Yardley, V.; Croft, S. L. A Comparison of the Activities of Three Amphotericin B Lipid Formulations against Experimental Visceral and Cutaneous Leishmaniasis. *Int. J. Antimicrob. Agents* **2000,** *13*, 243–248.
174. Ordo´n˜ez-Gutie´rrez, L.; Espada-Ferna´ndez, R.; Dea-Ayuela, M. A.; Torrado, J. J.; Bola´sFernandez, F, Alunda, J. M. *In vitro* Effect of New Formulations of Amphotericin B on Amastigote and Promastigote Forms of *Leishmania infantum. Int. J. Antimicrob. Agents* **2007,** *30*, 325–329.

175. Berman, J.; Bryceson, A. D.; Croft, S.; Engel, J.; Gutteridge, W.; Karbwang, J.; Sindermann, H.; Soto, J.; Sundar, S.; Urbina, J. A. Miltefosine: Issues to be Addressed in the Future. *Trans. R. Soc. Trop. Med. Hyg.* **2006,** *100*, 41–44.
176. Sundar, S.; Murray, H. W. Availability of Miltefosine for the Treatment of Kala-azar in India. *Bull. World Health Organ.* **2005,** *83*, 394–395.
177. Sundar, S.; Olliaro, P. L. Miltefosine in the Treatment of Leishmaniasis: Clinical Evidence for Informed Clinical Risk Management. *Ther. Clin. Risk. Manag.* **2007,** *3*, 733–740.
178. Cabrera-Serra, M. G.; Valladares, B.; Pin˜ero, J. E. *In vivo* Activity of Perifosine Against *Leishmania amazonensis*. *Acta. Trop.* **2008,** *108*, 20–25.
179. Wasunna, M. K.; Rashid, J. R.; Mbui, L.; Kirigi, G.; Kinoti, D.; Lodenyo, H.; Felton, J. M.; Sabin, A. J.; Albert, M. J.; Horton, J. A Phase II Dose-increasing Study of Sitamaquine for the Treatment of Visceral Leishmaniasis in Kenya. *Am. J. Trop. Med. Hyg.* **2005,** *73*, 871–876.
180. Sundar, S.; Jha, T. K.; Thakur, C. P.; Sinha, P. K.; Bhattacharya, S. K. Injectable Paromomycin for Visceral Leishmaniasis in India. *N. Engl. J. Med.* **2007,** *356*, 2571–2581.
181. Armijos, R. X.; Weigel, M. M.; Calvopin˜a, M.; Mancheno, M.; Rodriguez, R. Comparison of the Effectiveness of Two Topical Paromomycin Treatments Versus Meglumine Antimoniate for New World Cutaneous Leishmaniasis. *Acta. Trop.* **2004,** *91*,153–160.
182. Croft, S. L.; Sundar, S.; Fairlamb, A. H. Drug Resistance in Leishmaniasis. *Clin. Microbiol. Rev.* **2006,** *19*, 111–126.
183. Davis, A. J.; Kedzierski, L. Recent Advances in Antileishmanial Drug Development. *Curr. Opin. Investig. Drugs* **2005,** *6* (2), 163–169.

CHAPTER 3

DIAGNOSIS AND STRATEGIES TO CONTROL LEISHMANIASIS

CONTENTS

PART III DIAGNOSIS AND STRATEGIES TO CONTROL LEISHMANIANSIS

ABSTRACT

For diagnosis of leishmaniasis, various noninvasive tests, with various specificities and sensitivities, are available however; none have become popular in areas of endemicity. Only few are commercialized. However these commercialized diagnostics tests are expensive. In addition, they require skilled personnel, expensive equipment, and electricity, and are technically demanding. Therefore *Leishmania* analysis by splenic, marrow, or skin lesion still utilized as standard with its usual limitations. Tests such as DAT, rK39 strip test, KATEX, and a field-adaptable version of PCR can also be utilized potentially for the diagnosis of leishmaniasis.

3.1 INTRODUCTION

The diagnosis of visceral leishmaniasis (VL) is complex because its clinical features are shared by a host of other commonly occurring diseases, such as malaria, typhoid, and tuberculosis; many of these diseases can be present along with VL (in cases of coinfection); sequestration of the parasite in the spleen, bone marrow, or lymph nodes further complicates this issue. Laboratory diagnosis of leishmaniasis can be made by the following: (1) demonstration of parasite in the tissues of relevance by light microscopic examination of the stained specimen, in vitro culture, or animal inoculation; (2) the detection of parasite DNA in tissue samples; or (3) immunodiagnosis by the detection of parasite antigen in tissue, blood, or urine samples, by detection of nonspecific or specific antileishmanial antibodies (immunoglobulin), or by assay for *Leishmania*-specific cell-mediated immunity.

Various noninvasive tests, with various specificities and sensitivities, are available for the diagnosis of leishmaniasis (Table 3-1); however, none have become popular in the areas of endemicity. Very few are commercially available; generally speaking, they also are expensive, require skilled personnel, expensive equipment, and electricity, and are technically demanding. Parasite diagnosis by splenic, marrow, or skin lesion remains the "gold standard," with its usual limitations. Direct agglutination test (DAT) can be performed only in a few centralized laboratories that are equipped for the purpose (and have trained personnel); cost, multiple steps, incubation, and antigenic variations are limiting factors. In these healthy endemic controls, a combination of DAT (that shows low titers in healthy endemic controls) and polymerase chain reaction (PCR) may be helpful in defining the status of these patients. DAT is mainly used for *Leishmania* DNA and antibody detection in the sample of infected patient. Species-level identification can also be done by the analysis of amplified minicircle kinetoplast DNA (KDNA), by choosing primers from conserved regions of different *Leishmania* species' KDNA minicircles.[1,2] PCR–enzyme-linked immunosorbent assay (ELISA) technique using a primer that was able to identify 33 *Leishmania infantum* strains from 19 different zymodemes has been developed. A new latex agglutination test (KATEX) is used for detecting leishmanial antigen in the urine of patients with VL. DNA detection by PCR with LDI primer is used to detect *Leishmania* DNA with whole blood from VL and skin specimens from Post-kala-azar dermal leishmaniasis patients. The rK39 strip test has the potential to be used for diagnosis of VL under field conditions. Other tests, which are likely candidates for diagnosis and prognosis of leishmaniasis in the future, are KATEX and afield-adaptable version of PCR, which would be simple, inexpensive, and easily available.

TABLE 3-1 Various methods used for diagnosis of visceral leishmaniasis[9]

Various diagnosis test	Specifications
Antibody detection	Enzyme-linked immunosorbent assay (ELISA) with fucose-mannose ligand
	Western blotting
	Various immunodiagnostic methods
	Countercurrent immunoelectrophoresis
	Complementfixation test
	Immunodiffusion test
	Countercurrent immunoelectrophoresis
	Indirect hemagglutination
	IFA test indirect fluorescent-antibody (IFA) test
	Direct agglutination test (DAT)
	Rapid strip test with rK39
	ELISA with rK39 antigen (Recombinant antigen)
	ELISA with crude soluble antigen
	Napier's formol gel or aldehyde test
	Chopra antimony test (for nonspecific immunoglobulins)

TABLE 3-1 *(Continued)*

Various diagnosis test	Specifications
Classical methods	Parasite culture, microscopic examination of tissue smears (a spleen, liver, or lymph node tissue specimen)
	Various in vitro culturing practices for amastigotes and promastigotes is done for chemotherapeutic studies
	Isolation of blood to isolate the parasite of the amastigotes
Identification test	Analysis of amplified minicircle kinetoplast DNA (KDNA)
Culturing practices	The culture media used may be monophasic (Schneider's insect medium, M199, or Grace's medium) or diphasic (Novy-McNeal Nicolle medium and Tobies medium)
Skin testing.	Delayed-type hypersensitivity (DTH) or T-cell-mediated immunity is a group-specific immune response: Montenegro skin test (leishmanin skin test)
DNA detection method	DNA hybridization
	PCR
	KDNA of leishmanias
	LDI primer
	PCR–ELISA technique
	IFA
	Proteinase K-based PCR
	Restriction fragment length polymorphism analysis of the PCR-amplified minicircle of leishmanial DNA
	DAT
Antigen testing	Latex agglutination test (KATEX)

3.2 VARIOUS IDENTIFICATION AND CULTURING PRACTICES USED DURING THE DIAGNOSIS OF LEISHMANIASIS

Identification of species of the *Leishmania donovani* complex is particularly difficult, because morphologically the species are almost indistinguishable from each other. For species-level identification, a large amount of promastigotes is obtained by a culture of the organism and the species-specific isoenzyme pattern is analyzed by cellulose acetate electrophoresis.[3] Typing of washed live promastigotes by DAT with species-specific monoclonal antibodies is another highly sensitive taxonomic tool frequently utilized for this purpose.[4] Species-level identification can also be done by the analysis of amplified KDNA, by choosing primers from conserved regions of different

Leishmania species' KDNA minicircles.[1,2] Yet another method used for the identification of species of *Leishmania* is the analysis of the in vitro promastigotes-released antigenic factors, which are different for different leishmanial species.[5]

Cultures are required for: *Leishmania* strains can be maintained as promastigotes in artificial culture medium.

- Obtaining a sufficient number of organisms to use an antigen for immunologic diagnosis and speciation,
- Obtaining parasites to be used in inoculating susceptible experimental animals,
- In vitro screening of drugs, and
- Accurate diagnosis of the infection with the organism (as a supplement to other methods or to provide a diagnosis when routine methods have failed).

3.3 STRATEGIES TO CONTROL THE VECTOR IN LEISHMANIASIS

Leishmaniasis is the vector-borne disease transmitted by the Phlebotomine flies in the Old World and Lutzomyiain in the New World.[6] The vector of various leishmaniases world over belongs to order Diptera of class Insecta (Phylum Arthopoda). Fauna of Indian sub-zone is represented by 46 species, of these 11 belong to Phlebotomine species and 35 to sergentomyia species.[7] *Phlebotomus argentipesis* is the proved vector of kala-azar (VL) in India.[8] Control of VL mainly depends on its epidemiological features. In the zoonotic foci where carriers are involved and dogs are the main vertebrate host, the effective methods include the destruction of dogs and elimination of sandflies by environmental and chemical control. In India, Bangladesh, and Nepal where VL is anthroponotic, the only choice is chemical and environmental control. Best method to interrupt any vector-borne disease is to reduce man–vector contact. Many methods exist at present for leishmaniasis control, which can be used individually or in combination. The selection of method or the combination of methods depends on the type of the leishmaniasis to be controlled and also the method should be situation specific. In this article, attempts have been made to discuss the conventional and some latest technologies of vectors control measures being used worldwide.

Spraying method such as indoor residual spraying is a simple and cost-effective method of controlling endophilic vectors and dichlorodiphenyl-trichloroethane (DDT) remains the insecticide of choice for the control of leishmaniasis. However, resistance to insecticide is likely to become more widespread in the population especially in those areas in which insecticide has been used for years. In this context, the use of slow release emulsified suspension (SRES) may be the best substitute. In this review, spraying frequencies of DDT and new schedule of spray have been discussed. Role of biological control and environment management in the control of leishmaniasis has been emphasized. Allethrin (coil) 0.1% and 1.6% prallethrin (liquid) have been found to be effective repellents against *P. argentipes*, the vector of Indian kala-azar. Insecticide impregnated bednets is another area that requires further research on priority basis for the control of leishmaniasis. Role of satellite remote sensing for early prediction of disease by identifying the sandfly genic conditions cannot be undermined. In future, synthetic pheromons can be exploited in the control of leishmaniasis.

KEYWORDS

- **diagnosis tests**
- ***Leishmania***
- **kala-azar**
- **leishmaniasis**

REFERENCES

1. Sacks, D. L.; Kenny, R. T.; Kreutzer, R. D.; Jaffe, C. L.; Gupta, A. K.; Sharma, M. C.; Sinha, S.; Neua, P. F. V.; Saran. R. Indian Kala-azar Caused by *Leishmania tropica*. *Lancet* **1995,** *345*, 959–961.
2. Smyth, A. J.; Gosh, A.; Hassan, M. Q.; Basu, D.; De Bruijn, M. H.; Adhya, S.; Mallik, K. K.; Barker, D. C. Rapid and Sensitive Detection of *Leishmania* Kinetoplast DNA from Spleen and Blood Samples of Kala-azar Patients. *Parasitol.* **1992,** *105*, 183–192.
3. Kreutzer, R.D.; Grogl, M.; Neva, F.A.; Fryauff, D.J.; Magill, A.J.; Aleman-Munoz M.M. Identification and genetic comparison of leishmanial parasites causing viscerotropic and cutaneous disease in soldiers returning from Operation Desert Storm. *Am. J. Trop. Med. Hyg.* **1993,** *49*,357–363.
4. Jaffe, C. L.; Sarfstein, R. Species-specific Antibodies to *Leishmania tropica* (Minor) Recognize Somatic Antigens and Exometabolites. *J. Immunol.* **1987,** *139*, 1310–1319.
5. Ilg, T.; Stierhof, Y. D.; Wiese, M.; McConville M. J., Overath, P. Characterization of Phosphoglycan Containing Secretory Products of *Leishmania. Parasitol.* **1994,** *108*, 563–571.

6. Kalra, N. L.; Bang, Y. H. Manual on Control of Leishmaniasis. *WHO Tech. Rep. Ser.* **1990,** *797*, 26.
7. Sharma, U.; Singh, S. Insect Vectors of *Leishmania*: Distribution, Physiology and their Control. J. Vector. Borne. Dis. **2008,** 45 (4), 255–272.
8. Swaminath, C. S.; Short, H. E.; Anderson, L. A. P. Transmission of Indian Kala-azar to Man by the Bite of *P. argentipes*. *Indian J. Med. Res.* **1942,** *30*, 473–477.
9. Sundar S, Rai M. Laboratory Diagnosis of Visceral Leishmaniasis. *Clin. Diag. Lab. Immunol.* **2002,** 951–958.Table caption.

CHAPTER 4

IMMUNOMODULATORY AGENTS FOR LEISHMANIASIS

CONTENTS

PART IV POTENTIAL IMMUNOMODULATORY AGENTS FOR LEISHMANIASIS

ABSTRACT

World infectious protozoal disease known as Leishmaniasis causes clinical manifestations. The clinical extent ranges from self-healing cutaneous lesions to the fatal visceral form. Classical treatment of Leishmaniasis with pentavalent antimony is now limited by its toxicity and alarming increase in unresponsiveness. Current treatments particularly with modern antileishmanial drugs are unaffordable in many affected countries. In addition, vaccination-based approaches have not yet proved to be effective. Therefore chemotherapeutic agents are the last alternative. However, this requires the identification of novel drug targets. This chapter describes various strategies adopted by antileishmanian drugs against the leishmania-infected host immunity. In addition, various host immune signaling pathways that could be considered as potential drug targets for *Leishmania* chemotherapy are also described.

4.1 INTRODUCTION

The key pathogenic event in leishmaniasis is harboring of the causative *Leishmania* parasite within phagolysosomes of macrophages. Therefore, to establish infection, *Leishmania* invariably develop mechanisms to neutralize the microbicidal machinery of macrophages. Hence, the establishment of infection critically hinges on whether the balance tilts toward the host's ability to activate its armamentarium or the parasite's ability to escape or evade this host immune response. Macrophages are host cells for the parasite, but also importantly, sentinels of the immune system. The parasite interferes with the signaling system of the host, such that effector functions triggered by various cell surface receptors are either actively suppressed or are altered so as to result in immune suppression that will promote parasite survival. Therefore, our quest for antileishmanial drugs should focus on their direct parasiticidal and/or indirect immunomodulatory activity, achieved via restoration of impaired host signaling pathways. In this review, we have highlighted the participation of various immune cells, microbicidal molecules and altered signaling mechanisms in leishmaniasis, together with the influence of antileishmanial drugs on various immune cells such as neutrophils, macrophages, dendritic cells (DCs), and lymphocytes. The different immune mechanisms impacted upon include increased generation of reactive oxygen species (ROS) and reactive nitrogen species (RNS), activation of co-stimulatory molecules, and signaling pathways, for example, toll-like receptors (TLRs), mitogen-activated protein kinase (MAPK), Janus kinase/signal transducers and activators of transcription (JAK-STAT), protein kinase C (PKC), and translocation of NF-kB. Taken together, screening for compounds having the propensity to modulate the host defense signaling pathways alone or in combination with existing antileishmanial drugs[1] may well prove to be an effective immunochemotherapeutic strategy in leishmaniasis worthy of pharmacological consideration.

4.2 TARGETING OF HOST IMMUNITY BY ANTILEISHMANIAL DRUGS

Within the mammalian host, *Leishmania* reside as amastigotes in phagocytic cells that include neutrophils, macrophages, and DCs; therefore, an immunomodulatory compound could be potentially leishmanicidal by virtue of its potential to activate phagocytic cells.

4.2.1 *ROLE OF NEUTROPHILS*

The best characterized function of polymorphonuclear neutrophils (PMNs) is their preeminent role in phagocytosis and killing of invading microorganisms via the generation of ROS and release of lytic enzymes. Following entry of *Leishmania* into the mammalian host, PMNs are recruited immediately to the site of infection within 24 hours, implying that they possibly serve as host cells for leishmaniasis, the very early phase of infection.[2,3]

Neutrophils being inherently short-lived undergo apoptosis,[2] whereas *Leishmania* parasites are known to delay their apoptosis, possibly by interfering with production of ROS, which importantly facilitates their survival.[4,5] To trigger apoptosis, neutrophils utilize a MAPK signaling pathway, p38 MAPK being a key player.[6] Importantly, *Leishmania* parasites that enter macrophages via the uptake of infected, apoptotic PMNs then survive and multiply effectively.[2] Therefore, as neutrophils harbor and transport *Leishmania*, targeting pathogens residing in neutrophils should be taken into consideration when designing novel antileishmanial compounds. Therefore, it is tempting to extrapolate that a compound capable of increasing phagocytic activity and generating an oxidative burst within *Leishmania*-infected neutrophils would effectively eliminate parasites. Indeed, antimonials increase the phagocytic capacity of neutrophils along with an increased production of superoxide.[7] Berberine chloride also promoted parasite elimination via the enhancement of apoptosis in *Leishmania donovani*-infected neutrophils, subsequent to modulation of the MAPK pathways.[8]

4.2.2 MONOCYTES AND MACROPHAGES

To sustain infection, it is mandatory that *Leishmania* parasites should establish themselves in macrophages, but considering the potent antimicrobial functions of macrophages, the subject of how *Leishmania* survive is a subject of intense research.

4.2.2.1 PHAGOCYTOSIS

C3b is a complement protein that following binding to *Leishmania* surface glycoprotein gp63 increases parasite uptake into macrophages as gp63 cleverly converts C3b into iC3b, which then favors phagocytosis, yet prevents lytic clearance.[9] Antimonials,[7] *Pourouma guinensis* (Oleanolic acid[10]), and Diphyllin isolated from *Haplophyllum bucharicum* Litv[11] influence the phagocytic activity of macrophages as do CpG oligodeoxynucleotide (CpG ODN) and Miltefosine.[12]

4.2.2.2 ACIDIFICATION

Generally, following the fusion of the phagosome with the endosomal compartment, a significant drop in pH ensues. However, *Leishmania* produce a surface acid phosphatase that inhibits the oxidative burst within macrophages, and additionally is an active proton pump that keeps the intracellular pH close to neutral.[13] Tamoxifen similarly modulates the macrophage intravacuolar compartment by causing a rapid, long-lasting alkalinization.[14]

4.2.3 ROLE OF REACTIVE OXYGEN SPECIES AND REACTIVE NITROGEN SPECIES

As nitric oxide (NO) is an effector molecule critical for the elimination of intracellular *Leishmania* parasites, disease progression is ensured via the enhancement of Th2 responses that causes a deactivation of macrophages and a decreased production of NO. Therefore, parasite removal should entail the activation of infected macrophages by increased expression of inducible nitric oxide synthase (iNOS) to form NO.[15] During *Leishmania* infection, decreased expression or inactivation of iNOS may also be associated with increased activation of *arginase* as deprivation of L-arginine impairs *Leishmania major* specific T-cell responses.[16] Following parasite engulfment by macrophages, reduced nicotinamide adenine dinucleotide phosphate (NAD(P)H) *oxidases* are initially activated, which transfer the reducing equivalents from NAD (P)H to molecular oxygen leading to the formation of extremely reactive superoxide. These then react with parasite membrane phospholipids leading to increased permeabilization as also react with the pathogen's macromolecules such as DNA leading to strand breaks; However, when the infection is sustained, macrophages are deactivated causing a decreased production of superoxide, which is now beneficial for parasite survival.

4.2.4 ROLE OF DENDRITIC CELLS

The interaction of *Leishmania* parasites with DCs is complex, as depending upon the species of *Leishmania*, the DC subset and other exogenous stimuli involved, there can either be control of infection or disease progression.[17] The first study with murine skin DC implicated epidermal Langerhans cells as important cells for the detection, uptake, and transport of *Leishmania* to lymph nodes.[18] Dermal DCs efficiently incorporate parasites into vacuoles and are proposed to act as principal antigen-presenting cells (APCs) in leishmaniasis, whereas others suggest that lymph node-resident DCs are initiators of the immune response.[17] *Leishmania* have cleverly devised several strategies to avoid DCs, as in humans, *L. donovani* blocks the maturation of DC[19] and production of IL-12, essential for the initiation of a protective immune response. Accordingly, Miltefosine in turn can activate DCs[20] as also does Pyrazinamide via an increased secretion of pro-inflammatory molecules and an enhanced expression of co-stimulatory molecules.

4.2.5 LYMPHOCYTES

T lymphocytes are generally responsible for intracellular pathogen elimination whereas B lymphocytes eliminate extracellular bacteria. In order to eliminate *Leishmania*, the macrophage needs to be activated by antigen-specific T lymphocytes. This process may further control the secretion of interferon (IFN)-γ and upregulate production of NO from macrophages. Both CD4 and CD8 cells are required for resolving the infection, along with a balance between Th1 and Th2, preferably a Th1-skewed response.[5] Therefore, essential prerequisites of an effective immunomodulatory, anti-leishmanial drug should be its potential to tilt the Th1-Th2 imbalance in favor of Th1. Furthermore in VL, T cell proliferation is impaired possibly due to the loss of co-stimulatory molecule(s),[21] and so this too can be an additional target.

4.2.6 MACROPHAGE-DERIVED CYTOKINES AS A MEASURE OF IMMUNOMODULATORY ACTIVITY

The immunomodulatory potential of antileishmanial drugs has been established by measuring its influence on macrophage-derived cytokines, mainly IFN-γ, IL-12, TNF-α, and IL-10. IL-6 and IL-1β are potent pro-inflammatory cytokines involved in the generation of NO and macrophage activation which are increased by antimonials,[22] tannins, and related compounds,[23] such as also sage phenolics.[24] Chemokines, a superfamily of low molecular weight cytokines recruit distinct subsets of leukocytes and by activating them play an important role in leishmaniasis. Tumor necrosis factor (TNF)-α and interlukin (IL)-1β together with Macrophage inflammatory protein 1α (MIP-1α) regulate transport of *Leishmania* from infected sites to lymph nodes.[25] During leishmaniasis, IFN-γ together with macrophage chemotactic protein 1 (MCP-1) eliminate *L. major* while conversely, IL-4 antagonizes the production of MCP-1.[26] Essential oil and extracts from Xylopia discrete induced differential production of MCP-1 in leishmaniasis.[27] IL-8 is another chemokine that controls the early infection of *Leishmania* via the recruitment of neutrophils[28] and release of NO along with pro-inflammatory cytokines from macrophages[29]; super antigens (SAG) in fact induces IL-8 synthesis in patients with CL.[22] It has been shown that coincubation of *Leishmania* parasites with PMNs inhibits the CXC chemokine and IFN-γ inducible protein-10 (IP-10), accounting for its Th1 inhibiting activity.[28] Furthermore, as IP-10 and CXCL-10 induce natural killer (NK) cells,[25] it suggests that induction of chemokines within *Leishmania*-infected cells could also be an effective strategy.

4.2.7 *EFFECT ON CO-STIMULATORY MOLECULES*

T cell-mediated regulation of immune responses is intimately associated with co-stimulatory molecules present on APCs, as they can modulate the T-cell receptor–major histocompatibility complex (MHC) interaction. Among them, CD28 plays a pivotal role as their enhanced or diminished expression causes immune activation or anergy respectively[30] owing to their interaction with B7.1 (CD80) or B7.2 (CD86) present on monocyte/macrophages and/or B cells. In post-kala-azar dermal leishmaniasis (PKDL), an increased levels of circulating CD8 +28 lymphocytes confers immune anergy, evidenced by their nonproliferating nature that gets reversed following treatment.[31] The impaired expression of CD86 on monocytes as evidenced in PKDL was markedly increased following treatment with Miltefosine and SAG, in which the effect of Miltefosine being greater.[32] Pyrazinamide-enhanced expression of CD80 and CD86 in *Leishmania* infected BALB/C mice as did an aqueous extract of human placenta, evidenced by an increased expression of MHC molecules on APCs.

4.3 MODULATION OF SIGNALING EVENTS IN *LEISHMANIA* INFECTION; ROLE OF CHEMOTHERAPY

4.3.1 *EFFECT ON EXPRESSION OF CD40 AND MITOGEN-ACTIVATED PROTEIN KINASE SIGNALING PATHWAYS*

An important co-stimulatory molecule that determines the outcome of macrophage–*Leishmania* interactions is CD40 as the CD40–CD40L interaction helps increase the Th1 immune response.[33] With regard to *Leishmania* infection, CD40-mediated MAPKs have been reported to promote parasite survival by modulating the expression of IL-10 and IL-12 in macrophages.[34] MAPKs, a group of serine/threonine kinases are responsible for phosphorylation of cellular proteins which in turn triggers signals necessary for cell proliferation, differentiation, and survival.

4.3.2 *TOLL-LIKE RECEPTORS AND THEIR RESPONSIVENESS IN LEISHMANIA INFECTION*

TLRs have been identified as ancient receptors that are of critical importance for the initiation of an efficient immune response.[35] Innate immunity coordinates the inflammatory response to pathogens, wherein the contribution of TLRs is widely recognized. These TLRs are located either on the plasma membrane or within the endosomal membrane of macrophages, DCs, NK cells, and also T and B lymphocytes. Mammalian cells express up to 12 different TLRs[35] that share an intracellular domain, called Toll-IL-1R[35]; among them, some signal through the myeloid differentiation protein 88 (MyD88)[36] that ultimately leads to nuclear translocation of NF-κB and expression of pro-inflammatory cytokines that includes TNF-α, IL-12 along with iNOS, collectively causing host protection.

4.3.3 LEISHMANIA INFECTION AND EFFECT ON JAK-STAT PATHWAYS

Cytokines play a critical role in determining the nature of the host immune response in *Leishmania* infection as they trigger a signaling pathway through a cascade of intra-cytoplasmic proteins known as Janus Kinase and signal transducer and activator of transcriptions.[37] The biological effects of IFN-γ are dependent on the activation of STAT1 transcription factors as ligation of IFN-γ with IFN-γ receptor (IFN-γR) activates JAK1/JAK2 kinase, which then phosphorylates STAT-1; the STAT1 then translocates to the nucleus and further enhances the transcription of IFN-γ-induced genes.[38]

4.3.4 MODULATION OF NF-κB SIGNALING PATHWAYS BY LEISHMANIA

The NF-κB family includes five members of which p50, p65 (Rel A), and c-Rel, have been detected in macrophages, in which p50-p65 being the most common.[39]

4.3.5 ALTERATIONS OF HOST CELL KINASES AND PHOSPHATASE BY LEISHMANIA

PKC is a family of 10 isoenzymes involved in controlling the function of other proteins through phosphorylation of hydroxyl groups of their serine and threonine residues. PKCs play an important role in several signal transduction cascades and are activated by increased concentration of diacylglycerol

(DAG) or Ca^{2+}.[40] During *Leishmania* infection, the activation of PKC is inhibited and subsequent intracellular signaling, lipophosphoglycan being a key determinant, and also other glycosylinositol phospholipids.[41]

KEYWORDS

- **immunomodulation**
- ***Leishmania***
- **macrophage**
- **chemotherapy**
- **signaling pathways**

REFERENCES

1. El-On, J. Current Status and Perspectives of the Immunotherapy of Leishmaniasis. *Isr. Med. Assoc. J.* **2009,** *11*, 623–628.
2. Laskay, T.; van Zandbergen, G.; Solbach, W. Neutrophil Granulocytes as Host Cells and Transport Vehicles for Intracellular Pathogens: Apoptosis as Infection-promoting Factor. *Immunobiology* **2008,** *213*, 183–191.
3. Sunderkötter, C.; Kunz, M.; Steinbrink, K.; Meinardus-Hager, G.; Goebeler, M.; Bildau, H; Sorg, C. Resistance of Mice to Experimental Leishmaniasis is Associated with More Rapid Appearance of Mature Macrophages *in vitro* and *in vivo*. *J. Immunol.* **1993,** *151*, 4891–4901.
4. Laufs, H.; Müller, K.; Fleischer, J.; Reiling, N.; Jahnke, N.; Jensenius, J.C.; Solbach, W.; Laskay, T. Intracellular Survival of *Leishmania major* in Neutrophil Granulocytes After Uptake in the Absence of Heat-labile Serum Factors. *Infect. Immun.* **2002,** *70*, 826–835.
5. Aga, E.; Katschinski, D. M.; van Zandbergen, G.; Laufs, H.; Hansen, B.; Müller, K.; Solbach, W.; Laskay, T. Inhibition of the Spontaneous Apoptosis of Neutrophil Granulocytes by the Intracellular Parasite *Leishmania major*. *J. Immunol.* **2002,** *169*, 898–905.
6. Aoshiba, K.; Yasui, S.; Hayashi, M.; Tamaoki, J.; Nagai, A. Role of p38-mitogen-activated Protein Kinase in Spontaneous Apoptosis of Human Neutrophils. *J. Immunol.* **1999,** *162*, 1692–1700.
7. Muniz-Junqueira, M. I.; de Paula-Coelho, V. N. Meglumine Antimonate Directly Increases Phagocytosis, Superoxide Anion and TNF-alpha Production, but Only via TNF-alpha it Indirectly Increases Nitric Oxide Production by Phagocytes of Healthy Individuals, in vitro. *Int. Immunopharmacol.* **2008,** *8*, 1633–1638.

8. Saha, P.; Sarkar, A.; Bhattacharjee, S.; Hariharan, C.; Laskay, T.; Majumdar, S.; et al. Berberine Chloride Modulates the *MAP Kinase* Pathway in Host Cells to Mediate its Antileishmanial Activity. *Poster presentation, Society of Free Radical ResearchIndia*, Hyderabad, India, January 11–13, 2010
9. Brittingham, A.; Morrison, C. J.; McMaster W. R.; McGwire, B. S.; Chang, K. P.; Mosser, D. M. Role of the *Leishmania* Surface Protease gp63 in Complement Fixation, Cell Adhesion, and Resistance to Complement-mediated Lysis. *J. Immunol.* **1995,** *155*, 3102–3111.
10. Torres-Santos, E. C.; Lopes, D.; Oliveira, R. R.; Carauta, J. P.; Falcao, C. A.; Kaplan, M. A.; Rossi-Bergmann, B. Antileishmanial Activity of Isolated Triterpenoids from *Pourouma guianensis*. *Phytomedicine* **2004,** *11*, 114–120.
11. Di Giorgio, C.; Delmas, F.; Akhmedjanova, V.; Ollivier, E.; Bessonova, I.; Riad, E.; Timon-David, P. In vitro Antileishmanial Activity of Diphyllin Isolated from *Haplophyllum bucharicum*. *Planta. Med.* **2005,** *71*, 366–369.
12. Sane, S. A.; Shakya, N.; Haq, W.; Gupta, S. CpG Oligodeoxynucleotide Augments the Antileishmanial Activity of Miltefosine against Experimental Visceral Leishmaniasis. *J. Antimicrob. Chemother.* **2010,** *65*, 1448–1454.
13. Sharma, U.; Singh, S. Immunobiology of Leishmaniasis. *Indian J. Exp. Biol.* **2009,** *47*, 412–423 and references therein.
14. Miguel, D. C.; Yokoyama-Yasunaka, J. K.; Andreoli, W. K.; Mortara, R. A.; Uliana, S. R. Tamoxifen is Effective against *Leishmania* and Induces a Rapid Alkalinization of Parasitophorous Vacuoles Harbouring *Leishmania (Leishmania) amazonensis* Amastigotes. *J. Antimicrob. Chemother.* **2007,** *60*, 526–534.
15. Holzmuller, P.; Sereno, D.; Cavaleyra, M.; Mangot, I.; Daulouede, S.; Vincendeau, P.; Lemesre, J. L. Nitric Oxide-mediated Proteasome-dependent Oligonucleosomal DNA Fragmentation in *Leishmania amazonensis* Amastigotes. *Infect. Immunol.* **2002,** *70*, 3727–3735.
16. Munder, M.; Choi, B. S.; Rogers, M.; Kropf, P. L-arginine Deprivation Impairs *Leishmania major*-specific T-cell Responses. *Eur. J. Immunol.* **2009,** *39*, 2161–2172.
17. Soong, L. Modulation of Dendritic Cell Function by *Leishmania* Parasites. *J. Immunol.* **2008,** *180*, 4355–4360.
18. Moll, H.; Fuchs, H.; Blank, C.; Rollinghoff, M. Langerhans Cells Transport *Leishmania major* from the Infected Skin to the Draining Lymph Node for Presentation to Antigen-specific T Cells. *Eur. J. Immunol.* **1993,** *23*, 1595–1601.
19. Tejle, K.; Lindroth, M.; Magnusson, K. E.; Rasmusson, B. Wild-type *Leishmania donovani* Promastigotes Block Maturation, Increase Integrin Expression and Inhibit Detachment of Human Monocyte-derived Dendritic Cells–the Influence of Phosphoglycans. *FEMS. Microbiol. Lett.* **2008,** *279*, 92–102.
20. Griewank, K.; Gazeau, C.; Eichhorn, A.; von Stebut, E. Miltefosine Efficiently Eliminates *Leishmania major* Amastigotes from Infected Murine Dendritic Cells Without Altering Their Immune Functions. *Antimicrob. Agents Chemother*. **2010,** *54*, 652–659.
21. Nylén, S.; Gautam, S. Immunological Perspectives of Leishmaniasis. *J. Glob. Infect. Dis.* **2010**, *2*, 135–146.
22. Kocyigit, A.; Gur, S.; Gurel, M. S.; Bulut, V.; Ulukanligil, M. Antimonial Therapy Induces Circulating Proinflammatory Cytokines in Patients with Cutaneous Leishmaniasis. *Infect. Immun.* **2002,** *70*, 6589–6591.

23. Kolodziej, H.; Kayser, O.; Kiderlen, A. F.; Ito, H.; Hatano, T.; Yoshida, T.; Foo, L. Y. Proanthocyanidins and Related Compounds: Antileishmanial Activity and Modulatory Effects on Nitric Oxide and Tumor Necrosis Factor-alpha-release in the Murine Macrophage-like Cell Line RAW 264.7. *Biol. Pharm. Bull.* **2001,** *24*, 1016–1021.
24. Radtke, O. A.; Foo, L.Y.; Lu, Y.; Kiderlen, A. F.; Kolodziej, H. Evaluation of Sage Phenolics for Their Antileishmanial Activity and Modulatory Effects on Interleukin-6, Interferon and Tumour Necrosis Factor-alpha-release in RAW 264.7 cells. *Z. Naturforsch. C.* **2003,** *58*, 395–400.
25. Teixeira, M. J.; Teixeira, C. R.; Andrade, B. B.; Barral-Netto, M.; Barral, A. Chemokines in Host-parasite Interactions in Leishmaniasis. *Trends Parasitol.* **2006,** *22*, 32–40.
26. Ritter, U.; Moll, H. Monocyte Chemotactic Protein-1 Stimulates the Killing of *Leishmania major* by Human Monocytes, Acts Synergistically with IFN-gamma and Is Antagonized by IL-4. *Eur. J. Immunol.* **2000,** *30*, 3111–3120.
27. López, R.; Cuca, L. E.; Delgado, G. Antileishmanial and Immunomodulatory Activity of *Xylopia discreta*. *Parasite Immunol.* **2009,** *31*, 623–630.
28. van Zandbergen, G.; Hermann, N.; Laufs, H.; Solbach, W.; Laskay, T. *Leishmania* Promastigotes Release a Granulocyte Chemotactic Factor and Induce Interleukin-8 Release but Inhibit Gamma Interferon-inducible Protein 10 Production by Neutrophil Granulocytes. *Infect. Immun.* **2002,** *70*, 4177–4184.
29. Gupta, G.; Bhattacharjee, S.; Bhattacharyya, S.; Bhattacharya, P.; Adhikari, A.; Mukherjee, A.; Bhattacharyya Majumdar, S.; Majumdar, S. CXC Chemokine-mediated Protection Against Visceral Leishmaniasis: Involvement of the Proinflammatory Response. *J. Infect. Dis.* **2009,** *200*, 1300–1310.
30. Linsley, P. S.; Ledbetter J. A. The Role of the CD28 Receptor during T Cell Responses to Antigen. *Annu. Rev. Immunol.* **1993,** *11*, 191–212.
31. Ganguly, S.; Mukhopadhyay, D.; Das, N. K.; Chaduvula, M.; Sadhu, S.; Chatterjee, U.; Rahman, M.; Goswami, R. P.; Guha, S. K.; Modak, D.; Mallik, S.; Gonju, D.; Pramanik, N.; Barbhuiya, J. N.; Saha, B.; Chatterjee, M. Enhanced Lesional Foxp3 Expression and Peripheral Anergic Lymphocytes Indicate a Role for Regulatory T Cells in Indian Post-kala-azar Dermal Leishmaniasis. *J. Invest. Dermatol.* **2010,** *130*, 1013–1022.
32. Mukhopadhyay, D.; Das., N. K.; Roy, S.; Kundu, S.; Barbhuiya, J. N.; Chatterjee, M. Miltefosine Effectively Modulates the Cytokine Milieu in Indian Post Kala-azar Dermal Leishmaniasis. *J. Infect. Dis.* **2011,** *204*, 1427–1436.
33. Mathur, R. K.; Awasthi, A.; Wadhone, P.; Ramanamurthy, B.; Saha, B. Reciprocal CD40 Signals though p38MAPK and ERK-1/2 Induce Counteracting Immune Responses. *Nat. Med.* **2004,** *10*, 540–544.
34. Karin, M. Signal Transduction from Cell Surface to Nucleus in Development and Disease. *FASEB. J.* **1992,** *6*, 2581–2590.
35. Akira, S.; Uematsu, S.; Takeuchi, O. Pathogen Recognition and Innate Immunity. *Cell* **2006,** *124*, 783–801.
36. Medzhitov, R.; Preston-Hurlburt, P.; Kopp, E.; Stadlen, A.; Chen, C.; Ghosh, S.; Janeway, C. A. Jr. MyD88 Is an Adaptor Protein in the hToll/IL-1 Receptor Family Signaling Pathways. *Mol. Cell* **1998,** *2*, 253–258.
37. Wurster, A. L.; Tanaka, T.; Grusby, M. J. The Biology of Stat4 and Stat6. *Oncogene* **2000,** *19*, 2577–2584.
38. Boehm, U.; Klamp, T.; Groot, M.; Howard, J. C. Cellular Responses to Interferon-γ. *Annu. Rev. Immunol.* **1997,** *15*, 749–795.

39. Verma, I. M.; Stevenson, J. K.; Schwarz, E. M.; Van Antwerp, D.; Miyamoto, S. Rel/NFkappaB/I-kappaB Family: Intimate Tales of Association and Dissociation. *Genes Dev.* **1995,** *9*, 2723–2735.
40. Mellor, H.; Parker, P. J. The Extended Protein Kinase C Superfamily. *Biochem. J.* **1998,** *332*, 281–292.
41. Forestier, C-L, Gao, Qi, Boons, G-J. *Leishmania* lipophosphoglycan: how to establish structure-activity relationships for this highly complex and multifunctional glycoconjugate? *Front. Cell Infect. Microbiol.* **2014**, *4*, 193.

CHAPTER 5

AYURVEDIC TREATMENTS FOR LEISHMANIASIS

CONTENTS

PART V AYURVEDIC TREATMENTS FOR LEISHMANIASIS

ABSTRACT

Parasitic diseases that pose a threat to human life include leishmaniasis caused by protozoa of *Leishmania* species. Existing drugs have limitations due to deleterious side effects like teratogenicity and factors like cost and drug resistance, thus furthering the need to develop this area of research. Ayurved do believes in microorganisms and their role in disease, but emphasized more on body's response and occurrence of disease occurs only if the Bala is reduced. Several Ayurvedic therapies can be used against leishmaniasis by using several natural products in their sutable form. These natural products have long been providing important drug leads for infectious diseases. This chapter decribes the strength of Ayurveda by exploring the various natural products reported against *Leishmania*.

5.1 INTRODUCTION

A group of diseases caused by the obligate intracellular protozoa of the genus *Leishmania* are called as leishmaniases. It is a parasitic disease, which is endemic in several poor countries and presents as epidemics. There are three types of leishmaniasis: systemic or visceral (VL), cutaneous (Vivrita), and mucocutaneous leishmaniasis. VL is a deadly disease caused by the parasitic protozoa *Leishmania donovani* that are transmitted to humans by the bite of infected female sandfly, *Phlebotomus argentipes*. The amastigote form of the parasite invades the reticuloendothelial system of humans. Therefore systemic infection affects the whole immunity of the body. Major symptoms of systemic leishmaniasis are vomiting, scaly and dark epidermis, thinning hair, lengthy periods of fever, diarrhea, cough, night perspires, weight-loss, and abdominal pain. It is estimated that 350 million people in 88 countries are at the risk of developing the disease. About 500,000 people suffer from it worldwide. The estimated number of cases is about 100,000 distributed in India, Bangladesh, and Nepal. A total of 165 million people are estimated to be at risk. The reported number of cases is around 20,000 and number of deaths about 200 per year. Estimated number of cases is much higher. Bihar state is the worst affected with 33 districts endemic. It is also found in the neighboring states of West Bengal with 10 districts affected, Jharkhand with 5 districts endemic, and Uttar Pradesh with 4. In 1901, Leishman identified certain organisms in smears taken from the spleen of a patient who had died from *"dum-dum fever."* At the time "dum-dum," a town not far from Calcutta, was considered to be particularly unhealthy. The disease was characterized by general debility, irregular and repetitive bouts of fever, severe anemia, muscular atrophy, and excessive swelling of the spleen. Initially, these organisms were considered to be trypanosomes, but in 1903, Captain Donovan described them as being new. The link between these organisms and kala-azar was eventually discovered by Major Ross, who named them *L. donovani.* In 1929, Upendra Nath Brahmachari discovered *Urea Stibamine*, a treatment for VL, more commonly known as black fever. Due to his discovery, he was nominated for the Nobel Prize in Medicine. Although he failed to win the award, his discovery has led to the complete eradication of black fever throughout the world, with the exception of very few underdeveloped nations. The *Leishmania* genus had been discovered. The diagnosis of VL is complex because its clinical features are shared by a host of other commonly occurring diseases, such as malaria, typhoid, and tuberculosis. At present, the rk39 test kit is widely used. Diagnosis of leishmaniasis can be made by light microscopic examination of parasite in vitro culture, or animal inoculation,parasite DNA detection in tissue samples, immunodiagnosis, or by assay for *Leishmania*-specific cell-mediated immunity. Diagnosis in Ayurvedic science encourage the supplementation of antimony powder to the patient is suffering from ala-azar and confirms relief from the same. the patient is suffering from kala-azar confirms relief. In contrast to VL, cutaneous leishmaniasis mainly affects the skin and mucous membranes. The major symptoms are rashes, stomach problems, ulceration and erosion of mouth tissue, breathlessness, stuffy nose and nose bleeds, and swallowing difficulty.

In Ayurvedic science leishmaniasis is called as Kala Jwara and black disease in Assam. It is also called by different names such as kala-azar, black fever, dum dum fever, black disease, sandfly disease, and espundia. The symptoms are the onset of fever, anemia, and enlargement of the spleen. The spleen of a kala-azar patient is sometimes found to weigh 4–5 kg. White bllod cells (WBCs) are less in count. The fever (Jwara) continues for 3–6 weeks and it recurs always with the enlargement of liver and spleen along with black spots on feet and face. Jwara rises gradually but in 25 % of patient attack is sudden, the temperature reaching 104°C within a couple of hours. The fever attacks twice or thrice time in 24 hours. This is what it distinguishes from other intermittent fevers. It is regular and may leave the patient after 3–6 weeks. But it recurs and leads to enlargement of liver and spleen, the former less than latter.

There may be distension of stomach with emaciation associated with the pain in bones and legs. The appetite of the patient is generally not affected and that probably explains the long course of the disease. Ayurvedic herbal treatment for leishmaniasis depends upon the presentation of the disease and whether it is cutaneous or visceral. Ayurvedic herbal medicines that have a specific antiparasitic action are used in high doses and for prolonged periods in order to treat this condition. In addition, symptomatic treatment is required according to the presentations of symptoms. Medicines that act on the skin and mucous membranes, the respiratory tract as well as the gastrointestinal tract (GIT) are useful in the management of this condition.Ayurvedic medicines that act on the blood in the circulation and remove parasites as well as toxins and flush them through the GIT or the kidneys are especially useful in the management of this condition. In addition, immunomodulation is an important part of treatment, because it reduces treatment time, brings about a complete cure, prevents chances for a recurrence, and helps affected individuals to develop immunity to this infection. Depending upon the type and severity of infection, most individuals affected with leishmaniasis require Ayurvedic herbal treatment for periods ranging from 4 to 6 months, in order to obtain a complete cure from this condition. Immunomodulation may be required for a few months more. Sometimes there is a lot of confusion between kala-azar and Malaria but symptoms of both are so succinct that there is hardly any room of confusion. Following comparison will clearly remove misgivings, if any as far as confusion between kala-azar and malaria is concerned [adapted from vaidya (Shri) Tara Shankars legendry book entitled "*Kaya Chikitsa*"]. The differentiating features between malaria and kala-azar are highlighted in Table 5-1.

TABLE 5-1 Comparison between symptoms of malaria and kala-azar

Sr. No.	Malaria	Kala-azar
	Fever occurs on every 3rd or 4th day and occurs once in 24 hours	Fever is irregular
		Onset of fever is insidious or acute
	Fever starts with chills	No chills
	Enlargement generally of spleen but also rarely of liver	Mark enlargement of spleen and liver
	No such symptom	Complexation of whole body turns dark/ black/blue, erosion of strength and flesh, tongue is dirty

TABLE 5-1 *(Continued)*

Sr. No.	Malaria	Kala-azar
	Rare chance of tuberculosis	In chronic stage cough and tuberculosis also surface
	Bleeding never occurs	Occasional bleeding
	Partial loss of appetite	Appetite is normal
	Relief from quinine but harm from antimony	Relief from antimony but harm from quinine

5.2 AYURVEDIC PRESCRIPTIONS FOR LEISHMANIASIS

Lauha bhasmas is specially marked in cases of chlorosis and in anemia caused by malaria, kala-azar, chronic discharges, and repeated passive hemorrhage. Among the various preparations, *Navayasa lauha* is very useful and is very commonly used in all kinds of anemia. Preparation of *Navayasa lauha* is as follows:

Take of prepared iron nine parts, ginger, long pepper, black pepper, tuber of *Cyperus rotendus*, plumbago root each one part, powder and mix. The dose is 4 grains with honey. The dose is increased gradually in every second day by day 2 grains till the maximum dose of 16 grains is reached (*chakra-datt*). *Guduchyadi lauha*, is a similar preparation with the only difference that it contains *gulancha lohasava* is another similar preparations containing, besides above drugs, triphla, ajovan, and vavading, it is useful in anemic and diseases of spleen. Dose is half to 2 tolas. In secondary anemia from chronic intermittent fever, iron is very useful adjuvant to antipyretic drugs. *Vrihat sarva,-juara-hara-lauha, Visama jwarantaka-lauha*, and *Jaya mangala* rasa are well known preparations containing iron and are commonly used in bleeding and anemic diseases.[1] Other preparation that are recommended in Ayurveda are described later in this chapter.

5.2.1 AYURVEDIC MEDICINE 1

The modern medicine antimony preparations are used for treatment. Probably, it may have been influenced by Ayurveda because even in Ayurveda, antimony is used as *Shuddha Neelanjana* in the dose of 100 mg with *Praval Bhasma, Tamra Bhasma* each 100 mg along with *Yakrit Pleehodarari Loha*

(100 mg). Another remedy is *Shuddha Nilanjan* (100 mg) with *Amritaarishta* (1/2 ounce) with *Loha Bhasma* (100 mg) + *Katuki Churna* (40 grains) twice daily.

5.2.2 AYURVEDIC MEDICINE 2

The ingredients are as follows:

60 mg *Shuddha Nilanjan (antimony).*

60 mg *Mukta Bhasma.*

120 mg *Praval Bhasma.*

120 mg *Shuddha Swar nagairika.*

120 mg *Shankha Bhasma.*

Mix all of the above ingredients properly. Now you can take this mixture four times daily with honey.

5.2.3 AYURVEDIC MEDICINE 3

The ingredients are as follows:

60 mg *Tamra Bhasma.*

60 mg *Yakritaplihodaradilauha.*

Mix all of the above ingredients properly. Now this mixture can be taken two times daily, usually at midday and at night with honey.

5.2.4 AYURVEDIC MEDICINE 4

Take equal quantity (60 mg of each medicine) of *Praval Bhasma, Shanka Bhasma, Shudha Nilaanjan, or Surma* (Antimony), *Sona Geru* (*Swarna Gairik*) *Shuddha*, and *Mukta Bhasma.*

Total quantity: 300 mg

Dose: after every 4 hours with honey

5.2.5 AYURVEDIC HERBS AND MINERAL USED FOR LEISHMANIASIS

Shuddh Nilanjan (Antimony)

Mukta Bhasma

Parval Bhasma

Shuddha Swar Nagairika

Shankha Bhasma

Tamer Bhasma

Yakritplihodaradilauha

Tulsi Leaves

Geloy Satwa

Faulaad Lauha

5.2.6 DIET AND OTHER REGIMEN

Nourishing food such as milk, milk products, eggs, fruits, and vegetables should be given to keep the patient in maintaining his condition. Excessive physical exertion should be avoided.

5.3 AYURVEDIC FORMULATIONS SUITABLE FOR LEISHMANIASIS

The Ayurvedic treatment of leishmaniasis is aimed at treating the symptoms and preventing the complications of the disease, like disfiguration of the face; excessive bleeding; and fatal infections due to immune system damage. To promote the innate immunity, the supplementation of various hebs in their suitable combinations is necessary. For example, supplementation of a tea fortified with five herbs selected from Indian traditional medicine (Ayurveda) for their putative immune-enhancing effect (*Withania somnifera, Glycyrrhzia glabra, Zingiber officinale, Ocimum sanctum*, and *Elettaria cardamomum*) on innate immunity can be an effective method for the enhancement of natural killer (NK) cell activity under in vivo conditions. Regular consumption of the tea fortified with Ayurvedic herbs enhanced NK cell activity, which is an important aspect of the (early) innate immune response to infections. Similarly, there are various Ayurvedic formulation containing a mixture of suitable herbs that may possibly cure leishmaniasis (Table 5-2).

TABLE 5-2 Ayurvedic formulation suitable for the treatment of leishmaniasis

Purpose	Formulation
To treat the basic parasitic infection	Triphala-Guggulu, Sukshma-Triphala, Gandhak-Rasayan, Ras-Sindur, Malla-Sindur, Sameer-Pannag-Ras, and Ras-Manikya
To treat fever	Chandrakala-Ras, Kamdudha-Ras, Laxmi-Narayan-Ras, and Maha-Sudarshan-Churna
Vomiting and diarrhea	Laghu-Sutshekhar, Shankh-Vati, Sutshekhar-Ras, Praval-Panchamrut, and Kutaj-Ghan-Vati
Fatigue, weakness and loss of appetite can be treated	Laxmi-Vilas-Ras, Agnitundi-Vati, Arogya-Vardhini, and Panchamrut-Parpati
Cough and breathlessness	Tribhuvan-Kirti, Sitopaladi-Churna, Shwas-Kuthar-Ras, Pippali (*Piper longum*), Yashtimadhuk (*Glycerrhiza glabra*), Kantakari (*Solanum xanthocarpum*), Som (*Ephedra vulgaris*), Vasa (*Adhatoda vasaka*), and Kushtha (*Saussurea lappa*)
Ulcerations and erosions in the skin and mucous membranes	Panch-Tikta-Ghrut-Guggulu, Kanchnaar-Guggulu, Trayodashang-Guggulu, Maha-Manjishthadi-Qadha, Saarivadi-Churna, Manjishtha (*Rubia cordifolia*), Yashtimadhuk, Haridra (*Curcuma longa*), Amalaki (*Emblica officinalis*), and Mandukparni (*Centella asiatica*)
To prevent ulcers and erosions	Medicines like Panch-Tikta-Ghrut, Yashtimadhuk-Ghrut, Shatadhout-Ghrut, and a mixture of equal parts of honey and ghee can be applied on the ulcers and erosions.
	An ointment containing Manjishtha, Saariva (*Hemidesmus indicus*), Yashtimadhuk, Haridra, and Mandukparni can also be used for this purpose and is very effective.
To prevent excessive bleeding	Medicines like Vasa, Laxa (Purified wax), Naagkeshar (*Messua ferrea*), and Sphatik-Bhasma
To boost the immune system, help in early recovery and prevent serious, opportunistic infections	Medicines like Ashwagandha (*Withania somnifera*), Shatavari (*Asparagus racemosus*), Bala (*Sida cordifolia*), Naagbala (*Grewia hirsuta*), Tulsi (*Ocimum sanctum*), Bhrungraj (*Eclipta alba*), Abhrak-Bhasma, Trivang-Bhasma, Suvarna-Bhasma, Suvarna-Malini-Vasant, and Suvarna-Parpati
Spleen and liver enlargement	Copper, gold and chiefly iron supplementation, guduchi sativa (1/2 g), laksha churna, vidarikand, gaduchi, punarnava, kalmegh, bhuiamala, bhringraja, bibhitaki, khairsar, coral and pearl oxide

5.4 PREVENTION

Leishmaniasis is transmitted by the bite of sandfly in endemic areas. It is important to adopt an appropriate protection and prevent exposure to sandfly bites. Public health measures to reduce the sandfly population and animal reservoirs are equally important. The phlebotomus (sandfly) breeds in moist dirt, cracks, crevices, sides of drains, piles of rubbish, and all kinds of refuse. Therefore, it is important to keep compounds clean and walls in good condition. Dark, moist places should be ventilated and kept dry. Spraying of Flit or DDT is recommended on all possible breeding places.

5.5 POSSIBLE MECHANISMS

Nitric oxide (NO) is a messenger molecule that plays a role in your muscular and immune systems. NO signals the smooth muscles surrounding your blood vessels to relax and dilate, increasing blood flow and relieving disorders like angina and hypertension. NO also activates cells in your immune system. Some herbs can increase NO naturally and may be helpful in treating certain disorders. Consult your health-care provider before starting herbal treatment.

Herbs increase NO and benefit you in various ways. Some herbs trigger NO production and activate macrophages—a type of WBC involved in engulfing and digesting invading pathogens. Other herbs act as vasodilators by increasing NO in your vascular tissue. NO has a role to play in keeping you healthy, but excess NO can have serious side effects. Check with a knowledgeable practitioner for advice about the dosage and preparation of herbs that increase NO.

5.6 AYURVEDIC HERBS FOR LEISHMANIASIS

Various plants that are mentioned in Ayurveda have proven for antileshmanian affect are discussed later and mentioned in Table 5-3 as well.

5.6.1 KUMARI (ALOE VERA, ALOE BARBADENSIS)

A. vera, A. barbadensis (Kumara and Ghrit kumari), and other species are known to be having laxative and stomachic effect. This herb restores the

TABLE 5-3 Antileishmanian potential of Ayurvedic herbs and their respective formulations

Traditional name	Biological source and family, part used	Active pincipal/ mechanism of action	Ayurvedic dose/suitable formulation/use	Parasite	Results	Ref.
Ghrita Kumari	*Aloe vera* (Liliaceae), Leaf exudates	Induction of nitric oxide	100–500 mg daily, juice 10–100 mL every day, gel externally as needed for wound, regeneration of skin and other skin disorders	*L. donovani*	100 to 180 µg/mL	3, 87
Amla + Neem	*Emblica officinalis* (Euphorbiaceae) + *Azadirachta indica* (Maliaceae)	Immunomodulation	Grind guduchi with any of the mentioned herbs, twice a day, for skin disorders	*L. donovani*	Reduced Parasite load and pronounced delayed type hypersensitivity	8
Neem	*Azadirachta indica* (Maliaceae)	Potent lavicidal activity	5 % neem oil; 2% neem oil mixed in coconut or mustard oil	*Phlebotomus papatasi*	N, N-diethylphenyl acetamide and 5 % neem oil both showed similar repellant action	11, 12
Shatavari	*Asparagus racemosus* **(Liliaceae)**	Racemoside A	Taken in milk with Amla and Ashwgandha	*L. donovani* promastigotes	IC_{50} 1.15 and 1.31 µg/mL	14,15
Gaduchi + Cisplatin	*Tinospora cordifolia* (Menis-permaceae)	Enhancement in proliferation and differentiation of lymphocytes; induces Th1 type of immune response and Th2 moderate decline	250 gm Guduchi in 1 liter water for fever, joint pains, & skin disorders	*L. donovani*	Prevents damage (liver and kidney) induced by cisplatin	16
Brahmi	Bacopa monniera, (Scrophulariaceae) and madukparni *Centella asiatica (Apiaceae)*	Without any side effects Bacopasaponin C in all the vesicular forms was found to be very active	5–25 grains Brahmi powder + vaseline three times daily for treatment of various skin problems	*Leishmania* sp.	1.75 mg/kg body weight	18

TABLE 5-3 *(Continued)*

Traditional name	Biological source and family, part used	Active pincipal/ mechanism of action	Ayurvedic dose/suitable formulation/use	Parasite	Results	Ref.
Lehsun	*Allium sativum* (Liliaceae)	Immunomodulation	Mixture of Garlic and Asafoetida against leishmaniansis	*Leishmania* sp.	18.6 μg/mL against promastigote and 13.5 μg/mL against amastigote	20
Gurmar, madhunashini	*Gymnema sylvestre* leaves (Asclepiadaceae)	Gymnemagenol	400 mg /day extract	*L. major, L. aethiopica* and *L. tropica*	52% parasitic death at 1000 μg/mL concentration	30, 88
Bhringaraj/ bhangra	*Eclipta prostrate* (Asteraceae)	Dasyscyphin C	Fresh juice 5–10 mL (tid); leaf powder 3–5 g (bid)	*L. major, L. aethiopica,* and *L. tropica*	Good leishmanicidal activity at 1000 μg/mL concentration, IC_{50} 450 μg/mL; % of parasitic death: 73%	30, 27
Ashwagandha	*Withania somnifera (Solanaceae)*	Withafein and withanolide	Taken in milk with Amla and Ashwgandha	*L. donovani* promastigotes	IC_{50} 12.5 (promastigotes); 9.5 μg/mL (amastigote)	20
Kiratatikta	*Swertia chirata* (Gentianaceae)	Amarogentin	Root powder 0.5–2 g	*Leishmania* sp.	Liposomal and niosomal forms active then than the amarogentin	37
Saptaparna	*Alstonia scholaris* (Apocyanaceae)	Active leishmanicidal action against *Leishmania donovani*-infected hamsters	Fresh juice (svaras): 12–20 mL b.i.d; decoction of the bark 60–100 mL b.i.d; dried powder of bark: 0.75–1.5 g b.i.d; latex (locally)	*L. donovani*	Among 23 plants Saptaparna showed good activity	17
Atibala	*Abutilon indicum (Malvaceae)*	High NO production	Mahanarayan taila, Mahamanjishtadi taila	*L. donovani* promastigotes	500 mg/kg dose: 75% efficacy	41
Bandhuka	*Ixora coccinea* (Rubiaceae)	*In vitro* leishmanicidal activity	*Leishmania donovani*	*L. donovani*	IC_{50} (promastigotes): 7.33 and 7.89	43

TABLE 5-3 *(Continued)*

Traditional name	Biological source and family, part used	Active pincipal/ mechanism of action	Ayurvedic dose/suitable formulation/use	Parasite	Results	Ref.
Daaruharidra	*Berberis aristata* (Berberidaceae)	Alkaloid berberine (*In vitro* leishmanicidal activity)	Daaruharidra: enlargement of spleen, leprosy, rheumatism, fever, morning/evening sickness, snakebite, and so forth	*L. major* & *L. tropica* promastigotes	IC50 (50% inhibitory concentration) 2.1 to 26.6 μg/mL	46
Shaalaparni	*Desmodium gangeticum* (Leguminosae)	Gangetnin and desmodin (herb stimulates macrophages and nitric oxide production)	Root -5–10 g powder; 10–20 g for decoction	*L. donovani*	*n*-butanol fraction exhibited better efficacy than the ethanolic extract to the tune of 66.7+/-6.1%	85; 72
Kukarondh, Manjurukh	*Pluchea indica* (Asteraceae)	*In vitro* leishmanicidal activity	Leaf juice : dysentery; Root: antinflammatory, hepatoprotective effect	*L. donovani* promastigotes	Ethyl acetate fraction IC_{50}< 20 μg/mL	51
Holy basil	*Ocimum sanctum* (Lamiaceae)	Eugenol dimmers, ferulaldehyde and ulsoric acid (*Ocimum sanctum*)	3 tsp. of dry herb brewed in to the water per day, 3 cups of tulsi tea daily in cough condition or fever	*L. major*	13.6, 16.9, 0.9, 2.2 μg/ml	52
Liquorice	*Glycyrrhzia glabra* (Leguminosae)	18β-glycyrrhetinic acid (GRA) effect the upstreaming of *IκB kinase* and increases NO production was	Can be used as tea or taken as capsule (4000–5000 mg/day)	*L. donovani*	IC_{50}, 4.6 μg/mL (amastigote)	55
Erand	*Ricinus communis* (Euphorbiaceae)	*In vitro* leishmanicidal activity and low cytotoxicity towards murine monocytic cells	Massage with warm castor oil is good for pain	*L. donovani*	IC(50) = 126 ± 19.70	56

TABLE 5-3 *(Continued)*

Traditional name	Biological source and family, part used	Active pincipal/ mechanism of action	Ayurvedic dose/suitable formulation/use	Parasite	Results	Ref.
Sprikkaa	*Anisomeles malabarica* (Labiatae)	*In vitro* leishmanicidal activity	*Sprška:* use on the head and in cases of chronic catarrh. Highly recommended for all ailments Kapha and Vata.	*L. donovani*	184 ± 39.33 μg/mL	56
Sweet Annie	*Artemisia annua* (Asteraceae)	*n*-hexane fractions of *Artemisia annua* leaves (AAL) and seeds (AAS) causes cell-cycle arrest at the sub-G(0)/G(1) phase		*L. donovani* (amasti-gotes)	IC_{50} 6.6 and 5.05 μg/mL	58,
Sarapunkhah	*Tephrosia purpurea* (Fabaceae)	*In vitro* leishmanicidal activity without producing any toxic side effects	*Eclipta alba* +*Andrographis paniculata* + *P. kurroa* + *Tephrosia purpurea* + *trikatu in combination for hepatitis*	*L. donovani*	Antileishmanial activity at 50 mg/kg	60
Kalmegh	*Andrographis paniculata* (Acanthaceae)	Mannosylated Liposomes of Andrographoli reduced parasitic burden in the spleen as well as in reducing the hepatic and renal toxicity	Switradilepa	*Leishmania* sp.	Significant activity	63
Nirgundi	*Vitex negundo* (Verbenaceae)	Quercetin (down-regulation of ribonucleotide reductase ($P < 0.05$)	Nirgundi taila (body pain), Nirgundi kalpa, Vishgarbha taila Safuf fanjkisht	*L. donovani*	Repression of splenic parasite load from 75% to 95%	64, 36

TABLE 5-3 *(Continued)*

Traditional name	Biological source and family, part used	Active pincipal/ mechanism of action	Ayurvedic dose/suitable formulation/use	Parasite	Results	Ref.
Amara	*Mangifera indica* L. (Anacard-iaceae)	β-pinene (40.7%) and terpinolene (28.3%): *In vitro* leishmanicidal activity	It is used in a Rasayana *formula* (q.v.), clearing digestion and acidity due to pitta (heat)	*L. amazonensis* promastigote	IC50 39.1 and 23.0 μg/mL	67, 68
Parijat/ Parijatak	*Nyctanthes arbortristis* (Oleaceae)	Iridoid glucosides by the inhibition of trypano-thione reductase	Leaves-10–12 mL juice/day	*Leishmania* parasite	3.24±0.05 μM to 6.49±0.05 μM	69
Aragvadha	*Cassia fistula* (Leguminosae)	Clerosterol	Doasage fruit pulp 5-10 g powder	*L. chagasi*	IC_{50} 10.03 (intracellular amastigotes); IC_{50} 18.10 μg/mL (promastigote)	72, 73
Parpatta	*Fumaria parviflora* Lam. (Fumaraceae)	A novel compound N-octacosan 7β ol	Dose 1–3 g/day	*L. donovani*	GI_{50} = 5.35 μgmL^{-1}	74
Babunah	*Matricaria chamomilla* (Asteraceae)	Bisabolol	Roghan babunah: *Matricaria chamomilla (215 g)* + *Sesamum indicum* oil (4 L) = Pain killing effect	*L. infatum*	1000 and 500 μg/mL	75
Arjuna	*Terminalia arjuna* (Combretaceae)	Pentacyclic triterpenoid,	Bark powder : 1–3 g twice daily Arjunarista: 2–4 oz twice daily Bark decoction 2–4 oz twice daily	*L. donovani*	IC_{50} 3.51 μg/mL	77

TABLE 5-3 *(Continued)*

Traditional name	Biological source and family, part used	Active pincipal/ mechanism of action	Ayurvedic dose/suitable formulation/use	Parasite	Results	Ref.
Kutki or Katuka	Picrorrhiza kurroa (Plantaginaceae)	Picroliv + sodium stibogluconate + improved antileishmanialspotential with lesser side effects	Root-1–3 g or 3–6 g for purgative effect; yograj guggul, aryogyavardhini vati, katukadya lauha, tiktadi kath, tiktadya ghrita, punarnava mandur, amritarista	*L.donovani*	Effective conc: Picroliv (12.5 mg/kg)	78
Champa	*Plumeria bicolor* (Apocynaceae)	Plumericin and isoplumericin	-	*L.donovani* promastigotes	IC_{50} 21 and 14 μg/mL	80
Indan valerian	*Valeriana wallchii root* (**Valarianacea**)	Morphological degeneration, DNA fragmentation, externalization of phosphatidyl serine, and mitochondrial membrane depolarization in promastigotes	Relieves cold sensation on the skin and pain (shita prashamana and vedana sthapana)	*L. major* amastigotes	IC_{50} at ~ 3–7 μg/mL	82
Jukti	*Dregea volubilis* (Asclepediaceae)	Taraxerone	–	*L. donovani* promastigotes	IC_{50} 3.18 μg/mL	86

energy of youth; renew the nature of female; it is a main tonic for female reproductive system; and also nourishes the spleen, liver, blood, and skin. Therefore it is called as Kumari (meaning a young girl or virgin). *A. vera* is frequently utilized for the various GIT and skin ailments.[2] Aloe plant is called as the queen of the desert. There are various reports available on the active role of Aloe against leishmaniansis.[3–6] Dutta et al (2007a,b & 2008) reported the potential leishmanicidal activity facilitated through the induction of NO in *Leishmania*-infected macrophages and caspase-independent cell death in *L. donovani* promastigotes.[3–6]

5.6.2 AMLA (PHYLLANTHUS EMBLICA)

English: Emblic, Emblic Myrobalan, Indain Gooseberry.

Hindi: Amla

Ayurveda: Amlika, Dhatri, Amrtaphala, Dhatriphala, Adiphala, Shreephala, Seeduphala, Tishya, Vrishya, Sheetaphala, Amrita, Shiva, Divya, Dhara, Kolam, Shukti, Vasaya

Indian gooseberry is a small or average deciduous tree. It is one of three myrobalans which have been extensively used in traditional systems of Ayurveda, Siddha, Unani, and Tibetan system of medicine 1,000 years ago. Amla contains sufficient amount of vitamin C. It also contains iron, calcium, phosphorus, and nicotinic acid and high amount of tannins. Sairam (2000) said that Amla acts on the body to increase or decrease the *vata, pitta*, and *kapha* (the three humors). It rejuvenates and tones up tissue and strengthens the body vital organs.[7] According to him, it is a rasnaya and imparts vigor and vitality and cures excessive thirst, burning sensation, vomiting, diabetes, emaciation, anorexia, toxicity, fever, impurity of the blood, and bleeding of any origin. It improves the functions of liver systems. For skin problem, dried fine powder of Amla can be used as soap.

5.6.2.1 PRESCRIPTION (SUITABLE FOR KALA-AZAR)

Amla churna: 50 g

Milk/water: 2 cups

As a Rasanaya, it can be taken daily early in the morning to prevent and combat disease of serious nature. It increases the immunity and vital force.

5.6.2.2 ANTILEISHMANIA ACTIVITY

Herbal combinations of *Emblica officinalis* as well as *Azadirachta indica* significantly reduced the *Leishmania* parasite load in animals treated with herbal drugs.[8] It was proposed that immunomodulation by *E. officinalis* may boost up the antileishmanial activity of *A. indica*. In leishmaniasis, IgG2a and IgG1 kinetics indirectly reflect the Th1/Th2 responses. The relative production of these antibodies is used as a marker for the induction of protective (IgG2a-induced Th1-type) or deleterious (IgG1induced Th2-type) type of immune responses. The levels of IgG2a were greater in *E. officinalis*-treated animals as compared to the animals treated with *A. indica*. The delayed-type hypersensitivity responses directly correlate with the cell-mediated immune (CMI) responses that potentiate the infiltration of lymphocytes and macrophages into the infected tissue for the clearance of pathogen from infected. It was greater in animals treated with *E. officinalis* as compared to those treated with *A. indicia.*

Combination of Neem and Amla is already established and prescribed for skin disease in Ayrurvedic science. Take Guduchi five fingers long, mix either with guggal/neem/haldi/khadir/acacia catechu and amla (myrobalan). Grind Guduchi with any of the mentioned herbs, twice a day, for skin disorders.[9]

5.6.3 NIMBA

Neem is one of the most powerful plants grown in Asia and one of the most widely used. It is sometime called as "the village of pharmacy" as people will plant a tree for the neighbors to share the leaves, barks, and seeds. Ayurvedic text describes it as "*sarva roga nivarini*" (that keeps all the disease at bay) or Arishtha (reliever of disease). Actions: bitter, digestive, antipyretic, antiseptic, antiemetic, anthelmentic. Uses: parasites, skin disease (eczema, ringworm, urticarea), malaria, fever, cough, vomiting, nausea.[10] Neem oil applied on the exposed parts of the body in cream, vaseline, coconut oil, mustard oil, or burned in kerosene or applied on mats provides complete protection from mosquito and sandfly bites that transmit malaria and kala-azar. Ayurvedic use of neem is recommended for Neem oil for wound healing purposes. Internally it is recommended for anthelminthic, jaundice, inflammatory bowl desease (IBD), respiratory infections, and gynecological disorders. *A. indica* has shown to possess nonspecific immune-stimulatory activity. Neem acts by activating macrophages and also increases the expression of major histocompatibility complex-2 antigens indicating enhancement of their antigen-presenting ability. *Nimba arishtas* are the commercially available preparations of *A. indica.* A total of 5% both neem oil and *N, N*-diethylphenyl acetamide exhibited similar repellent action against the sandfly, *Phlebotomus papatasi.*[11] Furthermore, it was reported that the concentrations of 2% neem oil mixed in coconut or mustard oil provided 100% protection against *P. argentipes* throughout the night under field conditions; against *P. papatasi*, it repelled sandflies for about 7 hours in the laboratory.[12] Herbal combinations of *E. officinalis* as well as *A. indica* significantly reduced the *Leishmania* parasite load in animals treated with herbal drugs.[8]

5.6.4 SHATAVARI

Medicinal use of *Asparagus racemosus* (Shatavari) has been recorded in traditional systems of medicine such as Ayurveda, Unani, and Siddha. Shatavari meaning "she who possess a hundred husbands" is often considered as aphrodisiac. It is recommended in Ayurvedic texts for the prevention and treatments of gastric ulcers and dyspepsia, for threatened miscarriage and a galactogogue, and is known as "Rasayana" (a substance that promotes general physical and mental well-being by improving defense mechanisms and vitality).[13] Racemoside A isolated from *A. racemosus* showed significant activity against antimonial-sensitive (strain AG83) and -unresponsive (strain GE1F8R) *L. donovani* promastigotes, with IC_{50} values of 1.15 and 1.31 μ/mL.[14]

5.6.4.1 IMMUNITY BOOSTER

Prescription: Wash tubers of Shatavari, remove outer skin layer, and crush well, then collect extracted juice. Mix about half cup of this fresh juice in half cup of pure milk and add a teaspoon of sugar and boil on gentle fire for 5 minutes. It is frequently prescribed for people with fatique, poor appetite, anemia (taken in milk with amla and ashwgandha), chachexia, and chronic fatique immune deficiency syndrome.[15]

5.6.5 AMRITA OR GUDUCHI OR GILOE

Tinosopra cardifolia mature stem powder, the aqueous extract, the starch obtained from the stem by repeated washing of the crushed stem with water is used in Ayurveda for obesity, debility, hepatitis, dyspepsia, jaundice, and other liver disorders. It is an official drug in the Indian herbal pharmacopoeia, 1990, for its analgesic and antipyretic activity. Prescriptions those are favorable for its use in kala-azar.[9]

5.6.5.1 PRESCRIPTION 1

Juice of Mandukparni (brahmi): 1 teaspoon

Powder of Liquorice: 1/2 teaspoon

Juice of Guduchi: 1 teaspoon

Shankpushpi powder/juice: 1 teaspoon

5.6.5.2 PRESCRIPTION 2 (FEVER, JOINT PAINS, AND SKIN DISORDERS)

Guduchi churan: 250 g

Water: 1 L

Boil and reduce to half and sieve it. This water can be used for bleeding from any organ of the body, fever, itching, gout, and skin problems in the dose of 15–30 mL twice or thrice a day.

5.6.5.3 PRESCRIPTION 3 (SKIN DISEASES)

Take Guduchi five fingers long, mix either with Guggal/Neem/Haldi/Khadir (*Acacia catechu*) and Amla (Myrobalan). Grind Guduchi with any of the mentioned herbs, twice a day, for skin disorders.

5.6.5.4 PRESCRIPTION 4 (FEVER, ACHES, AND PAINS)

Giloy powder (*Tinospora cordifolia*): 1 teaspoon

Chireta (*Swertia chireta*): 1 teaspoon

Saunth (*Gingiber officinals*): 1 teaspoon

Water: 500 mL

Mix all together and boil on the mild heat till the water reduced to half. One ounce of the medicine after every 3–4 times a day, look after the weakness that occurs after the long illness.

Sachdeva et al., (2014) reported the potential combination of *T. cordifolia* with high dose Cisplatin in *L. donovani* treatment may be a critical remedy for the amelioration of adverse effects of Cisplatin.[16] Singha et al., (1992) explored the potential antileishmanian effects of extracts derived from traditional plants such as *sscholaris, Swertia Chirata, Tibouchina Semidecandra, T. cordifolia*, and *Nyctanthes arbortristis* against *L. donovani* in golden hamsters.[17]

5.6.6 BRAHMI (MANDUKPARINI)/GOTU KOLA

Brahmi denotes that this sattivic herb is "*buddhi vardhak*," or the enhancer of intellect and wisdom. The Sanskrit name Mandukparini refers to the leaves of the herb that resembles the claw of frog. According to the old classics, it is reported that in India, Brahmi (*Bacopa monniera*) and madukparni (*Centella asiatica*) or Indian pennywort are shown as one and same plant. Although, both are different but they both posses the same properties and uses. However, comparative study revealed that *B. monniera* is more useful then *C. asiatica*. Both types of plants mainly act on the brain tissue. The leaves have strong appearance to the human brain. It is highly important source of both modern and traditional system of medicine. The herb is recognized in Ayurveda for use as Rasnaya (Rejuvenation) purpose mentioned in the ancient treaties "*Charakra Samahita*.". Brahmi has been used in Ayurvedic medicine to improve the memory and intellect. It also helps to overcome anxiety, depression, and mental fatique; the drug also causes significant improvement in systems of nervousness, palpitation, headache, and insomnia. From several decades, Brahmi is used in traditional medicine for different types of skin diseases. A dose of 5 to 25 grains of Brahmi powder mixed with Vaseline, three times daily, internally as well as externally is used in the treatment of various skin problems. It is widely used in homeopathy for various skin disorders. Bacopasaponin C, an indigenous glycoside, was isolated from Indian medicinal plant *B. monniera* was proved for antileishmanial properties both in free and in various delivery modes, for example, niosomes, microspheres, and nanoparticle.[18]

5.6.7 RASONA (GARLIC)

Gralic (*Allium sativum* L. Liliaceae) is called as Rasona or one taste missing in old sanskrit texts. Rasona possess five of six tastes; it is sweet, salty, bitter, and astringent. However it is not sour, this is the missing flavor. Lehsun is a strength promoter, aphrodisiac, reduces the level of cholesterol and fat, soothes inflammation, and a sedative. It is widely used for cough, skin troubles, and chronic fever. Relieves breathing problems, heart ailments, and helps in recovery of fracture. Lehsun is used in rejuvenation therapy, which should be carried out during winter. Physical constitution should be very strong for this treatment, and body and mind of the patient should be prepared to accept the treatment that implies 15 g of garlic per day. Complications may include vomiting and fainting. Avoid garlic if you are pregnant, if you suffer from hyperacidity, or other symptoms of excess pita. The use of this spice has been found valuable in kala-azar, which is characterized by irregular fever, progressive anemia, and gradual increase in temperature. Mixture of garlic and asafoetida is one of the most popular and basic natural therapy, which is already recommended in Ayurveda against leishmaniansis. The small piece of asafoetida and one piece of garlic should be ground together. A drink made from the mixture should be taken once daily for a week in treating this disease. The same mixture can be applied as ointment over the spleen till it softens. Calcined garlic (bhasma) with honey is used externally for various skin disorders.[19] Reports explored the high antileishmanian activities of ashwagandha (withaferin A) and garlic consistently with 50% inhibitory concentration (IC_{50}) of 12.5 ± 4 and 18.6 ± 3 µg/mL against promastigotes whereas IC_{50} of 9.5 ± 3 and 13.5 ± 2 µg/mL against amastigote form, respectively.[20] Gamboa-Leon R et al. (2014) reported the administration of mixture of *Tridax procumbens* and *A. sativum* extracts increase ratio of IgG2a/IgG1, which raised the Th1-type immune response in mice infected with *Leishmania mexicana*. Administration of 37 mg/mL of garlic extract leads to the activation of amastigotes-infected macrophages.[21] In addition, Aqueous Garlic Extract (AGE) increased the level of interleukin (IL)-12 in *Leishmania*-infected cell lines significantly. It was also suggested that administration of garlic extract exerts cytotoxic effect on *Leishmania major*-infected cell line.[22] In addition, it was hypothesized that garlic can improve cellular immunity with raising the expression of interferon (IFN)-γ and of inducible nitric oxide synthase (iNOS) genes confirmed.[23] Immunomodulatory effect of garlic compounds was reported[24] in rodents infected *with L. major* and *L. donovani*. *L. mexicana* is the main causal agent of cutaneous leishmaniasis in the Yucatán Peninsula in Mexico.

A report suggested that garlic extract acts on both T cells and macrophages to stimulate IFN-γ production and NO synthesis for parasite (*L. mexicana*) killing.[25] Furthermore, it was reported that intraperitoneal injection of garlic extract (20 mg/kg) or its protein fraction (0.04 mg/kg) augments parasite engulfment and destruction of intracellular amastigotes by macrophages.[26] Because the mechanism of action for the garlic extract is apparently immunomodulatory, garlic compounds could be purified and tried as complementary medicine in the management of leishmaniases. These reports confirm that garlic (*A. sativum*) extract modulates immune responses.

5.6.8 BHRINGARAJ/BHANGRA (RULER THE HAIR) AND GURMAR

Eclipta prostrate, *Eclipta alba*, and *Eclipta erecta*. This is the main herb for liver, hair, and cirrhosis. It is a rejuvenative drug and helps in rejuvenation of hairs, liver, bones, kidneys, and pitta. The root powder is used for hepatitis and enlarged spleen and skin disorders.[27] By benefiting the liver and and aiding its detoxifying work, bhringraj makes a good herb for skin problems including utricaria, eczema, and psoriasis. It is also helpful in vitiligo. It reduces itching and inflammation and said to promote a lustrous complexion.[28]

5.6.9 GYMNEMA

Gymnema sylvestre (Gurmar, Madhunashini) leaves are traditionally used as medicine for the control of diabetes mellitus and stomach ache. *Susruta* has described this plant as a destroyer of madhumeha, the glycosuria and other urinary disorders. It neutralizes the excess sugar present in the body in diabetes mellitus. Its leaves afer mixing with castor oil are applied externally to swollen glands and enlarged spleen.[29] *G. sylvestre* leaves are traditionally used as medicine for the control of diabetes mellitus and stomach ache. They are also often used as a diuretic agent. The decoction of *Eclipta prostrata* leaves has long been used orally to control jaundice. Earlier reports from our laboratory revealed the antimicrobial activity of gymnemagenol and dasyscyphin C. Dasyscyphin C/gymnemagenol, saponins isolated from the leaves of *E. prostrata* and *G. sylvestre* showed good leishmanicidal activity at 1,000 μg/mL concentration against *L. major* promastigote.[30]

5.6.10 ASHWAGANDHA

Ashwagandha is in high esteem in Ayurveda because of its rejuvenative and antiaging property. It is being used traditionally in Ayurveda for lack of libido, fatique, mental problems, senile dementia, and recovery from prolonged illness and as a rasnaya (rejuvenator). The vital force that protects the human body and cure diseases is known as "*Bala*" in Ayurveda. The herbs that increase the *bala* of the body is "*Balya.*" In sushruta words, it is "*Brimhanam.*" In modern science, it is nutritious. Unani doctors call it "*Mussamin badan.*" One such herb which is "*Balya*" and "*Brimhanam*" in action is known as Ashwagandha.[9] Ashwagandha is renowned for its ability to impart vitality and sexual energy like a horse. The word Ashwgandha literally means the smell of the horse. The English name of the plant is winter cherry, is misleading, implying use of the fruit. In actual practice, the fruit is never used as it is harmful. The fresh root gives a smell of a horse. It is known as Indian ginseng. Apart from its immune modulation and aphrodisiac property, wealth of India (1950) reported its role in various skin and inflammatory disease (powder of Ashwagandha and saunth is grinded with a little hot water and then apply this paste over the affected area). To treat skin and inflammatory disorders, root powder in ghee, leaves in castor oil, or Narayana tail or Ashwagandha tail can also be applied over the affected area. It is an anabolic drug that increases the hemoglobin and red blood cell.[9] Its prescription for tubercular infection is as follows:

Ashwagandha powder (2 teaspoon) + Pippal powder (2 teaspoon) + Honey (4 teaspoon) + Mishri (4 teaspoon) + Ghee (4 teaspoon)

Mix and triturate well and take 1 teaspoonful twice a day, morning and evening. It strengthens the defense mechanisms (immunity and combat tubercular bacillus).

Reports explored the high antileishmanian activities of ashwagandha (withaferin A) and garlic consistently with 50% inhibitory concentration [IC(50)] of 12.5 ± 4 and 18.6 ± 3 μg/mL against promastigotes whereas IC(50) of 9.5 ± 3 and 13.5 ± 2 μg/mL against amastigote form, respectively.[20] A report suggested that the supplementation of *A. racemosus* and *W. somnifera* in combination at 200 mg/kg to *L. donovani*-infected BALB/c mice, which resulted in successful reduction of parasite load, but protective Th1 type of immune responses were also generated with normalization of biochemical and hematological parameters suggesting their potential as potent antileishmanial agents.[31] In addition, the supplementation of chemotype of

Withaferin A in *L. donovani*-infected hamsters significantly increased the mRNA expression of iNOS, IFN-γ, IL-12, and TNF-α but decrease in IL-4, IL-10, and Transforming growth factor (TGF)-β, an enhanced *Leishmania*-specific lymphoproliferative response (LTT) response as well as reactive oxygen species ROS, NO, and antileishmanial IgG2 levels was reported.[32] The protective and immunomodulatory activity of *W. somnifera* was reported with cisplatin for their potential in amelioration of adverse effects of cisplatin. Thus, this combination appears to offer a fruitful strategy for the treatment of VL.[33] Recent report suggested that in vitro treatment with withanolides resulted in morphological alterations from spindle to round shape and loss of flagella/cell integrity in *L. donovani* promastigotes. Moreover, it induced DNA nicks, cell cycle arrest at sub G0/G1 phase and externalization of phosphatidylserine in dose and time-dependent manner via increase in ROS and decrease in Ψm. Therefore withanolides induce apoptotic-like death through the production of ROS from mitochondria and disruption of Ψm in promastigotes of *L. donovani.*[34] Leishmanial protein kinase C has been identified as a potential target to develop drugs against leishmaniasis. In one report that suggested the tertiary structure of leishmanial *protein kinase C* using computational methods revealed the mode of inhibition of two reported natural compounds from *W. somnifera,* withaferin A and withanone.[35]

5.6.11 CHIRATTA

Swertia chirata in Ayurveda is known as *Kirata-tikta*. The drug is reported to be specific remedy for all types of fevers. Adecoction of entire plant is taken for curing chronic fever as a households remedy through out the country. It is laxative, dry, cooling, bitter, light, and overcomes *sannipata* type of fever, difficulty in breeting, homeopathy due to morbidity of *kapha* and *pitta*, burning sensation, cough, edema, thrist, skin diseases, fever, ulcer, and worms. It is also useful in acidity and liver complaints. There are several preperations such as *Kiratadi kwath, Sarwajwar-har louha, Phalatrikadi kwath*, and *Chandraparbha* vati are used for different kind of disorders.[36] A report suggested that amarogentin "an active bitter principal of Swertia *chirata*" in both liposomal and niosomal forms were found to be more active leishmanicidal agents than the free amarogentin. These reported formulations do not show any toxicity, thus can be used for the treatment of leishmaniasis.[37]

Alstonia scholaris bark (Saptaparna) of the tree has been reputed in Ayurveda for the treatment of periodic fever and Saptaparna skin diseases in India and in the Far East. The extract of the bark is used in the treatment of leprosy. It is popular remedy for diarrhea and dysentery. Echitamine and others are the active principals of this herb.[38] In 1992, Singha et al. explored the potential antileishmanian effects of extracts derived from traditional plants such as *Alstonia scholaris* against *L. donovani* in golden hamsters.[39]

5.6.12 ATIBALA

In Ayurveda, *Abutilon indicum* is called as atibala. *Bala* means strength in Sanskrit and this is an herb that provides it. It is used in Ayurveda, Unani, and Siddha. Plant used for abortion, fresh plant decoction is taken in gonorrhea, dysuria, metrorrhea, ash of the whole plant is applied on burns; leaves, flowers, and seeds decoction can be used in fever, colic, wounds, and ulcers. Root leaves and seeds are tonic for men. Contact therapy, roots tied to the waist of the pregnant women to prevent miscarriage, roots tied to the waist of the delivering mother for safe and smooth delivery.[40] *Mahanarayan taila* (bilva, ashwagandha, brihati, goshukra, sandalwood, manjishtha, kushtha, ela, musta, camphor, sesame oil) and mahamanjishtadi taila are the highly recommended formulation of atibala in Ayurveda.[41] One report suggested potential leishmanicidal activity of *n*-hexane and *n*-butanol fractions of methanol extract against *Leishmania* promastigotes and intracellular amastigotes. In addition, this report also suggested that these isolated fractions when administered in *L. donovani*-infected hamsters showed more than 75% efficacy.[42]

5.6.13 BANDHUKA

Ixora coccinea (Vetchie-Ixora, Sacred Ixora, Jungle flame) is a botanical name for Ratmal (Tamil name). In Ayurveda, it is called as *Bandhuka* and *Paranti*. This is regarded by Hindus as a sacred tree to Shiva and the word Iroxa itself is a corruption of Shiva or Ishvara by the Portugese. Traditionally its roots, leaves, and flowers are used for headache, boils, nausea, and sedative in hiccough, chronic ulcers, and skin desease. In Ayurveda, Bandhuka formulation is used for poisoned collyrium. Flowers have been used in Indian system of traditional medicine for dysentery, healing of ulcers. Leaf extract of *I. coccinea* showed potent inhibition against *L. donovani* promastigotes.[43–45]

5.6.14 DARUHARIDRA

Berberis aristata known as "*Daruharidra*" in Ayurveda is a versatile medicinal plant used singly or in combination with other medicinal plants for treating a variety of ailments such as jaundice, enlargement of spleen, leprosy, rheumatism, fever, morning/evening sickness, snakebite, and so forth. A major bioactive marker of this genus is an alkaloid berberine, which is known for its activity against cholera, acute diarrhea, amoebiasis, and latent malaria and for the treatment of oriental sore caused by *Leishmania tropica*. Although the roots of *B. aristata* are considered as the official drug (Ayurvedic Pharmacopoeia of India), the study revealed that different species of Berberis, namely. *B. asiatica*, *Berberis chitria*, and *Berberis lycium* are also used under the name of Daruharidra in different parts of the country. Gupta and Dikshit have shown that berberine is toxic to *L. tropica* in concentration as high as 1 in 80,000. Although powerful protoplasmic poisons such as quinine and emetine require about 80 times this concentration to produce the same effect, a decoction made from root was said to bring down the fever. Dried extract of root is called as Rasaut is used a purgative and blood purifier. Berebrine extract are also effective in healing oriental sore and malaria.

A recent report revealed that *Berberis vulgaris* extracts as well as berberine were effective in inhibiting *L. major* and *L. tropica* promastigotes growth in a dose-dependent manner with IC50 (50% inhibitory concentration) values varying from 2.1 to 26.6 μg/mL.[46] A complex interplay between *Leishmania* and macrophages influences parasite survival and necessitates disruption of signaling molecules, eventually resulting in impairment of macrophage function.[47] Recent report demonstrated the role of immunomodulatory Berberine chloride, highlighting the importance of MAPKs as an antiparasite target. The IC_{50} of Berberine chloride, a quaternary isoquinoline alkaloid was found to be 7.10 μM versus 2.54 μM for intracellular amastigotes and promastigotes. In *Leishmania*-infected macrophages, Berberine chloride caused a time-dependent activation of p38 MAPK along with deactivation of ERK1/2; addition of a p38 MAPK inhibitor SB203580 inhibited the increased generation of NO and IL-12p40 by Berberine chloride as also prevented its decrease of IL-10. Saha et al., (2009) reported the Berberine chloride role in triggering an apoptosis-like death followed by enhanced generation of ROS, thus meriting further pharmacological investigations.[48] Saha et al. (2009) also demonstrated the caspase-independent apoptosis to induce caspase activity and antileishmanial activity of Berberine chloride.[48]

Vennerstrom et al. (1990) suggested the potential role of various Berberine derivatives as antileishmanial drugs such as berberine and 8-cyanodihydroberberine, showed significant activity (greater than 50% suppression of lesion size) against *Leishmania braziliensis* panamensis.[49]

Manometric studies conducted by Ghosh et al. (1985) proved that Berberine had inhibitory action on both the endogenous and the glucose-stimulated respiration of amastigotes.[50] Berberine inhibited incorporation of [14C]adenine, [14C]uracil, and [3H]thymidine into nucleic acids, and of [14C]leucine into the protein of amastigotes, indicating an inhibitory action on macromolecular biosynthesis. Berberine also decreased deoxyglucose uptake.[50]

5.6.15 KUKARONDH (MANJURUKH)

Pluchea indica traditionally used as medicine for fever and inflammation in various regions of India. A root of *Pluchea indica* is having astringent, antipyretic, anti-inflammatory and hepatoprotective property. It was reported that ethyl acetate insoluble part showed maximum antileishmanian activity with IC < 20 μg/mL. In addition, significant antileshmanian activity of a thiopene derivative isolated from tissue cultured plant *P. indica* was also reported.[51]

5.6.16 TULSI

Tulsi, its very name holy basil certifies to its sacred nature. Holy basil is a major ingredient of many cough syrups. It is a good stress reliever and modern research has found to be good for respiratory problems, cold fever, and all types of cough. It has the strong propery of destroying the bacteria and insects and even it purifies the air around it. It has been scientifically proven that tulsi absorbs the positive ions and energizes the negative ions, and liperaes ozone from atmosphere. In Hindu mythology, it is believed that the messenger of god of death cannot approach a home where there is a tulsi plant. Recent report suggested its components potential against *Leishmania.* Eugenol dimmers, ferulaldehyde, and ulsoric acid and three newly discovered compounds showed stong antileishmnail activity against *Leishmania major*.[52]

5.6.17 TURMERIC

Turmeric (Curcuma longa) called as *haldi* in hind is having strong anti-inflammatory and wound healing properties and we are utilizing it for various skin disorders from several decades. Upon *Leishmania* infection, macrophages are activated to produce nitrogen and oxygen radicals simultaneously. It is well established that the infected host cells rely on NO as the major weapon against the intracellular parasite. Curcumin, the active principle of turmeric, is a scavenger of NO. A report proved that curcumin protects promastigotes and amastigotes of the visceral species, *L. donovani*, and promastigotes of the cutaneous species against leishmanicidal drugs. Curcumin, as an antioxidant, is capable of blocking the action of both NO and NO congeners on the *Leishmania* parasite and hence protect the parasite from antileishmanian drugs. Therefore application of turmeric on ulcers/lesions induced by leishmania parasite may aggrevate the symptom of desease.[53]

5.6.18 LIQUORICE (YASTIMADHU)

Glycyrrhiza glabra, popularly known as liquorice, is one of the most ancient medicinal plants and has long been used in traditional Chinese, Tibetan, Indian, and Arabian medicine for the treatment of pulmonary diseases and inflammatory processes. The medicinal value of liquorice root is defined by biologically active substances such as triterpene glycosides, phenolic compounds, oligosaccharides, polysaccharides, lipids, and so forth. The predominant bioactive components in liquorice root are licochalone A, glycyrrhetinic acid, and glycyrrhizic acid (GA). It was reported that GA treatment caused an enhanced expression of iNOS2 along with the inhibition of Cox-2 in *L. donovani*-infected macrophages. In addition, GA treatment in infected macrophages enhanced the expression of IL-12 and TNF-α, concomitant with a downregulation of IL-10 and TGF-β. GA increased macrophage effector responses via inhibition of Cox-2-mediated prostaglandin E2 release in *L. donovani*-infected macrophages. GA also decreased hepatic and splenic parasite burden and increased T-cell proliferation in *Leishmania*-infected BALB/c mice.[54] A report also suggested that the 18β-glycyrrhetinic acid treatment to mouse peritoneal macrophages infected with *L. donovani* promastigotes, activated the mouse immunity, thereby imparting resistance to reinfection. In addition, 18β-glycyrrhetinic acid showed its effects on some level of upstreaming of IκB kinase in the signaling pathway and induces the production of proinflammatory mediators through a mechanism that, at least in part, involves induction of NF-κB activation.[55]

5.6.19 SPRIKKAA AND ERAND: IN AYURVEDA

Anisomeles malabarica (Labiatae), which is also called as Sprikkaa in Ayurveda exterts some physiological actions such as antispasmodic, antipyretic, diaphoretic, emmenagogue, and antirheumatic. The oil is externally used as an embrocation in rheumatic arthritis. Castor oil plant "*arnica of ayurveda*" or Eranda (*Ricinus communis*) belonging to family Euphorbiaceae widely used in Ayurvedic, Chinese, and Western medicine. It helps to relieve constipation, pain relief, for wounds, boils and abscesses, joint pains, and enlarge lymph nodes. According to Ayurveda, a massage with warm castor oil is good for pain. Castor oil is the main treatment for Vata Dosha.[10] Zahir et al. (2012) reported that the leaf methanol extracts of *A. malabarica* and *R. communis* showed good antileishmanial activity (IC(50) = 126 ± 19.70 and 184 ± 39.33 μg/mL), respectively against promastigotes.[56] Report on *R. communis* and *Bougainvillea glabra* available for the control of vector (*P. papatasi*) of leishmaniasis. This report indicates that the planting high densities of *R. communis* and *B. glabra* in sand flies-endemic areas will reduce population sizes and reduce the risk of *L. major* infections.[57]

5.6.20 SWEET ANNIE

In the Chinese traditional medicine, *Artemisia annua* is used for centuries to treat fever. Chinese have reported the success at curing quinine-resistant malarial strains from the extract of *A. annua* (Sweet annie). Islamuddin et al. (2012) reported here that n-hexane fractions of *A. annua* leaves (AAL) and seeds (AAS) possess significant antileishmanial activity against *L. donovani* promastigotes, with GI_{50} of 14.4 and 14.6 μgmL^{-1}, respectively, and the IC_{50} against intracellular amastigotes was found to be 6.6 and 5.05 μgmL^{-1}, respectively.[58] Ganguly et al. (2006) reported the antipromastigote activity of an ethanolic extract of leaves of *A. indica*. *A. indica* showed a pronounced leishmanicidal activity in all the *Leishmania* strains studied, the IC50 ranging from 0.21 to 0.58 mg/mL, indicating its effectiveness in all three forms of leishmaniasis.[59]

5.6.21 SPRIKKAA AND ERAND

The actions of *A. malabarica* (Labiatae) are antispasmodic, antipyretic, diaphoretic, mmenagogue, and antirheumatic. The oil is externally used as an embrocation in rheumatic arthritis. Castor oil plant "*arnica of ayurveda*" or Eranda (*R. communis*) belonging to family Euphorbiaceae widely used in Ayurvedic, Chinese, and Western medicine. It helps to relieve constipation, pain relief, for wounds, boils and abscesses, joint pains, and enlarge lymph nodes. According to Ayurveda, a massage with warm castor oil is good for pain. Castor oil is the main treatment for Vata Dosha.[10] Zahir et al. (2012) reported that the leaf methanol extracts of *A. malabarica* and *R. communis* showed good antileishmanial activity (IC(50) = 126 ± 19.70 and 184 ± 39.33 μg/mL), respectively against promastigotes.[56]

5.6.22 SARAPUNKHAH

Tephrosia purpurea (Fabaceae), which is used in traditional remedies for the treatment of various skin desease; febrile attacks; and enlargement and obstruction of liver, spleen, and kidney. Recently, this drug was found to have significant antileishmanial activity, and has been extensively fractionated to locate the abode of activity.[60] *N*-butanol extract of *T. purpurea* showed consistent antileishmanial activity at 50 mg/kg against *L. donovani* infection in hamsters. The root is highly efficacious against fever, leprosy, skin disorders, and mainly in inflammation and enlargement of spleen and liver and hence name *Plihasatru* (pliha = spleen). The drug is having a potential in purifying the blood and overcomes the diseases due to morbid Kapha and Vata.[61]

5.6.23 KALMEGH

In Ayurvedic science, it is called as bhuinimb, kirata, mahateet. This herb is widely used in Ayurvedic and Chinese medicine. In Ayurveda, which calls it kalmegh (kings of bitter), it is used for the respiratory infections, flu bronchitis. Chinese medicine utilizes andrographis for fever and headache of colds and flu, tonsillitis, larynopharyngitis, bronchitis, and inflammation. Herb is an ideal candidate for prophylactic and therapeutic hepatoprotective herbal preperations. Kalmegh is the major constituent of the Ayurvedic drug "switradilepa" which is effective in treating vitiligo. If enlargement of spleen is due to kala-azar, alternate it with kalmegh 2 to 5 drops twice daily.[62] Recent reports suggested its action in reducing parasite load and toxicity.[63] Mannosylated liposomes loaded with an indigenous drug, andrographolide, a labdane diterpenoid isolated from Indian medicinal plant *Andrographis paniculata* were found to be most potent in reducing the parasitic burden in the spleen as well as in reducing the hepatic and renal toxicity.[63]

5.6.24 NIRGUNDI (VITEX NEGUNDO, FAMILY: VERBENACEAE)

The whole plant in Ayurveda is known as acrid, astringent, anthelmentic, bitter, stomachic and used to promote the growth of the hairs, eye disease, inflammation, leucoderma, and enlargement of spleen. It is also used in the asthma bronchitis and painful teething. Rheumatic patients are advised to have bath in water boiled with its leaves. The juice of the leaves is administered in the doses of 24 g every morning in the enlargement of spleen. Leaves are considered to be very effective in several inflammatory conditions like rheumatoid arthriris. In Assam (India) about 5 mL juice of its fresh leaves are mixed in a glass of lukewarm water and is administered twice a dayfor one week in chronic liver problems associated with loss of appetite.[36] The juice of leaves of *Leucas plukentii* is also added to make it more effective. In Andhra Pradesh, peoples take bath to reduce the pain in body. There are some reports yhat explore the leishmanicidal potential of *Nirgundi.*[36] Quercetin is one of the active components of *Vitex negundo,* having strong antimicrobial property. Recent report suggested that quercetin in combination with serum albumin increased the bioavailability of the flavonoid and proved to be of major advantage in promoting the effectiveness of Quercetin against *L. donovani.* In addition for improved leishmanicidal action, Quercetin in combination with serum albumin targets *ribonucleotide reductase* and interfere with the parasite's iron metabolism under in vivo conditions.[64] Recent study suggested potential role luteolin and quercetin in inhibiting the growth of *L. donovani* promastigotes and amastigotes in vitro, inhibiting DNA synthesis in promastigotes and promoted topoisomerase-II-mediated linearization of kDNA minicircles. The reported IC_{50} values of luteolin and quercetin were 12.5 and 45.5 μM, respectively. In addition these compounds have the potential to arrest cell cycle progression in *L. donovani* promastigotes, leading to apoptosis and reduced splenic parasite burden in hamster models.[65]

5.6.25 AMARA

Mangifera indica L. (Anacardiaceae), commonly known as Mango, is a large evergreen tree indigenous to Asia and found throughout the Indian subcontinent. According to the classical texts, amara is a cardiac tonic, promotes complexation, semen and strength, increases digestive power, cures urinary disease, and disorders caused by vitiated blood. It belongs to astringent group of drugs. Juice of ripe mango, added with honey was prescribed in enlargement of spleen (*vrindamaadhava, bhaavarakaasha*).[66] *M. indica* leaf extracts exhibited remarkable antileishmanial activity against *L. donovani* promastigotes in vitro.[67] Recent report suggested that essential oil of *M. indica* contains high amounts of β-pinene (40.7%) and terpinolene (28.3%). In addition, in this study it was reported that these components have potent leishmanicidal activity against promastigotes forms of *L. amazonensis*, showed IC50 (72 h) of 39.1 and 23.0 μg/mL, respectively.[68]

5.6.26 PARIJAT/PARIJATAK

Nyctanthes arbortristis also known as night jasmine recently reported for their active role in leishmaniasis. By the inhibition of *trypanothione reductase* (validated drug target enzyme of the *Leishmania* parasite) iridoid glucosides (isolated from *Nyctanthes arbortristis*) was shown to posses potent (3.24 ± 0.05 μM to 6.49 ± 0.05 μM) antileishmanial activity.[69] In earlier studies, it was suggested that these compounds led to an increase in ROS by inhibiting a crucial enzyme of redox metabolism of the parasite. Exact mechanism of iridoid glucosides was reported to increases ROS level that leads to oxidative stress, cell membrane damage, and at last apoptosis of *Leishmania* sp.[70]

5.6.27 ARAGVADHA

In Ayurveda, Aragvadha leaves are useful for various skin disorders and fresh fruit pulp is taken as best laxative.[71,72]

Common name: Amaltas

Ayurvedic actions: Kusthaghna alleviates skin disease, kandughna stop itching, sramsanottama the best bowel cleanser, jvaraghna reduces fever, raktapitta stops bleeding, anulomana directs vata downwards

Biomedical action: febrifuge, stops bleeding, improves digestion, prevent various skin disorders

A sterol, clerosterol from hexane extract of the fruits of Cassia fistula showed significant (50% (IC50) of 10.03 μg/mL and intracellular amastigotes demonstrated high susceptibility, with an IC50 of 18.10 μg/mL) antileishmanial activity against the promastigote form of *Leishmania* (*L. chagasi*).[73]

5.6.28 PARPATTA

Fumaria parviflora Lam. (Fumaraceae) is called by different name Parpatta (Ayurveda), tusha (Siddha), and shaahtara for *Fumaria officinalis* in Unani. It widely used in traditional as well as folkloric system of medicine from ancient. It is known for treating numerous ailments such as diarrhea, fever, influenza, blood purifier, and other complications. Parpatta alone or combined with Guduchi, Amla, Chandana, or Shunthi was prescribed for alleviating fever. This drug mainly used in fever, blood purification, and several disorders of liver. A novel compound N-octacosan 7β ol from *F. parviflora* showed significant antimicrobial activity against *L. donovani* promastigotes without having any adverse effect against mammalian macrophages.[74]

Babunah or babuni ke phul *(Matricaria chamomilla L.)* Asteraceae

In English it is called as Chamomile. Babunah or Chamomile is useful in trating rheumatic affections, where its extracted oil is rubbed in affected parts. It eases the pain of rheumatism and gout. Schnitzler et al., 1996 reported the strong antileishmnian activity chamomile extract on *L. mexicana.* Morales-Yuste et al. (2010) also reported the antileishmnian effect of chamomile with α-bisabolol was found to be totally inhibiting *Leishmania infatum* promastigotes at the concentration of 1000 and 500 μg/mL.[75]

5.6.29 ARJUN (ARJUNA)

Terminalia arjuna Roxb (Combretaceae) is commonly known as Arjjhan and Arjun in Bengal, India. It is highly recommended plant for cardiovascular diseases. The bark of this botanical has been shown to lower the blood pressure and heart rate. Ayurvedic physicians use Arjuna bark in the treatment of cardiac decompensation due to dearrangements of all three doshas, vata, pita, or kapha. Arjuna unusually has high content of calcium salts and not surprisingly it is prescribed for both internally and externally to heal the factures.[76] Recent report suggested its antileishmanial role of a pentacyclic triterpenoid isolated from leaves.[77] The methanol extract of the leaves of *Terminalia arjuna* constituting pentacyclic triterpenoid, ursolic acid demonstrated in vitro antileishmanial against promastigotes of *L. donovani.*

5.6.30 KUTKI OR KATUKA

Picrorhiza is a bitter herb traditionally used for both digestion and liver protection. It is one of the Ayurvedic most popular hepatoprotective herbs. *Aarogyavardhani* (herbo mineral preparation containing Picrorhiza as a major ingredient), phalatri kaadi kwaatha (decoction) and punarnavaadi are the most popular Ayurvedic formulations of Picrorhiza (frequently administered in viral hepatitis). Picrorhiza root extracts are widely used in India with no adverse effects being reported. Studies on the rhizome of *Picrorhiza kurroa*, was shown to boost the immune system and to have a specific action against the parasite *L. donovani*, which causes the tropical parasitic disease called leishmaniasis.[66]

Dosage and Administration: Picrorhiza does not easily release its components into water; therefore is not usually taken as a tea. It is usually administered as a standardized (4% kitkin) encapsulated powder extract. Typical adult dosage is 400–1500 mg/day, with dosages up to 3.5 g/day sometimes recommended for fevers. A dose of 3–4 g is recommended as antiperiodic and 0.6–1.2 g as a bitter tonic (CCRAS).

Recent report suggested that Picroliv, a standardized fraction from root and rhizome of *Picrorhiza kurroa*, consisting of iridoid glycosides induced a high degree of protection in golden hamsters against challenge infection with *L. donovani* promastigotes. Mittal et al. (1998) also suggested that a marked hepatoprotective effect of Picroliv and a significant antileishmanial activity implying that it can be utilized as an adjunct to chemotherapy or in combination therapy of kala-azar along with sodium stibogluconate, thus enhancing the efficacy of antileishmanials.[79]

5.6.31 CHAMPA

Plumeria bicolor, commonly known as "*Champa*" sometime called as temple tree in south of India. In Ayurvedic medicine, it is used to calm fear and anxiety and also to treat tremors and insomnia.[80] Plumericin (IC50 of 3.17 and 1.41μM) isolated from Plumeria bicolor showed potent against promastigote and amastigote forms of *L. donovani.*

Plumeria bicolor extract showed activity with the IC 50 of 21 ± 2.2 and 14 ± 1.6 μg/mL against promastigote and amastigote forms of *L. donovani*, respectively. Plumericin consistently showed high activity with the IC 50 of 3.17 ± 0.12 and 1.41 ± 0.03 μM whereas isoplumericin showed the IC 50 of 7.2 ± 0.08 μM and 4.1 ± 0.02 μM against promastigote and amastigote forms, respectively.

5.6.32 INDIAN VALERIAN

In Ayurveda, it is called as Tagara (*Valeriana wallchii*) and in Unani it is called as Jatamansi (*Valeriana jatamansi*). *V. jatamansi* can be used as substitute for Tagara. *V. wallchii* is mainly used for central nervous system disorders. In Ayurveda, it is used in delirium, insomnia, epilepsy, and in behavioral disorders.[81] *Valeriana wallchii* acts on nerve channels known for clearing out toxins from brain, joints, tissue, colon, and nerves. Recent report explored its potential use in kala-azar. Chloroform extract *Valeriana wallichii* root showed IC(50) at ~ 3–7 μg/mL against both the promastigotes and 0.3 μg/mL against *L. major* amastigotes. In addition to cytotoxicity, morphological degeneration, DNA fragmentation, externalization of phosphatidyl serine, and mitochondrial membrane depolarization in *L. donovani* promastigotes proved its potent antileishmanial activity.[82,83]

5.6.33 SALAPARNI

Desmodium, or *Desmodium gangeticum,* is a perennial herb native to India. Ayurvedic healers use it as a heart tonic, and to treat upper respiratory infections, worms, and indigestion. In addition, *Desmodium gangeticum* (Salaparni) root is having antipyretic, astringent, anticatarrhal, diuretic, anthelmintic, laxative, and nervine tonic actions.[72] The active ingredients include alkaloids, isoflavones, pterocarpans, sterols, and flavonoids, and the plant has immunomodulatory, smooth muscle relaxant, anti-inflammatory, and antileishmanial actions. In 1992, extracts of 11 plants used in Nigerian traditional medicine have been evaluated for possible antileishmanial activity using a radiorespirometric microtest technique.[73] Out of these 11 plants extracts, five plants including *D. gangeticum* were found to be active against

Leishmania strain at 50 μg/mL. Mishra et al. (2005) reported the antileishmanial and immunomodulatory activities of glycosphingolipid (cerebroside) isolated from *D. gangeticum.*[84] It was also found that the herb stimulates macrophages and NO production. Its effect on the immune system enhanced in vitro resistance against infection by the parasite known as *L. donovani*, which causes the deadly disease leishmaniasis. In addition, a report on antileishmanian activity on *D. gangeticum* demonstrated the prophylactic and therapeutic efficacy of n-butanol fraction against *Leishmania* infection.[85]

5.6.34 JUKTI

Dregea volubilis (Linn. f.) Benth ex. Hook f. Syn: *Wattakaka volubilis* (Linn. f.) Stapf; *Marsedenia volubilis* (Cooke) belongs to the family Asclepiadaceae and is commonly known as "Jukti" in Bengal. The parts of the plant are used traditionally as medicines. The juice of the plant is used as a sternutatory and the leaves are employed in the treatment of boils and abscesses. The roots and tender stalks are used as emetic and expectorant. A pentacyclic triterpenoid compound designated as taraxerone reported for its in vitro antileishmanial activity against promastigotes of *L. donovani.*[86]

5.7 OTHER PLANTS

5.7.1 KANTALA/PIPPLAI/BHRINGRAJ

Agave Americana (Kantala or barakhawar or Ramban, Kantala) also known as American aloe, which is an edible gum and therefore become part of the certain Ayurvedic formulations. Plant contains active steroidal saponins that are responsible for most of the potent activities.

Piper longum or pipplai is an aromatic climber which has been used in various Ayurvedic formulations as an appetizer, stimulant, anticolic, antitussive, and immunostimulant. It is mainly effective in various respiratory disorders, for example, asthma.

Eclipta alba (Bhringraj or Bhangra) is a rejuvenating herb that rejuvenates hairs, teeth bones, kidney, and liver. This is the main herb for hairs and cirrhosis.[27]

5.7.2 NEEM, KUMARI, ERAND

Coriandrum sativum, fresh herb is known as cilantro or Chinese parsley and is a favorite in Mexican food. The essential oil is produced from the seed, is an antidote to food, very decongesting to the liver and is a great reducer of fire and heat in the body. It is thought to be an aphrodisiac because of its phyto-estrogen content.

Rondon et al. (2011)[6] reported that *A. vera, C. sativum,* and *R. communis* fractions are effective against *L. infantum* promastigotes and did not differ from the positive control pentamidine ($p > 0.05$). *R. communis* ethyl acetate and chloroform fractions, as well as the *C. sativum* methanol fraction, were the most effective against amastigotes and did not differ from the positive control amphotericin B ($p > 0.05$).

Ayurveda or Ayurvedic medicine is a Hindu system of traditional medicine native to India and a form of alternative medicine. The earliest literature on Indian medical practice appeared during the Vedic period of India, that is in the mid second millennium B.C.E. Ayurveda stresses the use of plant-based medicines and treatment. Ayurvedic herbal treatment thus has a significant role in the management and treatment of leishmaniasis. Various reports explored the antileishmanian activities of Indian traditional plants.

5.8 UNANI TREATMENT

In Unani medicine, berries were used in the treatment of jaundice, enlargement of spleen, and kala-azar. Whereas there are some established formulations that are prescribed in Ayurveda:

Qurs Shifa with Aab Kasini sabz, Aab Shitrah each 50 mL and mix in Sikanjabeen bazoori 20 mL two times daily.

Qurs Tabasheer with Sharbat Habbul aas 20 mL two times daily.

Gul surkh 20 g, Zarshak 10 g, Tukhm Khayareen, Tukhm Khurfa each 2 g, Revand chini, Tabaseer, Luk magsool, Kaffor qaisoori, Usharah afsanteen, Saffron, Airsa, sambal ul taib each 3 g, Usharah Gafis 2 g, make powder and use this powder 6 g two times with Aab kasini sabz, Aab shahitrah each 50 mL and Sikanjabeen bazoori 20 mL.

Habbe Sammul far is also very effective in this fever.

Berberine: In Unani medicine, berries (Daarhalda, Zarishk) were used in the treatment of jaundice, enlargement of spleen, and the whole drug as a cholgougue, stomachic, laxative, and antiseptic. Berberine is a bitter-tasting, yellow, plant alkaloid with a long history of medicinal use in Chinese and Ayurvedic medicine. Berberine has been found to possess antimicrobial properties, and there is limited evidence of anti-inflammatory properties as well. The benefits of berberine in the treatment of leishmaniasis are widely accepted. Berberine is thought to be equally efficacious as the standard drug treatment for cutaneous leishmaniasis, antimonite (sulfide mineral), although limited study of this treatment probably limits its widespread use. Human study has also assessed the use of berberine in combination with pyrimethamine in the treatment of chloroquine-resistant malaria. Well-designed clinical trials are still required (www.dramitdutta.com).

KEYWORDS

- **Ayurveda**
- **natural product**
- ***Leishmania***
- **medicinal plant**
- **ayurvedic formulation**

REFERENCES

1. Board of Consultants and Engineers. *Handbook on Unani Medicines with Formulae, Processes, Uses and Analysis*, 1st ed.; National Institute of Industrial Research: New Delhi, India, 2003.
2. Feily, A.; Namazi, M. R. *Aloe vera*in Dermatology: A Brief Review. *G. Ital. Dermatol. Venereol.* **2009,** *144* (1), 85–91.
3. Dutta, A.; Mandal, G.; Mandal, C.; Chatterjee, M. *In vitro* Antileishmanial Activity of *Aloe vera* Leaf Exudate: A Potential Herbal Therapy in Leishmaniasis. *Glycoconj. J.* **2007,** *24* (1), 81–86.
4. Dutta, A; Bandyopadhyay, S.; Mandal, C.; Chatterjee, M. *Aloe vera* Leaf Exudate Induces a Caspase-independent Cell Death in *Leishmania donovani* Promastigotes. *J. Med. Microbiol.* **2007,** *56* (Pt 5), 629–636.
5. Dutta, A.; Sarkar, D.; Gurib-Fakim, A.; Mandal, C.; Chatterjee, M. *In vitro* and *in vivo* Activity of Aloe *vera* Leaf Exudate in Experimental Visceral Leishmaniasis. *Parasitol. Res.* **2008,** *102* (6), 1235–1242.
6. Rondon, F. C.; Bevilaqua, C. M.; Accioly, M. P.; Morais, S. M.; Andrade-Junior, H. F.; Machado, L. K.; Cardoso, R. P.; Almeida, C. A.; Queiroz-Junior, E. M.; Rodrigues, A.

C. *In vitro* Effect of *Aloe vera, Coriandrum sativum* and *Ricinus communis* Fractions on *Leishmania infantum* and on Murine Monocytic Cells. *Vet. Parasitol.* **2011,** *178* (3-4), 235–240.
7. Sairam, T. V. *Home Remedies*; Penguin: United Kingdom, 2000; p 1.
8. Kaur, S.; Kaur, G.; Sachdeva,H.; Kaur, J. In vivo Evaluation of the Antileishmanial Activity of Two Immunomodulatory Plants, *Emblica officinalis* and *Azadirachta indica* in balb/c Mice. *International J. Ayurved. Herbal Med.* **2013**, *3* (1), 1066–1079.
9. Ghai, C. M. *Health Rejuvenation and Longevity Through Ayurveda*; Deep and Deep Publications:New delhi, India, 2004; pp 114–121.
10. Khalsa, K. P. S.; Tierra, M. *The Way of Ayurvedic Herbs: The Most Complete Guide to Natural Healing and Health with Traditional Ayurvedic Herbalism*, 1st ed.; Lotus Press: Silver Lake, WI, 2008; 161–162.
11. Srinivasan, R.; Kalyanasundaram, M. Relative Efficacy of DEPA and Neem Oil for Repellent Activity against *Phlebotomus papatasi*, the Vector of Leishmaniasis. *J. Commun. Dis.* **2001,** *33* (3), 180–184.
12. Sharma, V. P.;Dhiman, R. C. Neem Oil as a Sand Fly (Diptera: *Psychodidae*) Repellent. *J. Am. Mosq. Control Assoc.* **1993,** *9* (3), 364–366.
13. Braun, L.; Cohen M. *Herbs and Natural Supplements Inkling: An Evidence-Based Guide*, 3rd ed.; Elsevier Health Sciences: Amsterdam, Netherlands,2010.
14. Dutta, A.; Ghoshal, A.; Mandal, D.; Mondal, N. B.; Banerjee, S.; Sahu, N. P.; Mandal, C. Racemoside A, an Anti-leishmanial, Water-soluble, Natural Steroidal Saponin, Induces Programmed Cell Death in *Leishmania donovani. J. Med. Microbiol.* **2007,** *56* (Pt 9), 1196–1204.
15. Winston, D.; Maimes, S. *Adaptogens: Herbs for Strength, Stamina, and Stress Relief*; Healing Arts Press: Rochester, VT, 2007, pp 118–120
16. Sachdeva, H.; Sehgal, R.; Kaur, S. *Tinospora cordifolia* as a Protective and Immunomodulatory Agent in Combination with Cisplatin against Murine Visceral Leishmaniasis. *Exp. Parasitol.* **2014,** *137*, 53–65.
17. Singha U. K.; Guru P. Y.; Sen A. B.; Tandon J. S. Antileishmanial Activity of Traditional Plants against *Leishmania donovani* in Golden Hamsters. *Pharmaceutical Biol.* **1992,** *30* (4), 289–295
18. Sinha, J.; Raay, B.; Das, N.; Medda, S.; Garai, S.; Mahato, S. B.; Basu, M. K. Bacopasaponin C: Critical Evaluation of Anti-leishmanial Properties in Various Delivery Modes. *Drug Deliv.* **2002,** *9* (1), 55–62.
19. Bakhru, H. K. *Indian Spices & Condiments as Natural Healers*; Jaico Publishing House: Mumbai, India, 2001.
20. Sharma, U.; Velpandian, T.; Sharma, P.; Singh, S. Evaluation of Anti-leishmanial Activity of Selected Indian Plants Known to Have Antimicrobial Properties. *Parasitol. Res.* **2009,** *105* (5), 1287–1293.
21. Gamboa-Leon, R.; Vera-Ku, M.; Peraza-Sanchez, S. R.; Ku-Chulim, C.; Horta-Baas, A.; Rosado-Vallado, M. Antileishmanial Activity of a Mixture of *Tridax procumbens* and *Allium sativum* in Mice. *Parasite* **2014,** *21*, 15.
22. Gharavi, M.; Nobakht, M.; Khademvatan, S.; Fani, F.; Bakhshayesh, M.; Roozbehani, M. The Effect of Aqueous Garlic Extract on Interleukin-12 and 10 Levels in *Leishmania major* (MRHO/IR/75/ER) Infected Macrophages. *Iran J. Public Health.* **2011,** *40* (4), 105–111.
23. Gharavi, M.; Nobakht, M.; Khademvatan, S. H.; Bandani, E.; Bakhshayesh, M.; Roozbehani, M. The Effect of Garlic Extract on Expression of INFγ and Inos Genes in Macrophages Infected with *Leishmania* major. *Iran J. Parasitol.* **2011,** *6* (3), 74–81.

24. Wabwoba, B. W.; Anjili, C. O.; Ngeiywa, M. M.; Ngure, P. K.; Kigondu, E. M.; Ingonga, J.; Makwali, J. Experimental Chemotherapy with *Allium sativum* (Liliaceae) Methanolic Extract in Rodents Infected with *Leishmania major* and *Leishmania donovani*. *J. Vector Borne Dis.* **2010,** *47* (3), 160–167.
25. Gamboa-León, M. R.; Aranda-González, I.; Mut-Martín, M.; García-Miss, M. R.; Dumonteil, E. In vivo and in vitro Control of *Leishmania mexicana* due to Garlic-induced NO Production. *Scand. J. Immunol.* **2007,** *66* (5), 508–514.
26. Ghazanfari, T.; Hassan, Z. M.; Ebtekar, M.; Ahmadiani, A.; Naderi, G.; Azar, A. Garlic Induces a Shift in Cytokine Pattern in *Leishmania major*-infected BALB/c Mice. *Scand J. Immunol.* **2000,** *52* (5), 491–495.
27. Tirtha, S. S. S. *The Ayurveda Encyclopedia: Natural Secrets to Healing, Prevention, and Longevity*, 2nd ed. Ayurveda Holistic Center Press: Chicago, IL, 2007.
28. Anne McIntyre, F. N. I. M. H. *Herbal Treatment of Children: Western and Ayurvedic Perspectives*, 1st ed.; Butterworth-Heinemann: Oxford, United Kingdom, 2005.
29. Dhiman, A. K.; Kumar, A. *Ayurvedic Drug Plants*; Daya Books: New Delhi, India, 2006; p 598.
30. Gopiesh, K. V.; Krishnan, K.; Giulia, G. Leishmanicidal Activity of Saponins Isolated from the Leaves of *Eclipta prostrata* and *Gymnema sylvestre*. *Indian J. Pharmacol.* **2009,** *41*, 32–35.
31. Kaur, S. D.; Chauhan, K. M.; Sachdeva, H. Protection against Experimental Visceral Leishmaniasis by Immunostimulation with Herbal Drugs *Withania somnifera* and *Asparagus racemosus*. *J. Med. Microbiol.* 2014.
32. Tripathi, C. D.; Gupta, R.; Kushawaha, P. K.; Mandal, C.; Misra Bhattacharya, S.; Dube, A. Efficacy of *Withania somnifera* Chemotypes NMITLI - 101R, 118R and Withaferin A against Experimental Visceral Leishmaniasis. *Parasite Immunol.* **2014,** *36* (6), 253–265.
33. Sachdeva, H.; Sehgal, R.; Kaur, S. Studies on the Protective and Immunomodulatory Efficacy of *Withania somnifera* along with Cisplatin against Experimental Visceral Leishmaniasis. *Parasitol. Res.* **2013,** *112* (6), 2269–2280.
34. Chandrasekaran ,S.; Dayakar, A.; Veronica, J.; Sundar, S.; Maurya, R. An in vitroSs-tudy of Apoptotic Like Death in *Leishmania donovani* Promastigotes by with Anolides. *Parasitol. Int.* **2013,** *62* (3), 253–261.
35. Grover, A.; Katiyar, S. P.; Jeyakanthan, J.; Dubey, V. K.; Sundar, D. Blocking Protein Kinase C Signaling Pathway: Mechanistic Insights into the Anti-leishmanial Activity of Prospective Herbal Drugs from *Withania somnifera*. *BMC. Genomics* **2012,** *13*, S20.
36. Dhiman, A. K. *Ayurvedic Drug Plants*; Daya Publishing House: New Delhi, India, 2007; pp 103–104.
37. Medda S.; Mukhopadhyay, S.; Basu, M. K. Evaluation of the in-vivo Activity and Toxicity of Amarogentin, an Antileishmanial Agent, in Both Liposomal and Niosomal Forms. *J. Antimicrob. Chemother.* **1999,** *44* (6), 791–794.
38. Panda, H. *Medicinal Plants: Cultivation and Their Uses*; National Institute of Industrial Research: New Delhi, India, 2002.
39. Singha, U. K.; Guru P. Y.; Sen, A. B.; Tandon, J. S. Antileishmanial Activity of Traditional Plants against *Leishmania donovani* in Golden Hamsters. *Pharmaceutical Biol.* **1992,** *30*, 289–295.
40. Quattrocchi, U. *CRC World Dictionary of Medicinal and Poisonous Plants: Common Names, Scientific Names, Eponyms, Synonyms, and Etymology*; CRC Press: Boca Raton, FL, 2012; p 13.

41. Khare, P.; Rastogi P.; Gupta, S.; Maurya, R.; Dube, A. *In vitro* and *In vivo* Efficacy of a New Herbaceous Indian Plant- Abutilon indicum Against *Leishmania donovani* Infection. *Am. J. Phytomed. Clin. Therapeutics* **2014,** *1*, 134–139.
42. Frawley, D.; Ranade, S.; Lele, A. *Ayurveda and Marma Therapy: Energy Points in Yogic Healing*; Lotus Press: Silver Lake, WI, 2003.
43. Naskar, M., Bhattacharya, S., Biswas, M. Antileishmanial effect of *Ixora coccinea* leaf extracts on the *in vitro* growth of *Leishmania donovani* promastigotes. *J. Adv. Pharm. Edu. Res.* **2013,** 3, 471–474.
44. Pullaiah, T. *Encyclopedia of World Medicinal Plants*, 1st ed.; Daya Books: New Delhi, India, 2006; p1165.
45. Srivastava, S.; Rawat. A. K. S. Quality Evaluation of Ayurvedic Crude Drug Daruharidra, Its Allied Species, and Commercial Samples from Herbal Drug Markets of India. *Evid. Based Complement. Alternat. Med.* **2013,** *2013*, 472973.
46. Mahmoudvand, H.;Ayatollahi Mousavi, S. A.; Sepahvand, A.; Sharififar, F.; Ezatpour, B.; Gorohi, F.; Saedi Dezaki, E.; Jahanbakhsh, S. Antifungal, Antileishmanial, and Cytotoxicity Activities of Various Extracts of *Berberis vulgaris* (Berberidaceae) and Its Active Principle Berberine. *ISRN Pharmacol.* **2014,** *2014*, 602436.
47. Saha, P.; Sen, R.; Hariharan, C.; Kumar, D.; Das, P.; Chatterjee, M. Berberine Chloride Causes a Caspase-independent, Apoptotic-like Death in *Leishmania donovani* Promastigotes. *Free Radic. Res.* **2009,** *43* (11), 1101–1110.
48. Saha, P.; Bhattacharjee, S.; Sarkar, A.; Manna, A.; Majumder S.; Chatterjee M. Berberine Chloride Mediates its Anti-leishmanial Activity via Differential Regulation of the Mitogen Activated Protein Kinase Pathway in Macrophages. *PLoS One.* **2011,** *6* (4), e18467.
49. Vennerstrom, J. L.; Lovelace, J. K; Waits, V. B.; Hanson, W. L.; Klayman, D. L. Berberine Derivatives as Antileishmanial Drugs. *Antimicrob. Agents. Chemother*. 1990, *34* (5), 918–921.
50. Ghosh, A.K.; Bhattacharyya, F. K.; Ghosh, D. K. *Leishmania donovani*: Amastigote Inhibition and Mode of Action of Berberine. *Exp. Parasitol.* **1985,** *60* (3), 404–413.
51. Kundu, A.; Goswami, S.; Chatterjee, T. K. Antileishmanial Effect of Tissue Cultured *Pluchea indica* Root Extracts, Pitc – 2 (a Thiophen Derivative) and ItsDderivative on the in vitro Growth of *Leishmania donovani* Promastigotes. *J. Sci.* **2014,** *4*, 259–262.
52. Suzuki, A.; Shirota, O.; Mori, K.; Sekita, S.; Fuchino, H.; Takano, A.; Kuroyanagi, M. Leishmanicidal Active Constituents from Nepalese Medicinal Plant Tulsi (*Ocimum sanctum* L.). *Chem. Pharm. Bull.* **2009,** *57* (3), 245–251.
53. Chan M. M.; Adapala, N. S; Fong, D. Curcumin Overcomes the Inhibitory Effect of Nitric Oxide on *Leishmania*. *Parasitol. Res.* **2005,** *96* (1), 49–56.
54. Bhattacharjee, S.; Bhattacharjee, A.; Majumder, S.; Majumdar, S. B.; Majumdar, S. Glycyrrhizic Acid Suppresses Cox-2-mediated Anti-inflammatory Responses during *Leishmania donovani* Infection. *J. Antimicrob. Chemother.* **2012,** *67* (8), 1905–1914.
55. Anindita, U.; Biswas, A.; Das, T.; Das, P. K. 18β-Glycyrrhetinic Acid Triggers Curative Th1 Response and Nitric Oxide Up-Regulation in Experimental Visceral Leishmaniasis Associated with the Activation of NF-κB. *J. Immunol.* **2005,** *15* (175), 1161–1169.
56. Zahir, A. A.; Rahuman, A. A.; Pakrashi, S.; Ghosh, D.; Bagavan,A.; Kamaraj, C.; Elango, G.; Chatterjee, M. Evaluation of Antileishmanial Activity of South Indian Medicinal Plants against *Leishmania donovani*. *Experimental parasitol.* **2012,** *132* (2), 180–184.
57. Kaldas, R. M.; El Shafey, A. S.; Shehata, M. G.; Samy, A. M.; Villinski, J. T. Experimental Effect of Feeding on *Ricinus communis* and *Bougainvillea glabra* on the Development

of the Sand Fly *Phlebotomus papatasi* (Diptera: Psychodidae) from Egypt. *J. Egypt. Soc. Parasitol.* **2014,** *44* (1), 1–12.

58. Islamuddin, M.; Farooque A.; Dwarakanath, B. S. Sahal, D.; Afrin, F. Extracts of *Artemisia annua* Leaves and Seeds Mediate Programmed Cell Death in *Leishmania donovani*. *J. Med. Microbiol.* **2012,** *61*, 1709–1718.
59. Ganguly S.; Bandyopadhyay, S.; Bera, A.; Chatterjee, M. Antipromastigote Activity of an Ethanolic Extract of Leaves of *Artemisia indica*. *Indian J. Pharmacol.* **2006,** *38*, 64–65.
60. Sharma, P.; Rastogi, S.; Bhatnagar, S.; Srivastava, J. K.; Dube, A.; Guru, P. Y.; Kulshrestha, D. K.; Mehrotra, B. N.; Dhawan B. N. Antileishmanial Action of *Tephrosia purpurea* Linn, Extract and its Fractions against Experimental Visceral Leishmaniasis. *Drug Development Res.* **2003,** *60* (4), 285–293.
61. Sivarajan, V. V.; Balachandran, I. *Ayurvedic Drugs and Their Plant Sources*; Oxford & IBH Pub. Co: Oxford, United Kingdom, 1994.
62. Mathur, K. N. *Systematic Materia Medica of Homoeopathic Remedies*, 1st ed.; Jain Pub Pvt Ltd: Uttar Pradesh, India, 2002.
63. Sinha, J.; Mukhopadhyay, S.; Das, N.; Basu M. K. Targeting of Liposomal Andrographolide to *L. donovani*-Infected Macrophages *in vivo*. *Drug Delivery* **2000,** *7* (4), 209–213.
64. Sen G.; Mukhopadhyay S.; Manju R.; Biswas, T. Quercetin Interferes with Iron Metabolism in *Leishmania donovani* and Targets Ribonucleotide Reductase to Exert Leishmanicidal Activity. *J. Antimicrob. Chemother.* **2008,** *61* (5), 1066–1075.
65. Mittra, B.; Saha, A.; Chowdhury, A. R.; Pal, C.; Mandal, S.; Mukhopadhyay, S.; Bandyopadhyay S.; Majumder, H. K. Luteolin an Abundant Dietary Component Is a Potent Anti-leishmanial Agent that Acts by Inducing Topoisomerase II-mediated Kinetoplast DNA Cleavage Leading to Apoptosis. *Mol. Med.* **2000,** *6*, 527–541.
66. Khare C. P. *Indian Herbal Remedies: Rational Western Therapy, Ayurvedic and Other Traditional Usage, Botany*; Springer: New Delhi, India, 2004.
67. Haldar, N.; Basu, S.; Bhattacharya, S.; Pandey, J. N.; Biswas, M. Antileishmanial Activity of *Mangifera indica* Leaf Extracts on the in vitro Growth of *Leishmania donovani* Promastigotes. *Elixir. Pharmacy* **2012,** *46*, 8189–8191.
68. Ramos, H.S.; Moraes, M. M.; Nerys, L. L.; Nascimento, S. C.; Militão, G. C.; de Figueiredo, R. C.; da Câmara, C. A.; Silva, T. G. Chemical Composition, Leishmanicidal and Cytotoxic Activities of the Essential Oils from *Mangifera indica* L. var. Rosa and Espada Eduardo. *Biomed. Res. Int.* **2014,** *2014*, 734946.
69. Shukla, A. K.; Patra, S.; Dubey, V. K. Deciphering Molecular Mechanism Underlying Antileishmanial Activity of *Nyctanthes arbortristis,* an Indian Medicinal Plant. *J. Ethnopharmacol.* **2011,** *134* (3), 996–998.
70. Shukla, A. K.; Patra, S.; Dubey, V. K. Iridoid Glucosides from *Nyctanthes arbortristis* Result in Increased Reactive Oxygen Species and Cellular Redox Homeostasis Imbalance in *Leishmania* Parasite. *Eur. J. Med. Chem.* **2012,** *54*, 49–58.
71. Sebastian, P. *Ayurvedic Medicine: The Principles of Traditional Practice*; Jessica Kingsley: London, United Kingdom, 2013.
72. Khare, C. P. Indian Medicinal Plants: An Illustrated Dictionary. Springer: New Delhi, India, 2007; 128–129
73. Sartorelli, P.; Andrade, S. P.; Melhem, M. S.; Prado, F. O.; Tempone, A. G. Isolation of Antileishmanial Sterol from the Fruits of *Cassia fistula* Using Bioguided Fractionation. *Phytother. Res.* **2007,** *21* (7), 644–647.

74. Jameel, M.; Islamuddin, M.; Ali, A.; Afrin, F.; Ali, M. Isolation, Characterization and Antimicrobial Evaluation of a Novel Compound N-octacosan 7β ol, from *Fumaria parviflora* Lam. *BMC. Complement Altern. Med.* **2014**, *14*, 98.
75. Morales-Yuste, M.; Morillas-Márquez, F.; Martín-Sánchez, J.; Valero-López, A.; Navarro-Moll, M.C. Activity of (-)alpha-bisabolol against *Leishmania infantum* Promastigotes. *Phytomedicine* **2010,** *17* (3–4), 279–281.
76. Gerson, S. *The Ayurvedic Guide to Diet and Weight Loss: The Sattva Program*, 1st ed.; Lotus Press: Silver Lake, WI, 2002; pp 390–391.
77. Biswas, M.; Ghosh, A. K.; Haldar, P. K. Anti-leishmanial and Anti-cancer Activities of a Pentacyclic Triterpenoid Isolated from the Leaves of *Terminalia arjuna* Combretaceae. *Tropical J. Pharmaceutical Res.* **2010,** *9* (2), 135–140.
78. Puri, A.; Saxena, R. P.; Sumati, Guru, P. Y.; Kulshreshtha, D. K., Saxena, K.C.; Dhawan, B. N. Immunostimulant Activity of Picroliv, the Iridoid Glycoside Fraction of *Picrorhiza kurroa*, and its Protective Action against *Leishmania* donovani Infection in Hamsters. *Planta Med.* **1992,** *58*, 528–532.
79. Mittal, N.; Gupta, N.; Saksena, S.; Goyal, N.; Roy, U.; Rastogi, A. K. Protective Effect of Picroliv from *Picrorhiza kurroa* against *Leishmania donovani* Infections in *Mesocricetus auratus. Life Sci.* **1998,** *63* (20), 1823–1834.
80. McMahon, C. *Monograph: Frangipani* (*Plumeria alba*) [Online]; Posted July 5, 2011. http://www.whitelotusblog.com/2011/07/monograph-frangipani-plumeria-alba.html (accessed June 28, 2012.
81. Tyler, V. M.; Premila, M. S. *Ayurvedic Herbs: A Clinical Guide to the Healing Plants of Traditional Indian Medicine*, 1st ed.; Routledge: New York and London, 2012.
82. Ghosh, S.; Debnath, S.; Hazra, S.; Hartung, A.; Thomale, K.; Schultheis, M.; Kapkova, P.; Schurigt, U.; Moll, H.; Holzgrabe, U.; Hazra, B. *Valeriana wallichii* Root Extracts and Fractions with Activity against *Leishmania* spp. *Parasitol. Res.* **2011,** *108* (4), 861–871.
83. Iwu, M. M.; Jackson, J. E.; Tally, J. D.; Klayman, D. L. Evaluation of Plant Extracts for Antileishmanial Activity Using a Mechanism-based Radiorespirometric Microtechnique (RAM). *Planta Med.* **1992,** *58* (5), 436–441.
84. Mishra, P. K.; Singh, N.; Ahmad, G.; Dube, A.; Maurya, R. Glycolipids and Other Constituents from *Desmodium gangeticum* with Antileishmanial and Immunomodulatory Activities. *Bioorg. Med. Chem. Lett.* **2005,** *15* (20), 4543–4546.
85. Singh, N.; Mishra, P. K.; Kapil, A.; Arya, K. R.; Maurya, R.; Dube, A. Efficacy of *Desmodium gangeticum* Extract and its Fractions against Experimental Visceral Leishmaniasis. *J. Ethnopharmacol.* **2005,** *98* (1-2), 83–88.
86. Biswas, M.; Mandal, N.; Bikash, Palit P.; Ghosh, A. K.; Bannerjee, S.; Haldar P. *In vitro* Anti-Leishmanial and Anti-Tumour Activities of a Pentacyclic Triterpenoid Compound Isolated from the Fruits of Dregea *volubilis* Benth Asclepiadaceae Kanti Tropical. *J. Pharmaceutical Res.* **2009,** *8* (2), 127–131.
87. Feily, A.; Namazi, M. R. *Aloe vera* in Dermatology: A Brief Review. *G. Ital. Dermatol. Venereol.* **2009,** *144* (1), 85–91.
88. Chun-Su Y.; Bieber, E. J. *Textbook of Complementary and Alternative Medicine*; CRC Press: Boca Raton, FL, 2002; p 271.

CHAPTER 6

PHYTOTHERAPY FOR LEISHMANIASIS

CONTENTS

PART VI PHYTOTHERAPY FOR LEISHMANIASIS

ABSTRACT

Plants have been used medicinally throughout history. Before the beginning of the 19th century, many herbs were considered conventional medicines and were included in medical curricula and formularies. Plants and their extracts have been used traditionally against different pathologies, and in some poor regions they are the only therapeutic source for treatments and the presence of specific active secondary metabolites can be accounted for amelioration of clinical status of suffering individual. Leishmaniasis is one of the neglected tropical diseases prevalent in various developing nations. The information available is very limited in a number of countries so the first in-depth exercise is better to estimate the real impact of leishmaniasis and its approaches to cure. This chapter highlights the current status of antileishmanial drugs along with an insight to herbal and marine moieties for which antileishmanial activity has been documented. Since most of the natural products were biocompatible and safe to use with few impact of side effects, the evaluation of these natural exudates or extracts and their active constituents is a logical way of approaching for new drugs to treat leishmaniasis.

6.1 INTRODUCTION

According to World Health Organization (WHO), leishmaniasis is one of the 17 neglected tropical diseases in the world. Leishmaniasis is a zoonotic infection caused by the parasite belongs to the various speciesof *Leishmania*, family Trypanosomatidae that causes a wide spectrum of clinical manisfestation in humans. Leishmaniasis is transmitted by certain sandfly species namely, Lutzomyiain the new world and Phlebotomusin the old world. Traditionally, leishmaniasis has been classified in three different clinical forms, cutaneous leishmaniasis (CL), mucocutaneous leishmaniasis (MCL), and visceral leishmaniasis (VL). CL, which causes skin sores, is themost common form of leishmaniasis. In case of MCL, parasite spreads from the skin and causes sores in the mucous membranes of the nose (most common location), mouth, or throat. VL, also known as kala azar (black fever), in which the skin of patient may become darkened. It is caused by *Leishmania donovani*, where the parasite migrates to the vital organs such as bone marrow, liver, and spleen, which may leads to death in 20 months if left untreated. As per WHO, an estimated 20,000–40,000 deaths were occurring every year due to leishmaniasis. Currently, it is considered to be endemic in 88 countries, of which 72 are developing nations. Plants and animals have a broad range of molecules which can be explored for different medical and biotechnological applications. In spite a high number of compounds purified from plants and animal secretions, currently only a few pharmaceutical products have been developed from these natural products. This is in part due the important role of medicinal chemistry, which synthesizes new compounds from previously designed ones. The extracts or secondary metabolites presented in plants that might be capable of modifying these pathological conditions can be attractive candidates in the development of new chemotherapeutical against leishmaniasis. Various medicinal plants and their antileishmanial potential are highlighted in Table 6-1.

6.2 NATURAL PLANT PRODUCTS

Many natural products exhibit antiparasitic properties and are highly selective in their mode of action. However, some of those products also show undesirable properties such as high toxicity, poor solubility, low bioavailability, less than average efficacy at moderate doses, and unsuitability for oral or topical application [5–13]. Nevertheless, the diversity of antiparasitic plant extracts and herbal remedies offers a plethora of interesting and innovative lead structures for new antileishmanial compounds. One of the main sources of new compounds is metabolites derived from plants. This vast group contains several products with leishmanicidal activity that includes quinones, alkaloids, terpenes, saponins, phenolic derivatives, and other metabolites. Unfortunately, most of those compounds do not meet the requirements for drug development due to their lack of in vivo activity or high cytotoxicity, requiring chemical modifications to the basic compound. The most promising antileishmanial compounds are some of the alkaloids, such as benzoquinolizidine alkaloids, the terpenes: diterpenoids and sesquiterpenes, and phenolics (e.g., neolignans or naphthoquinones). Chalcones constitute another group of natural products with leishmanicidal properties with antileishmanial activities demonstrated for berberine and licochalcone A[5–13].

Recently, novel compounds with leishmanicidal activity belonging to the above mentioned groups have been identified. These include manzamine alkaloids, triterpenoids, and compounds isolated from medicinal plants of the Ivory Coast or ferns. A triterpenoid saponin extract from the Vietnamese plant *Maesa balance* containing a mixture of six oleane triterpene saponins, exhibited

TABLE 6-1 List of various medicinal plants and their anti-leishmanian potential

Plant name	Family	Extracts	Part used	Chemical components	Native place	Pathogenic strain	IC50	Ref.
Acacia nilotica (Acacia)	Mimosaceae	ME	Husk	Poly hydroxyl compounds	India	*L. donovanii*	IC_{50}< 8 μg/mL against promastigotes	1
Ambrosia miratima (**Nigeria** hausa)	Astraceae	ME	AS	Poly hydroxyl compounds	India	*L. donovanii*	IC_{50}< 8 μg/mL against promastigotes	1
Anisomeles malabarica (Irattaippeymarutti, malabar catmint)	Lamiaceae	ME, ACE	L	NI	India	*L. donovanii*	IC_{50}126 ± 19.70 μg/mL against promastigotes	2
Ocimum basilicum (Basil)	Lamiaceae	ME, ACE	L	Rosmarinic acid	India	*L. donovanii*	ND	2
Ricinus communis (Aamanakku)	Euphorbiaceae	ME, ACE	SE	NI	India	*L. donovanii*	IC_{50}184 ± 39.33 μg/mL against promastigotes	2
Gloriosa superb (Nobhi-kkodi)	Liliaceae	ME, ACE	FL	NI	India	*L. donovanii*	ND	2
Jurinea dolomiaea (Nazar zeal)	Asteraceae	ME, EAE	R	Saponins, cardiac glycosides, phenolics	Pakistan	*L. tropica*	IC_{50}10.9; 5.3 μg/mL)	3
Asparagus gracilis (Sha gandal)	Asparagaceae	ME	AP	Flavonoids, phenolics	Pakistan	*L. tropica*	IC_{50}12.6 to 36.6 μg/mL	3
Sida cordata (Simak)	Malvaceae	ME, EAE	WP	Flavonoids, phenolics	Pakistan	*L. tropica*	IC_{50}9.2 to 259.1 μg/mL	3
Stellaria media (Gander)	Caryophyllaceae	ME, EAE	WP	Anthraquinones, phloba-tannins	Pakistan	*L. tropica*	IC_{50}36.4 to 185.9 μg/mL	3

TABLE 6-1 *(Continued)*

Plant name	Family	Extracts	Part used	Chemical components	Native place	Pathogenic strain	IC50	Ref.
Allamanda schottii	Apocynaceae	DCM	R, S, L	Plumericin, (0.3, 0.04 μg/mL) plumieride ursolic acid	Brazil	*L. amazonensis, L. brasiliensis*	IC_{50}14.0, 2.0 μg/mL	4
Eugenia umbelliflora	Myrtaceae	HXE	FR	Eugenial A	Brazil	*L. amazonensis, L. brasiliensis*	IC_{50}14.3,5.7 μg/mL	4
Garcinia achachairu	Clusiaceae	ME	SE	Guttiferone A (10.4 μg/mL)	Brazil	*L. amazonensis*	IC_{50}35.9 μg/mL	4
Rapanea ferruginea	Myrsinaceae	EE	FR, L, B	Myrsinoic acid B (6.1 μg/mL)	Brazil	*L. brasiliensis*	IC_{50}24.1 g/mL	4
Solanum sisymbriifolium	Solanaceae	HXE, EAE	AP	Cilistol A (6.6 and 3.1 μg/mL), cilistadiol	Brazil	*L. amazonensis, L. brasiliensis*	IC_{50}33.8 and 20.5 μg/mL	4
Vanillosmopsis arborea	Asteraceae	EO	Stems	α-bisabolol against promastigotes (4.95 μg/mL); intracellular amastigotes (10.70 μg/mL)	Brazil	*L. amazonensis*	Intra-cellular amastigotes (IC_{50} 12.58 μg/mL); Pro-mastigotes (IC_{50} 7.35 μg/mL)	5
Hura crepitans	Euphorbiaceae	EE	L	Crepitin (phytohemagglutinin)	Cuba	*L. amazonensis*	IC_{50} 16.4 μg/mL	6
Bambusa vulgaris	Bambusinae	EE	L	Alkaloids, tannins, phenolics, glycosides, saponins, flavonoids	Cuba	*L. amazonensis*	IC_{50}60.5 μg/mL	6

TABLE 6-1 *(Continued)*

Plant name	Family	Extracts	Part used	Chemical components	Native place	Pathogenic strain	IC50	Ref.
Simarouba glauca	Simaroubaceae	EE	L	Glaucarrubin	Cuba	*L. amazonensis*	IC_{50}47.5 µg/mL	6
Albizia gummifera	Leguminosae	EE	L	Spermine alkaloids	Kenya	*L. donovanii*	IC_{50}10 µg/mL	7
Abrus schimperi	Fabaceae	EE	L	Amorphaquinone (0.63 µg/mL), pendulone (0.43 µg/mL)	Kenya	*L. donovanii*	IC_{50}10 µg/mL (extract of flavanquinones)	7
Albizia schimperiana	Leguminosae	EE	L	5,14-dimethylbudmunchiamine L1 (1.2 µg/mL), 6-hydroxybudmunchiamine K (3.4 µg/mL), 5-normethylbudmunchiamine K (0.8 µg/mL) and 6-hydroxy-5-normethylbudmunchiamine K (2.1 µg/mL)	Kenya	*L. donovanii*	IC_{50}10 µg/mL (macrocyclic spermine alkaloids)	7
Sphaeranthus bullatus	Compositae	EE	L	Carvotacetone derivatives	Kenya	*L. donovanii*	IC_{50}10 µg/mL	7
Suregada procera	Euphorbiaceae	EE	L	Diterpenoid	Kenya	*L. donovanii*	IC_{50}10 µg/mL	7
Triclisia sacleuxii	Menispermaceae	EE	L	Alkaloid	Kenya	*L. donovanii*	IC_{50}10 µg/mL	7
Pittosporum viridiflorum	Pittosporaceae	EE	L	Triterpenoid saponin, pittovirid-oside	Kenya	*L. donovanii*	IC_{50}10 µg/mL	7

TABLE 6-1 *(Continued)*

Plant name	Family	Extracts	Part used	Chemical components	Native place	Pathogenic strain	IC50	Ref.
Warbugia stuhlmanii	Canellaceae	EE	L	Flavonoid,kaempferol	Kenya	*L. donovanii*	IC_{50}10 μg/mL	7
Clerodendrum eriophyllum	Verbenaceae	EE	L	Abietane, diterpenoids	Kenya	*L. donovanii*	IC_{50}taxodione (0.08 μg/mL), ferruginol (4 μg/mL), 6-hydroxysalvinolone (3.2 μg/mL), uncinatone (0.2 μg/mL)	7
Cupressus sempervirens	Cupressaceae	EE	FR	Terpene (Ferruginol, sugiol, taxodione)	Yemen and Saudi Arabia	*L. infantum, L. donovani*	IC_{50}6-deoxytaxodione (11-hydroxy-7, 9(11), 13-abietatrien-12-one) [0.077 μg/mL], taxodione [0.025 μg/mL]	8, 48
Costus arabicus	Zingiberaceae	ME	R	-	Yemen and Saudi Arabia	-	IC_{50}27.3 μg/mL	8
Vernonia leopoldii	Asteraceae	ME	L, FL	-	Yemen and Saudi Arabia	-	IC_{50}27.3 μg/mL	8
Chrozophora oblongifolia	Euphorbiacea	ME	L, S	-	Yemen and Saudi Arabia	*L. infantum*	IC_{50}27.3 μg/mL	8
Grewia erythraea	Tiliaceae	ME	L, S	Terpenoids	Yemen and Saudi Arabia	*L. infantum*	IC_{50}24.1 μg/mL	8
Lavandula dentata	Labiatae	ME	L, FL	-	Yemen and-Saudi Arabia	*L. infantum*	IC_{50}20.3 μg/mL	8

TABLE 6-1 *(Continued)*

Plant name	Family	Extracts	Part used	Chemical components	Native place	Pathogenic strain	IC50	Ref.
Plectranthus barbatus	Labiatae	ME	L, S	-	Yemen and Saudi Arabia	*L. infantum L. chagasi*	IC_{50}24.1, 54.5 µg/mL	8
Vernonia leopoldii	Asteraceae	ME	L, F	Stigmastane-type steroids (vernoguinosterol and vernoguinoside)	Yemen and Saudi Arabia	*L. infantum*	IC_{50}27.3 µg/mL	8
Austroplenckia populnea	Celastraceae	HAE	B	Pentacyclic triterpenes populnoic acid, populnoate (52 µg/mL), stigmast-5-en (18 µg/mL)	Brazil	*L. donovani*	-	9
Baccharis dracunculifolia	Asteraceae	Green propolis HAE	L	Uvaol (15.0 µg/mL), acacetin (18.0 µg/mL), ermanin (40.0 µg/mL), ursolic acid (3.7 µg/mL), hautriwaic acid lactone (7.0 µg/mL)	Brazil	*L.donvani*	IC_{50}49 µg/mL	10
Bixa orellana L.	*Bixaceae*	HAE	WP	Bixin, norbixin	Cuba	*L. amazonensis*	2 fractions (IC_{50}12.9, 12 µg/mL)	11
Bixa orellana L.	*Bixaceae*	EO	SE	Ishwarane (18.6%) and geranylgeraniol (9.1%)	Cuba	*L. amazonensis*	IC_{50}8.5 µg/mL	49
Periploca aphylla.	*Asclepiadaceae*	ME	L,S	Cardenolides and pregnane glycosides	Yemen and Saudi Arabia	*L. infantum*	IC_{50}6.0 µg/mL	12
Caralluma sinaica	*Asclepiadaceae*	ME	L	Pregnane glycosides penicilloside E	Yemen and Saudi Arabia	*L. infantum*	IC_{50}8.1 µg/mL	12

TABLE 6-1 *(Continued)*

Plant name	Family	Extracts	Part used	Chemical components	Native place	Pathogenic strain	IC50	Ref.
Iris germanica	*Iridaceae*	ME	R	Iso-flavonoids	Yemen and Saudi Arabia	*L. infantum*	IC_{50}32.2 μg/mL	12
Phoenix dactylifera	*Arecaceae*	ME	SE	Flavonoids, tannins, glycosides, cardiac glycosides, steroids	Yemen and Saudi Arabia	*L. infantum*	IC_{50}32.5 μg/mL	12
Prosopis juliflora	*Leguminosae*	ME	FR	Flavonoids, alkaloids, saponins, phenols	Yemen and Saudi Arabia	*L. infantum*	IC_{50}35.3 μg/mL	12
Albizia lebbeck	*Leguminosae*	ME	FR, S	Spermine alkaloids including budmunchi-amine K	Yemen and Saudi Arabia	*L. infantum*	IC_{50}50.8 μg/mL	12
Punica granatum	*Punicaceae*	ME	FR	Ellagic acid and punicalagin	Yemen and Saudi Arabia	*L. infantum*	IC_{50}> 64.0 μg/mL	12
Calophyllum rivulare	*Clusiaceae*	EAE, ME	L	Pyranochromanone ac-ids and amento-flavone	Brazil	*L. amazonensis*	IC_{50}95.1 μg/mL (pro-mastigote), 20.6 μg/mL (amastigote)	13
Aloe Secundiflora	Aloeaceae	AE, ME	L	Flavanoids, tannins	Kenya	*L. major*	IC_{50}279.488, 42.824 μg/mL	14
Melia azedarac	*Melia azedarac*	AE	Green and ripe FR	Phenolic compounds	Pakistan	*L. tropica*	Green FR (LC_{50} = 0.41 μg/mL) Ripe FR (LC_{50}: 8227.51 μg/mL)	15
Satureja khuzestanica Jamzad	*Lamiaceae*	EE,ME	L	Triterpenes	Iran	*L. major*	0.3And 0.6 mg/mL	16

TABLE 6-1 *(Continued)*

Plant name	Family	Extracts	Part used	Chemical components	Native place	Pathogenic strain	IC50	Ref.
Tridax procumbens	*Asteraceae*	_	WP	_	_	*L. mexicana*	0.48 μM	17
Urechites andrieuxii	*Apocynaceae*	ME	L,R	Cholest-4-en-3-one, cholest-5,20,24-trien-3β-ol	Mexico	*L. mexicana*	Cholest-4-en-3-one 0.03 μM	17
Desmodiumgangeticum	*Fabaceae*	EE	WP	Glycolipids (glycosphingolipid or cerebroside, amino-glucosyl glycerolipid)	India	*L. donovan*	_	17
Pseudelephantopus spicatus	*Asteraceae*	E	L,AP	Hirsutinolides, ursolic acid	Chayahuita in Peru	*L. amazonensis*	0.2, 0.37and 0.99 μM	17
Himatanthussucuuba	*Apocynaceae*	EE	S,B	Spirolactoneiridoids (plumericin and its isomer isoplumeric)	_	*L. amazonensis*	IC_{50}5 μg/mL	17
Azadirchta indica	*Meliaceae*	EE DCM, CE	S,B,L	Limonoids, azadirachtin	Brazil	*L. amazonensis*	IC_{50}38, 3.9, 1.2 μg/mL (promastigotes), IC_{50}9.8, 1.1, 0.6 μg/mL for (amastigotes)	17, 50
Azadirchta indica	*Meliaceae*	EE, DCM	Nut tegument	Limonoids, azadirachtin	Brazil	*L. amazonensis*	IC_{50}2.7, 2.1 μg/mL (promastigotes) and IC_{50}0.4, 0.6 μg/mL for (amastigotes)	17,50
Maytenus senegalensis	*Celasteraceae*	EE	R, B	Pristimerin	Khartoum.	*L. major*	IC_{50}6.8 μg/mL	17

TABLE 6-1 *(Continued)*

Plant name	Family	Extracts	Part used	Chemical components	Native place	Pathogenic strain	IC50	Ref.
Pseudocedrela kotscifye	*Meliaceae*	crude extract	R, B	Kotschyins phragmalin-type limonoid orthoacetates	Malian	*Leishmania donovani*	_	17
Balanites aegyptiaca	*Balanitaceae*	ME	SE, S, B	Diosgenin	Sudanese plants	*L. major* (promastigotes)	Moderate biological activity	17
Eucalyptus globulus	*Myrtaceae*	ME	L	Terpenoids	Sudanese medicinal plants	*L. major*	IC_{50}78 µg/mL	17
Acanthospermum hispidum	*Asteraceae*	EE	AP	Ursolic acid, oleanolic acid	Bolivia	*L. amazonensis*	IC_{50}11.1 µg/mL	17, 19
Cymbopogon citratus	*Poaceae*	EO	L	Citral	_	*L. amazonensis*	IC_{50}1.7 µg/mL	17, 51
Peschiera australis	*Apocynaceae*	CE	S	Bis-indole alkaloids, coronaridine (12.5 µg/mL against promastigote)	Brazil	*L. amazonensis*	IC_{50} 2.6 µg/mL	17, 52
Peschiera australis var. heurkii	*Apocynaceae*	EE	L	alkaloids conodurine, gabunine, conoduramine	Bolivia	*L. amazonensis*	Significant activity in refrence with glucantime	17,52
Lantana ukambensis	*Verbenaceae*	EE	S, L	_	_	*L. amazonensis*	NT	17

TABLE 6-1 *(Continued)*

Plant name	Family	Extracts	Part used	Chemical components	Native place	Pathogenic strain	IC50	Ref.
Chondodendron tomentosum Curare	*Menisperma-ceae*	HXE	L	Chondrocurine, cycleanine	Peru	*L. infatum*	% Growth inhibition at 400 µg/mL: 96%	17, 53
		CE	B, L	Chondrocurine, cycleanine	Peru	*L. infatum*	% Growth inhibition at 100 µg/mL: B(93%) and L (44%)	
		ACE	Mixed extract (B, L)	Chondrocurine, cycleanine	Peru	*L. infatum*	% Growth inhibition at 100 µg/mL: 100%	
Cedrela odorata L	*Meliaceae*	HXE, CE	B	_	Peru	*L. infatum*	% Growth inhibition at 100 µg/mL: HXE (95.9) and CE(100)	17, 53
Pentacalia desiderabilis	*Asteraceae*	CE	L	Jacaranone	Brazil	*L. chagasi, L. braziliensis, L. amazonensis*	IC_{50}17.22, 12.93, 11.86 µg/mL	17
Drimys brasiliensis Miers	*Winteraceae*	HE	S, B	Sesquiterpene polygodial	Brazil	*Leishmania* spp.	Activity range (22–62 µg/mL)	17
Polyalthia longifolia	*Annonaceae*	EE	L	16α-Hydroxycleroda-3,13 (14) Z-dien-15,16-olide	India	*L. donovani*	IC_{50}8.04 ± 0.40 $\mu g \cdot mL^{-1}$	17
Valeriana wallichii	*Valerianaceae*	CE	R	_	India	*L. major, L. donovani*	IC_{50}3-7 µg/mL against both the promastigotes and 0.3 µg/mL against *L. major* amastigote	17

TABLE 6-1 *(Continued)*

Plant name	Family	Extracts	Part used	Chemical components	Native place	Pathogenic strain	IC50	Ref.
Aristoloquia pilosa	*Aristolochiaceae*	*HXE*	S, L	_	Peru	*L. infatum*	% Growth inhibition at 100 μg/mL: stem (37.8) and leaf (40.8)	53
Brunfelsia grandiflora	*Solanaceae*	*HAE*	S, L	_	Peru	*L. infatum*	% Growth inhibition at 800 μg/mL: stem (99) and leaf (98)	53
Brunfelsia grandiflora	*Solanaceae*	*CE*	S, L	_	Peru	*L. infatum*	% Growth inhibition at 100 μg/mL: stem (88) and leaf (69)	53
Tabebuia serratifolia	*Bignoniaceae*	*CE*	B	Naphthoquinones, lapachol, and lapachone	Peru	*L. infatum*	% Growth inhibition at 100 μg/mL: 90.5	53
Tradescantia zebrina	*Commeliaceae*	*HXE*	*AP*		Peru	*L.infatum*	% Growth inhibition at 800 μg/mL: 96.4 ± 1.2	53
Zamia ulei	*Zamiaceae*	*HXE*	*S*	Cycasin	Peru	*L.infatum*	% Growth inhibition at 400 μg/mL: 72.2 ± 1.3	53
Alstonia scholaris						*L. donovani*		18
Swertia Chirata,						*L. donovani*		18
Tibouchina Semidecandra,						*L. donovani*		18
Tinospora cordifolia						*L. donovani*		18

TABLE 6-1 *(Continued)*

Plant name	Family	Extracts	Part used	Chemical components	Native place	Pathogenic strain	IC50	Ref.
Nyctanthes arbortristis				Iridoid glucosides		*L. donovani*		18
Acanthospermum hispidum	Asteraceae	DCM	AP	SesquiterpeniC lactones	South of Benin	*L. mexicana*	IC_{50}11.1 μg/mL	19
Carpolobia lutea	Polygalaceae	DCM	AP	Polyphenols	South of Benin	*L. mexicana*	IC_{50}31.1 μg/mL	19
Keetia leucantha	Rubiaceae	DCM	L, TW	Ursolic and oleanolic acids	South of Benin	*L. mexicana*	IC_{50}21.2 and 23.5	19
Jatropha multifida	*Euphorbiaceae*	ME	B	Lathyrane diterpenoids, multifidone and multifidinol	*Nigeria*	*L. donavoni*	Multifidone IC_{50}4.69, IC_{50}6.22	20
Ampelocera edentula	*Ulmaceae*	ME	B	Tetralone	Bolivian Plant	*L. amazonensis*	4-hydroxy-1-tetralone (50 mg/kg) was more effective than Glucantime (112 mg/kg).	21
Echinacea purpurea	Asteraceae	EE	SE	_	Iran	*L. major*	Effective concenteration of crude extract is 50 mg/mL	22
Nepeta praetervisa	*Lamiaceae*	ME	L	_	Pakistan	*L. major*	IC_{50}24.41 μg/mL	23
Melodinus eugeniifolus	Apocynaceae	EE, HX	B, L	_	Malaysia	*L. donovani*	IC_{50}(159.9 μg/mL and 270.3 μg/mL)	24

TABLE 6-1 *(Continued)*

Plant name	Family	Extracts	Part used	Chemical components	Native place	Pathogenic strain	IC50	Ref.
Warburgia ugandensis	Canellaceae	HX, DCM, EAE; ME	B	_	Kenya	*L. major*, *L. donovani*	Extracts orally resulted in a reduction of the size of lesions when compared with the intraperitoneal injection	25
Piper auritum	Piperaceae	EO	AP	Safrol	Cuba	*L. major*, *L. mexicana*, *L. braziliensis*, *L. donovani*	IC_{50} value of 22.3 ± 1.8 µg/mL	26
Juniperus excel	Cupressaceae	DEF, ME	BR	Alkaloids, flavonoids, phenols, saponins, diterpenes	Pakistan	*L. major*	IC_{50}11.9 µg/mL	27
Hedera helix	Araliaceae	EE	L	Saponin complex (hederasaponin)	Iran	*L. major*, *L. infantom*, and *L. tropica*	20% concentration of extract reduces amastigotes counts (mean ± SD) of the skin lesions	28
Peganum harmala	Zygophyllaceae	HAE	AP, S	Alkaloids	Iran	L. major	IC_{50}(59.4 µg/mL)	29
Ixora coccinea	Rubiaceae	ME, EAE	L		India	*L. donovani*	IC_{50} (promastigotes): 7.33 and 7.89	30

TABLE 6-1 *(Continued)*

Plant name	Family	Extracts	Part used	Chemical components	Native place	Pathogenic strain	IC50	Ref.
Eclipta prostrata	Asteraceae		L	Dasyscyphin C	India	*L. major, L. aethiopica, L. tropica*	IC_{50} (promastigotes): 450 μg/mL	31
Gymnema sylvestre	Asclepiadaceae	ME	L	Gymnemagenol	India	*L. major, L. aethiopica, L. tropica*	IC_{50}(promastigotes): 965 μg/mL	31
Aloe vera	Liliaceae	ME, leafy exudates	L	-	Pakistan	*L. tropica a* and *L. donovani*	Maximum percent growth inhibition (*L. tropica*-induced cutaneous) at 100 μg/mL; 6.0 μg/mL for *L. donovani*	32
Asparagus racemosus,	Liliaceae		FR	Racemoside A		*Leishmania donovani* (promastigote and amastigotes)	IC_{50} 1.15 and1.31 μg mL (promastigote); 0.17 and 0.16 μg mL^{-1} (amastigotes)	54
Tamarix aphylla	Tamaricaceae		B	-	Pakistan	*L. tropica*	Maximum percent growth inhibition (cutaneous)at 100 μg/mL	32

TABLE 6-1 *(Continued)*

Plant name	Family	Extracts	Part used	Chemical components	Native place	Pathogenic strain	IC50	Ref.
Agave americana	Agavaceae	DW	L	-	India	*L. donovani*	Significant promastigotes killing ($p = 0.00098$) in comparison with phytohemagglutinin and amphotericin B ($p < 0.03$).	33
Azadirachta indica	Meliaceae	Oil, DW	L, B, SE	-	India	*L. donovani*	Significant promastigotes killing ($p = 0.00098$) in comparison with phytohemagglutinin and amphotericin B ($p < 0.03$).	33
Eclipta alba	Asteraceae	DW		-	India	*L. donovani*	Significant promastigotes killing ($p = 0.00098$) in comparison with phytohemagglutinin and amphotericin B ($p < 0.03$).	33
Phaseolus vulgaris L.	Papilionaceae	DW	PHA-P		India	*L. donovani*		33

TABLE 6-1 *(Continued)*

Plant name	Family	Extracts	Part used	Chemical components	Native place	Pathogenic strain	IC50	Ref.
Piper longum L.	Piperaceae	Eth	Spike		India	*L. donovani*	Significant promastigotes killing ($p = 0.00098$) in comparison with phytohemagglutinin and amphotericin B ($p < 0.03$).	33
Anisomeles malabarica	Lamiaceae	ACE, ME	L		South India	*L. donovani* promastigotes	IC(50) = 126 ± 19.70	34
Ricinus communis	Euphorbiaceae	ACE, ME	L		South India	*L. donovani* promastigotes	IC(50) = 184 ± 39.33 μg/mL	34
Allium sativum	Alliaceae		Bulb	Allicindiallyl thiosulfinate = 2-Propene-88 1-sulfinothioic acid S-2-propenyl ester		*L. donovani and L. infantum* promastigotes	Inhibitory concentrations (10–30 μM)	35
Albizia zygia	Mimosaceae	ME	S,B	Saponins	Cameroon	*L. donovani*		36
Allanblackia monticola	Clusiaceae	ME	FR	Xanthones, benzophenones, flavonoids	Cameroon	*L. donovani*		36
Harungana madagascariensis	Clusiaceae	ME	SE	Anthraquinones, xanthones, biflavonoids, coumarins, anthrones derivatives	Cameroon	*L. donovani*		36

TABLE 6-1 *(Continued)*

Plant name	Family	Extracts	Part used	Chemical components	Native place	Pathogenic strain	IC50	Ref.
Rauvolfia macrophylla	Apocynaceae	ME	S,B	E-seco indole, sarpagan, heteroyohimbine, yohimbine, 18-hydroxyyohimbine, indolohomotropane types	Cameroon	*L. donovani*		36
Stereospermum kunthianum	Bignoniaceae	ME	S,B	Lignan, phenolic, iridoid glycosides	Cameroon	*L. donovani*		36
Symphonia globulifera	Clusiaceae	ME	L	Prenylated xanthones, benzophenones	Cameroon	*L. donovani*		36
Chenopodium ambrosioides	Chenopodiaceae	HAE	L	Flavonoids, Terpenoids	Brazil	*Leishmania amazonensis*	Intralesional (dissemination of infection) administeration is more effective then oral	37
		Essential oil	L	Ascaridole, carvacrol and caryophyllene oxide	Cuba	*L. amazonensis*	Ascaridole exhibited the better antileishmanial activity	55
Copaifera L. genus (ten sp.)	Fabaceae	Copaiba oil	TR	*Sesquiterpenes* copaene, bergamotene, caryophyllene *Diterpenes* copalic, kaurenoic, hardwickiic	Brazil	*Leishmania amazonensis*	Hydroxycopalic acid and methyl copalate: 2.5 and 6.0 μg/mL (proma-stigotes); pinifolic and kaurenoic: 3.5 and 4.0 μg/mL(amastigote)	38

TABLE 6-1 *(Continued)*

Plant name	Family	Extracts	Part used	Chemical components	Native place	Pathogenic strain	IC50	Ref.
Hyptis lacustris A. St.-Hil. ex Benth.	Lamiaceae	EE	L	Essential oils	Peru	*Leishmania*	IC50 < 10 μg/mL	39
Calea montana Klat.	Asteraceae	EE	L	Chromanones	Peru	*L. amazonensis*	IC50 < 10 μg/mL	39
Carica papaya L.	Caricaceae	EE	L	Papain	Peru	*L. amazonensis*	IC50 < 10 μg/mL	39
Piper dennisii Trel	Piperaceae	EE	L	Chalcones, amides and prenylated aromatic acid derivatives	Peru	*L. amazonensis*	IC50 < 10 μg/mL	39
Begonia parviflora	Begoniaceae	EE	L		Peru	*L. amazonensis*	18.1 ± 8.2	39
Piper crassinervium	Piperaceae	EE	L		Peru	*L. amazonensis*	25.8 ± 3.2	39
Phytolacca rivinoides	Phyotlacaceae	EE	FR		Peru	*L. amazonensis*	26.3 ± 7.2	39
Phthirusa stelis	Viscaceae	EE	L		Peru	*L. amazonensis*	28.5 ± 2.4	39
Phoradendron crassifolium	Loranthaceae	EE	L		Peru	*L. amazonensis*	14.2 ± 4.1	39
Oreocallis grandiflora	Proteaceae	EE	L		Peru	*L. amazonensis*	23.7 ± 4.2	39

TABLE 6-1 *(Continued)*

Plant name	Family	Extracts	Part used	Chemical components	Native place	Pathogenic strain	IC50	Ref.
Munnozia hastifolia	Asteraceae	EE	B	Dehydrozaluzanin-C	Peru	*L. amazonensis*	14.1 ± 0.5	39
Mansoa alliacea	Bignoniaceae	EE	B		Peru	*L. amazonensis*	21.8 ± 9	39
Jacaranda copaia	Bignoniaceae	EE	B	n quinone derivatives jacaranone and triterpene	Peru	*L. amazonensis*	16.5 ± 4.5	39
Hedyosmum lechleri	Chloranthaceae	EE	L		Peru	*L. amazonensis*	17.9 ± 5.1	39
Euphorbia heterophylla L.	Euphorbiaceae	EE	L		Peru	*L. amazonensis*	25.6 ± 7.7	39
Columnea guttata Poepp.	Gesneriaceae	EE	L		Peru	*L. amazonensis*	28.8 ± 4.3	39
Hedychium coronarium J. König	Zingiberaceae	EE	R	Diterpene (coronarin D)	Peru	*Leishmania*	IC_{50}< 10 μg/mL	39
Cestrum racemosum Ruiz & Pav.	Solanaceae	EE	L	Saponins	Peru	*amazonensis*	IC_{50}< 10 μg/mL	39
Renealmia alpinia (Rottb.)	Zingiberaceae	EE	Rz	Labadanes terpenes, aryl-heptanoids	Peru	*Leishmania*	IC_{50}< 10 μg/mL	39
Renealmia thyrsoidea	Zingiberaceae	EE	Rz		Peru	*L. amazonensis*	10 ± 0.8	39

TABLE 6-1 *(Continued)*

Plant name	Family	Extracts	Part used	Chemical components	Native place	Pathogenic strain	IC50	Ref.
Lantana sp.	Verbenaceae	EE	L		Peru	*L. amazonensis*	IC_{50}< 10 μg/mL	39
Solanum peruvianum	Solanceae	EE	AP		Peru	*L. amazonensis*	14.2 ± 4.2	39
Rollinia mucosa	Annonaceae	EE	L		Peru	*L. amazonensis*	25.2 ± 0.4	39
Zanthoxylum rhoifolium	Rutaceae	50% HAE	B, L		Brazil	*L. amazonensis*		40
Schinus terebinthifolius		HAE			Brazil	*L. amazonensis*		40
Napoleona vogelii	Lecythidaceae	AE	S,B	Alkaloids, tannins and saponins	Republic of Congo	*L. infantum*	5.66	41
Quassia africana	Simaroubaceae	AE	R,B	Quassinoids	Republic of Congo	*L. infantum*	5.04	41
Musanga cecropioides	Leguminosae	AE	S,B	Saponins, tannins, anthraquinones, alkaloids, steroids, triterpenes, flavonoids	Republic of Congo	*L. infantum*	6.35	41
Massularia acuminata	Rubiaceae	AE	S,B	Alkaloids, saponins, anthraquinones, flavonoids and tannins	Republic of Congo	*L. infantum*	6.96	41

TABLE 6-1 *(Continued)*

Plant name	Family	Extracts	Part used	Chemical components	Native place	Pathogenic strain	IC50	Ref.
Harugana madagascariensis	Clusiaceae	AE	Sb	Xanthones, anthrone derivatives, steroids, terpenes, alkaloids, coumarins, flavonoids, anthraquinones and tannins	Republic of Congo	*L. infantum*	20.32	41
Enantia chlorantha	Annonaceae	AE	Sb		Republic of Congo	*L. infantum*	10.08	41
Autranella congolensis	Sapotaceae	AE	Sb	Saponins, tannins and phlobatannins, flavonoids, cardiotonic glycosides and terpenes	Republic of Congo	*L. infantum*	20.32	41
Tetrapleura tetraptera	Leguminosae	AE	Fr	Triterpenoid glycosides, coumarins, flavonoids and tannins	Republic of Congo	*L. infantum*	12.70	41
Scorodophloeus zenkeri	Leguminosae	AE	Sb	Flavonoids, tannins, terpenes, steroids and alkaloids	Republic of Congo	*L. infantum*	9.51	41
Polyalthia suaveolens	Annonaceae	AE	Rb	Terpenes, tannins, flavonoids and saponins	Republic of Congo	*L. infantum*	8.00	41
Piptadeniastrum africanum	Leguminosae	AE	Sb	Saponins, tannins, flavonoids and leucoanthocyans	Republic of Congo	*L. infantum*	6.01	41

TABLE 6-1 *(Continued)*

Plant name	Family	Extracts	Part used	Chemical components	Native place	Pathogenic strain	IC50	Ref.
Leucas Cephalotes (Dronapuspi)	Lamiaceae	CE	WP	-	India	*L. donovani*	3.61	42
Viola canescens	Violaceae	PEE	WP	Epi-oleanolic acid	India	*L. donovani*	0.4	42
Nyctanthes arbortris-tis L.	Oleaceae		S, L, FL	Iridoid glucosides	India	*Leishmania* parasite (Amastigotes)	Trypanothione reductase (TryR), a validated drug target enzyme of the *Leish-mania* parasite	43
Annona coriacea	Annonaceae		L	(*E*)-caryophyl-lene, δ-cadinene1(9, 4 μg/mL)	brazil	*L.chagasi, L.braziliensis, L. mazonensis*	3.24 ± 0.05 μM to 6.49 ± 0.05 μM	44
Piper sanguineispicum Trel.	Piperaceae	EE EE	L S	Chalcones	Peru	*L. amazonensis*	<10 15 ± 1	45
Cybianthus anthurio-phyllus Pipoly	Myrsinaceae	EE	L,R	Maesasaponins	Peru	*L. amazonensis*	12 ± 1	45
Desmodium axillare	Fabaceae	EE	Aerial parts		Peru	*L. amazonensis*	17 ± 2.5	45
Clibadium sylvestre (Aubl.) Baill.	Asteraceae	EE	L	Cunaniol or ichthyothereol	Peru	*L. amazonensis*	15.7 ± 2	45
Piper loretoanum	Piperaceae	EE	L	Chalcones	Peru	*L. amazonensis*	13.6 ± 0.6	45

TABLE 6-1 *(Continued)*

Plant name	Family	Extracts	Part used	Chemical components	Native place	Pathogenic strain	IC50	Ref.
Calotropis gigantean	Asclepiadaceae	ME	AP	-	Iran	*L. major*	IC_{50} of 0.18 and 0.17 mg mL^{-1}	46
Pluchea carolinensis	Asteraceae	EE HXE	L.A	Kaempf-erol, myricetin, quercetin	Cuba	*L. amazonensis*	30.4 ± 1.2 54.5 ± 4.8	47
Nuphar lutea	Nymphaeaceae	HAE	L	Sesquiterpene thioalkaloids containing (thionupharidines)	Israel	*L. major*	0.25, 0.5 mg/mL	48

Seed: SE; L: Leaves; R: Root; S: Stem; AP: Aerial partS; WP: Whole plant; Trunks: TR; TW: Twigs; FR: Fruits; FL:Flowers;B: Bark; BR: BERRIES; L.A: L. amazonensis; L.M: *L. major;L.I: Leishmania* infantum; L.D: *Leishmania donovani; LMX: Leishmania mexicana, L.B: Leishmania braziliensis* ; L.T: *L. tropica; Prm: Promastigote; Amastigote: Am; ethanolic extract: EE; Methanolic extract: ME; hrdroalcoholic extract: HAE: Aqueous extract: AE; Chloroform extract: CE; Ethyl acetate fraction: EAF; petroleum ether extract: PEE; ACE: ACETONE EXTRACT; DEF: Diethyl ETHER fraction; ESSENTIAL OIL: EO; HX: hexane; DCM:* dichloro-methane.

antileishmanial activity in vitro and in vivo in mice. A further study in golden hamsters investigating the antileishmanial properties of a single component of the extract maesabalide III demonstrated a 94.2% reduction in liver amastigote burden when using a single 0.8 mg/kg dose at 28 days postinfection. Although not protective, the treatment was comparable to a single dose of amphotericin B at 5 mg/kg. Some leishmanicidal compounds, such as carboline alkaloids, are extremely toxic to mammalian cells, whereas others belonging to the same group are devoid of toxicity but are ineffective against promastigotes, making them unsuitable as lead compounds. Antileishmanial activity has also been demonstrated by compounds synthesized from a banana plant in response to fungal infection or an aqueous onion extract able to inhibit parasite growth in vitro. So far, none of the natural products have been evaluated in clinical studies, although some of these have been in use for centuries as part of folk remedies. Most of the natural products are still at the experimental research stage and, in most cases, their mechanisms of action are yet to be determined. Therefore, it seems unlikely that these compounds will reach clinical application in the near future. Moreover, most of the studies focus on screening for new antileishmanial products rather than optimization of the selectivity and activity of already known compounds. Plants are clearly a potential source of new antiprotozoal drugs. The biological activity of plant extracts has been attributed to compounds belonging to diverse chemical groups including alkaloids, flavonoids, phenylpropanoids, steroids, and terpenoids. To obtain an herbal medicine or an isolated active compound, different research strategies can be employed, among them, investigation of the traditional use, the chemical composition, the toxicity of the plants, or the combination of several criteria.

6.2.1 MECHANISMS OF ACTION OF PLANT-DERIVED COMPOUNDS

Several promising antileishmanial compounds have been reported over the past few years based on their comparable efficacy with established antileishmanial drugs, using standard in vivo models. Once a promising candidate is identified, toxicology studies of those are then necessary to establish that the compound of interest possesses an adequate therapeutic index. In addition, it is also valid to study the putative mechanism(s), as for example, kinetoplastid topoisomerase (I and II) are potential targets based on their structural differences with human type I DNA topoisomerases, making the enzyme an attractive target for chemotherapeutic intervention. Topoisomerase inhibitors fall into two general categories namely (1) compounds that stimulate the formation of covalent enzyme–DNA complexes or topoisomerase poisons (class I inhibitors) and (2) products that interfere with enzymatic functions of the enzyme or class II inhibitors. Another potential target is the parasite mitochondrion because of its unique structure and function compared to its mammalian host; maintenance of the mitochondrial trans-membrane potential is essential for the survival of cells and study of mitochondrial trans-membrane potential has become a focus of apoptosis regulation. Another aspect is exploiting metabolic differences that completely distinguishes from the host and thereby generates the putative role of biochemical targets like glycolytic enzymes, sterols, purine, pyrimidine, cysteine proteases, protein kinases, fumarate reductases, and polyamine biosynthesis pathways of parasites. *Leishmania* possess a unique relatively weak trypanothione-dependent antioxidant system in which the ubiquitous glutathione/glutathione reductase system is replaced by parasite-specific trypanothione (T[SH2]) and trypanothione reductase (TryR). The dithiol trypanothione is composed of gluthathione and spermidine and is the key molecule for the synthesis of DNA precursors, detoxification of hydroperoxides, and sequestration/export of thiol conjugates. Different rate limiting enzymes that play a major role in trypanothione biosynthesis include glutamylcysteine synthase, ornithine decarboxylase (ODC) necessary for the synthesis of gluthathione and spermidine, respectively along with trypanothione synthase. Therefore, these rate limiting enzymes can act as good chemotherapeutic targets. Trypanothione reductase is a key enzyme in the redox metabolism of *Leishmania* responsible for the transfer of reducing equivalents from the NADP+/NADPH couple from T[SH]2 enzymes of the tryparedoxin peroxidase (TryP) family. Therefore enzymes of the trypanothione-dependent antioxidant system are potential antitrypanosomal drug targets. Moreover, absence of catalase and classical glutathione peroxidases in *Leishmania* renders the parasite more susceptible to free radical-mediated apoptosis. As leishmaniasis is associated with immunological dysfunction of T cells, natural killer cells and in particular, incapacitation of macrophages that ultimately leads to the establishment of the parasite, experimental approaches have included developing antileishmanial compounds capable of recovering the Th1 immune response, via activation of macrophages, through enhanced release of nitric oxide (NO). Phytoconstituents isolated from plants that have shown potent antileishmanial activity include phenolics such as aurones, lignans, chalcones, flavonoids, isoflavonoids, saponins, quinones, alkaloids, tannins, terpenoids, iridoids, terpenes, oxylipins, and miscellaneous sources of plant secondary metabolites (Table 6-2. Chalcones licochalcone A, an oxygenated chalcone isolated from the roots of Chinese plant liquorice alters the ultrastructure

TABLE 6-2 List of various antileishmanian compounds from macroalga, sponges, sea anemones, and sea stares

Plant name	Family and Phylum	Extracts and C.C	Native place	Pathogen	IC50	Ref.
			MACROALGAE			
Canistrocarpus cervicornis	Dictyotaceae, Phaeophyta	ME (4-Ace-toxydo-lastane)	Brazil	*L. amazonensis*	2.0 μg/mL (*prm*), 12.0 μg/mL (*ax am*), 4.0 μg/mL (*int am*)	57
Caulerpa racemosa	Caulerpaceae, Chlorophyta	EE	Pakistan	*L. major*	34.0 μg/mL	58
Ulva fasciata	Ulvaceae, Chlorophyta	EE	Pakistan	*L. major*	50 μg/mL	58
Caulerpa faridii	Caulerpaceae, Chlorophyta	EE	Pakistan	*L. major*	37.5 μg/mL	58
Codium flabellatum	Codiaceae, Chlorophyta	EE	Pakistan	*L. major*	34.0 μg/mL	58
Laurencia pinnatifida	Rhodomelaceae, Rhodophyta	EE	Pakistan	*L. major*	6.25 μg/mL	58
Melanothamnus afaqhusainii	Rhodomelaceae, Rhodophyta	EE	Pakistan	*L. major*	32.6 μg/mL	58
Gracilaria corticata	Gracilariaceae, Rhodophyta	EE	Pakistan	*L. major*	37.5 μg/mL	58
Scinaia Hatei	Scinaiaceae, Rhodophyta	EE	Pakistan	*L. major*	14.1 μg/mL	58
Codium iyengarii	Codiaceae, Chlorophyta	EE	Pakistan	*L. major*	60.4 μg/mL	58
Scinaia indica	Scinaiaceae, Rhodophyta	EE	Pakistan	*L. major*	59.6 μg/mL	58
Ulva rigida	Ulvaceae, Chlorophyta	EE	Pakistan	*L. major*	65.6 μg/mL	58
Ulva reticulate	Ulvaceae, Chlorophyta	EE	Pakistan	*L. major*	64.7 μg/mL	58
Botryocladia leptopoda	Rhodymeniaceae Rhodophyta	EE	Pakistan	*L. major*	60.8 μg/mL	58

TABLE 6-2 *(Continued)*

Plant name	Family and Phylum	Extracts and C.C	Native place	Pathogen	IC50	Ref.
Centroceras clavulatum	Ceramiaceae, Rhodophyta	EE	Pakistan	*L. major*	57.8 μg/mL	58
Cladophora rupestris	Cladophoraceae, Chlorophyta		England.	*L. donovani*	12.0–20.2 μg/mL	59
Codium fragile ssp. tomentosoides	Codiaceae, Chlorophyta		England	*L. donovani*	12.0–20.2 μg/mL	59
Ulva intestinalis	Ulvaceae, Chlorophyta		England	*L. donovani*	12.0–20.2 μg/mL	59
Ulva lactuca	Ulvaceae, Chlorophyta		England	*L. donovani*	12.0–20.2 μg/mL	59
Cladophora socialis	Cladophoraceae, Chlorophyta		England	*L. donovani*	12.0–20.2 μg/mL	59
Bryothamnion Iriquetrum	Rhodomelaceae, Rhodophyta	AE, HAE	Span	*L. amazonensis*	GI < 100 μg/mL	60
Halimeda opuntia Chlorophyta	Halimedaceae, Macroalga	AE, HAE	Span	*L. amazonensis*	GI < 100 μg/mL	60
Osmundea pinnatifida Macroalgae	Rhodomelaceae, Rhodophyta	EE (Scutellarein 4'-methyl ether, 4-Methoxy pyran)	Pakistan	*L. major*	6.25 μg/mL	66
Codium tomentosum Macroalgae	Codiaceae, Chlorophyta	Ethyl acetate and hydoalcoholic extract	France	*L. donovani*	16 μg/mL	67
Ulva lactuca	Chlorophyta Ulvaceae	Ethyl acetate and hydoalcoholic extract	Normandy coast in northern France	*L. donovani*	13 μg/mL	67

TABLE 6-2 *(Continued)*

Plant name	Family and Phylum	Extracts and C.C	Native place	Pathogen	IC50	Ref.
Ulva clathrata	Chlorophyta Ulvaceae	Ethyl acetate and hydoalcoholic extract	Normandy coast in northern France	*L. donovani*	15 μg/mL	67
Bifurcaria bifurcata	Sargassaceae, Heterokontophyta	EAE (Diterpenoids)	Normandy coast in northern France	*L. donovani*	3.8 μg/mL	67
Dictyopteris polypodioides	Dictyotaceae, Heterokontophyta	EAE	Normandy coast in northern France	*L. donovani*	10.8 μg/mL	67
Dictyota dichotoma	Dictyotaceae, Heterokontophyta	EAE	Normandy coast in northern France	*L. donovani*	8.8 μg/mL	67
Dilsea carnosa	Dictyotaceae Dumontiaceae	EAE	Normandy coast in northern France	*L. donovani*	0 9.5 μg/mL	67
Gracilaria corticata	Gracilariaceae, Rhodophyta	Hot AE	Southwest of Iran	*L. major*	≤38 μg/mL	68
Gracillaria salicornia	Rhodophyta Gracilariaceae	Hot AE	Southwest of Iran	*L. major*	≤46 μg/mL	68
Sargassum oligocystum	Sargassaceae, Heterokontophyta	Hot AE	Southwest of Iran	*L. major*	≤78 μg/mL	68
Gracilaria corticata	Gracilariaceae, Rhodophyta	Cold AE	Southwest of Iran	*L. major*	>65 μg/mL	68

TABLE 6-2 *(Continued)*

Plant name	Family and Phylum	Extracts and C.C	Native place	Pathogen	IC50	Ref.
Gracillaria salicornia	Gracilariaceae, Rhodophyta	Cold AE	Southwest of Iran	*L. major*	>74 μg/mL	68
Sargassum oligocystum	Sargassaceae, Heterokontophyta	Cold AE	Southwest of Iran).	*L. major*	>105 μg/mL	68
Caulerpa Sertularioides	Caulerpaceae, Chlorophyta		Southwest of Iran).	*L. major*	>125 μg/mL	68
Laurencia microcladia	Rhodophyta Rhodomelaceae	Organic extracts (Terpenes, polyphenol)	Gulf of Mexico & Caribbean coast	*L. mexicana*	16.3 μg/mL	69
Dictyota caribaea	Dictyotaceae Phaeophyta	Diterpene	Gulf of Mexico and Caribbean coast	*L. mexicana*	24.4 μg/mL	69
Turbinaria turbinata	Sargassaceae Phaeophyta	Sulfated fucans	Gulf of Mexico and Caribbean coast	*L. mexicana*	10.9 μg/mL	69
Lobophora variegata	Dictyotaceae, Phaeophyta	Polyciclic macrolide	Gulf of Mexico and Caribbean coast	*L. mexicana*	49.9 μg/mL	69
Solieria filiformis	Solieriaceae, Rhodophyta	SPs	Brazil	*L. amazonensis*	EC50 137.4 μg/mL; CC50: 99.8 μg/mL	70
Botryocladia occidentalis	RhodymeniaceaeRho-dophyta	SPs	Brazil	*L. amazonensis*	EC50: 63.7 μg/mL; CC50: 27.3 μg/mL	70
Caulerpa racemosa	Caulerpaceae, Chlorophyta	SPs	Brazil	*L. amazonensis*	EC50 value: 34.5 μg/mL; CC50 49.3 μg/mL	70

TABLE 6-2 *(Continued)*

Plant name	Family and Phylum	Extracts and C.C	Native place	Pathogen	IC50	Ref.
Gracilaria caudata	Gracilariaceae, Rhodophyta	SPs	Brazil	*L. amazonensis*	CC50: 73.2 µg/mL	70
Haliclona exigua	Demospongia Halicloniidae	ME	india	*Leishmania donovani*	18.6 µg/ml (*pro*), 47.2 µg/ml (*am*)	71
		CE (in vivo)			45 +/- 10.2% inhibition at 500 mg/kg	
		n-Butanol (insoluble) fraction, Aragus-pongin C			8 µg/ml (*pro*), 31.2 µg/ml (*int am*); *In vivo* 43.9 +/- 5.1% inhibition at < 250 mg/kg	
			SEA ANEMONES			
Bunodosoma granulifera	Actiniidae Cnidaria	AE,HAE	Span	*L. amazonensis*	GI >100 µg/mL	60
Physalia physalis Animalia	Physaliidae, Cnidaria	AE, HAE	Span	*L. amazonensis*	GI >100 µg/mL	60
			SPONGE			
Sarcotragus sp.	Ircinidae, Porifera	DCME	Coast of Tunisia	*L. major*	IC50 1.39 to 264.67 µg/ml	61
Ircinia spinosula Sponge	Ircinidae, Porifera	DCME	Coast of Tunisia	*L. major*	IC50 1.39 to 264.67 µg/ml	61
Dragmaxia undata Sponge	Ircinidae, Porifera	16-methyl-11-heptadecenoic acid	Colombian Caribbean sponge	*L. donovani*	165.5 µM	62

TABLE 6-2 *(Continued)*

Plant name	Family and Phylum	Extracts and C.C	Native place	Pathogen	IC50	Ref.
Ircinia campana Sponge	Irciniidae, Porifera	ME Epidioxysterols	Colombian marine sponge	*L. V. panamensis.*	CE 50: 25.7μg / ml	63
Neopetrosia sp. Sponge	Petrosiidae, Porifera	Lipophilic extract Renieramycin A	Japanese marine sponge	*La/egfp promastigotes*	0.2 μg/mL	64
			SEA STAR			
Echinaster echinophorus	Echinasteridae, Echinodermata	ME	Cuba	*L. amazonensis*	62.9 μg/mL (pro), 37.5 μg/mL(*am*)	65

PRM: promastigote; amastigote: AM; ethanolic extract: EE; methanolic extract: ME; hrdroalcoholic extract: HAE: aqueous extract: AE; chloroform extract: CE; ethyl acetate fraction: EAF; petroleum ether extract: PEE; ACE: acetone extract; DEF: diethyl ether fraction; essential oil: EO; HX: hexane; DCM: dichloro-methane of parasite mitochondria and causes inhibition of mitochondrial dehydrogenases, more specifically, an inhibition of fumarate reductase in the parasite respiratory chain. Furthermore, as the IC50 in amastigotes was lower than promastigotes, the activation of macrophages has been proposed as an additional mechanism. Kayser and Kiderlen (2001) studied 20 naturally occurring chalcones wherein their anti-parasitic activity appeared to increase in the presence of oxysubstituents and methoxy group whereas the introduction of hydrophilic substitutes reduced their leishmanicidal activity.

6.2.1.1 FLAVONOIDS

Flavonoids are widely distributed in the plant kingdom and a search for their anti-parasitic activity has yielded compounds such as luteolin isolated from *Vitex negundo* and quercetin derived from *Fagopyrum esculentum*. Luteolin has been shown to inhibit the synthesis of parasite DNA via inhibition of topoisomerase II-mediated linearization of kDNA minicircles, culminating in arresting of cell cycle progression; the scenario was similar with regard to quercetin. In addition, quercitin (aglycone) can chelate iron, which translates into a decreased availability of the iron-dependent ribonucleotide reductase, a rate limiting enzyme for DNA synthesis. In addition, its combination with SSG enhanced parasite removal as compared to quercetin treatment alone. A leafy extract of *Kalanchoe pinnata* (Crassulaceae, Kp), rich in flavonoids exhibited antileishmanial activity, by increasing the generation of reactive nitrogen intermediates that was further enhanced by the addition of IFN. Kp also exhibited reduced delayed type hypersensitivity (DTH) responses in *Leishmania*-infected mice and further studies revealed that quercetrin, a flavonoid isolated from Kp was one of the contributory phytoconstituents. An EtOH extract of *Piper betle* L. triggered mitochondria-mediated apoptosis in *Leishmania* parasites as also a eugenol rich PB-BM (methanolic extract) showed antileishmanial efficacy that occurred via enhanced production of reactive oxygen species that triggered apoptosis. Parasites treated with an IC50 concentration of guaianolide from *Tanacetum parthenium* (L.) Schultz Bip showed morphological changes. Saponins studies with hederin and hederin isolated from *Hedera helix* as also hederacolchiside A1 isolated from *Hedera colchic*a exhibited strong anti-proliferative activity, attributed to their ability to react with *Leishmania* membranes, induce a decrease in membrane potential and ultimately cause loss of membrane integrity.

6.2.1.2 QUINONES

Plant secondary compounds like plumbagin isolated from *Pera benensis* exhibited its effectivity via increased generation of free radicals in parasites; however, its ability to induce mammalian topoisomerase II mediated DNA cleavage suggests its potential cytotoxicity toward host cells, Diospyrin is another napthoquinone isolated from *Diospyros montana* (Ebenaceae) that also exhibited antileishmanial activity via free radical generation, inhibition of DNA topoisomerase I leading to an apoptosis-like cell death in promastigotes; however its efficacy in amastigotes has not been studied.

6.2.1.3 ALKALOIDS

Alkaloids have been abundantly used against leishmaniasis and include Berberine chloride isolated from Berberis aristata, that inhibits amastigote respiration by targeting mitochondrial enzymes, as also interferes with the macromolecular biosynthesis of amastigotes. More recent studies have revealed that Berberine chloride triggers a free radical-mediated, caspase-independent apoptosis-like death in promastigotes. In infected neutrophils, Berberine chloride induces apoptosis via generation of an oxidative burst that translated into a reduction in parasite load whereas in infected macrophages, it modulated mitogen-activated protein kinases (MAPKs), regulatory enzymes for apoptosis and inflammation. It caused increased phosphorylation of p38 MAPK and concomitant reduction in extracellular signal-related kinase, ERK1/2, thus highlighting MAPKs as a potential chemotherapeutic target in leishmaniasis. A superficial fluid of an EtOH fraction (AF3) containing alkaloids coronaridine (7%) and voacangine (53%) isolated from leaves of Tabernaemontana catharinensis has been shown to have leishmanicidal activity, independent of NO production in macrophages. However, a partially purified alkaloid fraction (NUP) extracted from *Nuphar lutea*, exhibited leishmanicidal activity that was both directly cytotoxic to parasites and via activation of nuclear factor (NF) of infected macrophages leading to elevated production of NO. Activity of the julocrotine, a glutarimide alkaloid from *Croton pullei* var. glabrior, was studied in *Leishmania amazonensis* wherein it caused morphological changes in promastigotes, such as swelling of the mitochondrion, chromatin condensation, presence of membranous structures near the Golgi complex, and appearance of vesicular bodies in the flagellar pocket.

6.2.1.4 LIGNANS

Diphyllin isolated from *Haplophyllum bucharicum* (Rutaceae) displayed anti-proliferative activity in promastigotes by interacting with macromolecules, resulting in cell cycle arrest in the S-phase. However, in amastigotes, its activity was related to its ability to prevent parasite attachment to macrophages and their subsequent entry.

6.2.1.5 TANNINS

In an extensive study by Kolodziej et al. (2001a,b); a series of proanthocyanidins and structural analogs were shown to exert an immunomodulatory activity, as they increased release of NO along with enhancement of expression of pro-inflammatory cytokines in host cells namely tumor necrosis factor-alpha (TNF) and interferon gamma (IFN). Similarly, polyphenol containing extracts and phenols, flavan-3-olgallocatechin tannins also upregulated mRNA expression of TNF, IFN, inducible NO synthase (iNOS), IL-1, IL-12, and IL-18 in *Leishmania*-infected macrophages.

6.2.1.6 TERPENOIDS

Monoterpenes like linalool isolated from leaves of *Croton cajucara* (Euphorbiaceae), effectively increased the production of NO in *Leishmania*-infected macrophages, along with directly targeting the parasite as evidenced by mitochondrial swelling and alterations in the organization of nuclear and kinetoplast chromatin. With regard to studies with sesquiterpene lactones like artemisinin and its derivatives, it has been proposed that the presence of an endoperoxide bridge within the compound selectively enhances generation of free radicals in the parasite; iron has been shown to play a critical role in inducing the observed apoptosis in parasites. In addition, artemisinin increased production of NO and mRNA expression of iNOS to levels present in uninfected macrophages and enhanced the release of Th1 cytokines (IFN) suggesting that artemisinin is directly parasiticidal and indirectly exerts an immunomodulatory activity. Dihydrobetulinic acid, an abundantly occurring triterpene showed antileishmanial activity via targeting of DNA topoisomerases (both I and II) and preventing DNA cleavage, ultimately inducing apoptosis in *L. donovani*. Terpenes like ursolic acid and oleanolic acid isolated from *Pourouma guinensis* also inhibited parasitic growth, but did not induce production of NO in macrophages and instead influenced the phagocytic activity of macrophages. A water soluble 18_-glycyrrhetinic acid (GRA) isolated from *Glycyrrhizza glabra* L. (Licorice) exhibited antileishmanial activity via triggering a curative Th1 cytokine response, concomitant with enhanced production of NO. 16-Hydroxycleroda- 3,13(14)Z-dien-15,16-olide, a clerodane diterpene isolated from an ethanolic extract of *Polyalthia longifolia* inhibited parasite DNA topoisomerase I by directly interacting with the enzyme, terminating in an apoptotic mode of cell death.

6.2.1.7 OXYLIPIN

An oxylipin 3(S)-16, 17-didehydrofalcarinol isolated from *Tridax procambens* (Asteraceae) showed direct parasiticidal effect, independent of NO production in macrophages. An aqueous extract (momordicatin) isolated from *Momordica charantia* inhibited iron-containing parasite superoxide dismutase (SOD), without affecting host SOD. As SOD is a key enzyme for attenuating oxidative stress, its inhibition would lead to increased generation of free radicals, that would be deleterious for the parasite, especially as it is known to have an inefficient antioxidant system. An EtOH extract and butanol fraction isolated from *Tinospora sinensis* induced an oxidative burst in macrophages by increasing production of ROS and NO resulting in parasite killing. *Himatanthus sucuuba* Latex (Apocynaceae) or HsL enhanced the generation of NO and TNF along with inhibition of TGF within macrophages.

6.2.1.7 MISCELLANEOUS

G3, isolated from *Withania somnifera* (withaferin A, steroidal lactone) exerted its parasiticidal activity via inhibition of protein kinase C (PKC), a central event for the induction of apoptosis following stabilization of the topoisomerase I–DNA complex. A plant extract isolated from *Allium sativum* L. (Garlic) was proposed to act via multiple targets as it effectively disturbed thiol homeostasis, disrupted the plasma membrane integrity and increased release of Th1 pro-inflammatory cytokines. The addition of SSG improved the activity of garlic possibly due to their synergistic immunomodulatory properties enhancing the protective Th1 response.

6.3 MARINE SOURCES

In addition to plant-based products, various naturalproducts are also derived from marine sources that are listed in Table 6-3.

TABLE 6-3 List of anti-leishmanian compounds obtained from fungi, cyanobacteria and mushroom

Plant name	Family	Extract or chemical comp.	Percentage inhibition	Native place	Pathogen	Ref
			FUNGI			
Pleurotus flabellatus	Pleurotaceae Basidiomycota			Brazil	*L. amazonensis*	72
Nothopanus hygrophanus	Polyporaceae Basidiomycota			Brazil	*L. amazonensis*	72
L. strigosus	Polyporaceae Basidiomycota			Brazil	*L. amazonensis*	72
Irpex lacteus	Steccherinaceae Basidiomycota			Brazil	*L. amazonensis*	72
Gymnopilus areolatus	Cortinariaceae Basidiomycota			Brazil	*L. amazonensis*	72
Nigrospora sphaerica (endophytic fungus)	Trichosphaeriaceae	Aphidicolin, 3-deoxy-aphidicolin	Aphidicolin 1 for *L. braziliensis* (0.37 M) and *L. major* (0.17 M); 3-deoxy-aphidicolin gor *L. braziliensis* (2.28 M), *L. major* (0.95 M)	Egypt	*L. braziliensis, L. major (prm)*	73
Aspergillus fungi	Aspergillosis	HAE, ACE (kojic acid)		-	*L. amazonensis*	74
Hypocrella bambusae	Clavicipitaceae	Hypocrellins A and B		Yunnan, People's Republic of China	*L. donovani*	75
Edenia sp	Pleosporaceae	Palmarumycin, preussomerin		Republic of Panama	*L. donovani*	76

TABLE 6-3 *(Continued)*

Plant name	Family	Extract or chemical comp.	Percentage inhibition	Native place	Pathogen	Ref
Drechslera rostrata	Pleosporaceae	di-2-ethylhexyl phthalate 1,8-dihydroxy-3-methoxy-6-methyl-anthraquinone	28.8 µg/mL	Riyadh 11495, KSA	*L. major*	77
Eurotium tonpholium	Eurotiaceae	di-2-ethylhexyl phthalate 1,8-dihydroxy-3-methoxy-6-methyl-anthraquinone	28.2 µg/mL	Riyadh 11495, KSA	*L. major*	77
Cell walls of fungi	Oxidation with NaOCl and NaBr	Chitosan (C-6 oxidized chitosan)	125 µg/mL		*L. infantum*	14
Edenia gomezpompae	Pleosporaceae	EA	%GI: 96.0 % on malt extract	Panamanian	*L. donovani*	83
Penicillium paxilli	Trichocomaceae	EA	%GI: 92.9% on Czapek Dox.	Panamanian	*L. donovani*	83
Diaporthe sp.	Trichocomaceae	EA	%GI: 98.66% on Czapek Dox.	Panamanian	*L. donovani*	83
Aspergillus sp.	Diaporthaceae	EA	%GI: 77.2% on Czapek Dox.	Panamanian	*L. donovani*	83
Diaporthe phaseolorum	Diaporthaceae	EA	%GI: 80% on Czapek Dox.	Panamanian	*L. donovani*	83
Nectria mauritiicola	Nectriaceae	EA	%GI: 97.2% on Czapek Dox.	Panamanian	*L. donovani*	83

TABLE 6-3 *(Continued)*

Plant name	Family	Extract or chemical comp.	Percentage inhibition	Native place	Pathogen	Ref
Mycosphaerella stromatosa		EA	%GI: 96.8% on Czapek Dox.	Panamanian	*L. donovani*	83
Edenia gomezpompae fungi	Pleosporaceae	EA	%GI: 96.0% on Czapek Dox.	Panamanian	*L. donovani*	83
			CYANOBACTERIA			
Lyngbya aestuarii	Cyanobacteria		15 mg/mL	India	*L. donovain*	78
Aphanothece bullosa	Cyanobacteria		24.0 mg/mL	India	*L. donovain*	78
Lyngbya majuscula		Dragonamide E				79
marine cyanobacterium, cf. Oscillatorla s	Cyanobacteria	Coibacins A-D		Panamanian		80
Cyanobacterium Oscillatoria nigro-Wiridis	Cyanobacteria	Viridamides A		Netherlands	*L. mexicana*	81
			MUSHROOMS			
Agaricus blazei	Agaricaceae Brazilian	AE, β-D-glucans, glycoproteins, cerebrosides, polysaccharides, steroids, ergosterol, and graxs acids	67.5, 65.8, 56.8 μg/mL (*pro*), and 115.4, 112.3, 108.4 μg/mL (*am*)	Brazil	*L. amazonensis L. major, L. chagasi*	82

- *4-Acetoxydolastane*, (4R, 9S, 14S)-4α-acetoxy-9β,14α- dihydroxy-dolast-1(15),7-diene is a diterpene isolated from the Brazilian brown alga *Canistrocarpus cervicornishas* exhibited antileishmanial activity with an IC50 of 2.0 and 4.0 μg/mL for promastigote and intracellular amastigote forms of *L. amazonensis*, respectively. It was also reported that the compound was 93 times less toxic to the macrophage than to the protozoan parasite.
- *Araguspongin C,* a marine alkaloid obtained from then-butanol fraction of Haliclona exiguainhibited the growth of promastigotes and amastigotes with 35.4%–61.2% and21.6%–48.6% efficacy respectively at concentrations of 50–100 μg/mL.
- *Coscinamide B*, 8,9-dihydrocoscinamide B, a marine alkaloid synthesized from a marine sponge, *Coscinoderma* sp.,has shown 99–100% inhibition against promastigotes and 97–98% inhibition against amastigotes forms of *L. donovani* at a concentration of 10 μg/mL.
- *Elatol,* a sesquiterpene, isolated from Brazilian red seaweed, Laurencia dendroideaelicited marked antileishmanial activity against *L. amazonensis* with an IC50 value of 4.0 μM and 0.45 μM for promastigotes and intracellular amastigote forms, respectively.
- *Holothurin B*, a triterpene glycoside isolated from the coral reef sea cucumber *Actinopyga lecanora* showed marked antileishmanial activity against the *L. donovani.*The glycoside effectively inhibited the growth of promastigotes and amastigotes with 47–82 % and 57–78 %, respectively at a concentration of 50–100 μg/mL.
- *Renieramycin A*, an active substance of a marine sponge *Neopetrosia spalso* elicited a dose-dependent inhibition against *L. amazonensis* with an IC50value of 0.2 μg/mL. The aqueous, dichloromethane and ethyl acetate extracts of two marine sponges *Ircinia spinosula* and *Sarcotragus* sp., obtained from the Tunisian coastline displayed prominent antileishmanial activity against the promastigotes of *L. major.*

6.4 MISCELLENOUS SOURCES

In addition to terrestrial plants and marine sources, natural antileishmanian adrugs are also obtained from certain fungal, cyanobacteria, and mushroom sources (Table 6-4).

TABLE 6-4 List of various secondary metabolites synthesized by plants having anti-leishmanian activity

Active component	Occurrence	Parasite	IC_{50}/standard	Ref.
		ALKALOIDS[87]		
Acivicin	-	*L. donovani*	-	85
Ajmalicine	*Rauwolfia canescens, R. vomitoria* (Apocynaceae)	*L. major*	0.57 µg/mL	86
Allopurinol	Purine analogue	*L. donovani*	75µM	
Ancistroealaine A	*Ancistrocladus ealaensis* (Ancistrocladaceae)	*L. donovani*	4.1 µg/mL	
Ancistroealaine B	*Ancistrocladus ealaensis* (Ancistrocladaceae)	*L. donovani*	10.0 µg/mL	
Ancistrocongolines B	*A. congolensis* (Sapotaceae)	*L. donovani*	18.8 µg/mL	
Ancistrocongolines C	*A. congolensis* (Sapotaceae)	*L. donovani*	19.3 µg/mL	
Ancistrolikokine D	*A. likoko* (Ancistrocladeceae)	*L. donovani*	5.9 µg/mL	
Ancistroealaine A	*A. tanzaniensis* (Sapindaceae)	*L. donovani*	1.8 µg/mL	
Ancistroealaine B	*A. tanzaniensis* (Sapindaceae)	*L. donovani*	1.6 µg/mL	
Ancistrocladidine	*A. tanzaniensis* (Sapindaceae)	*L. donovani*	2.9 µg/mL	
Ancistrogriffithine A	*A. griffithii* (Anisophylleaceae)	*L. donovani*	3.1 µg/mL	
Ancistrogriffithine C	*A. griffithii* (Anisophylleaceae)	*L. donovani*	18.3 µg/mL	
Annomontine	Annona foetida (Annonaceae)	*L.braziliensis*	34.8 µg/mL	88
Anonaine	*U.guatterioides, Annona spinescens* (Annonaceae)	*L.amazonesis*	1.07 µg/mL	89

TABLE 6-4 *(Continued)*

Active component	Occurrence	Parasite	IC_{50}/standard	Ref.
Antioquine	*Guatteria boliviana* (Annonaceae)	*L.amazonensis*	-	
Argentinine	*Guatteria goudotiana, Guatteria foliosa* (Annonaceae)	*L. donovani*	-	
Aristeromycin	-	*L. donovani*		
Aurones	*Gomphrena agrestis* (Amaranthaceae)	*L. donovani*	1.4 μg/mL	
Benzoxazol-2(3H)-one	*Acanthus illicifolius* (Acanthaceae)	*L. donovani*	-	
Berbamine	*Berberis crataegina, B. heteropoda, B. iliensis* (Berberidaceae)	*L. amazonensis*	-	
Berberine	*Berberis aristata* (Berberidaceae)	*L. donovani*	2.5 μg/mL (IC75)	
Bracteoline	*Annona spinescens* (Annonaceae)	*L. amazonensis*	-	
Buchtienine	*Kopsia Griffithii* (Apocynaceae)	*L. donovani*	-	
Camptothecin	*Camptotheca acuminata* (Nyssaceae)	*L. donovani*	EC50 3.2 μM	90
Chimanine B	*Galipea longiflora* (Rutacea)	*L. amazonensis*	IC90:50 μg/mL	91
Chimanine D	*Galipea longiflora* (Rutacea)	*L. amazonensis*	IC90:50 μg/mL	92
Conoduramine	*Peschiera vanheurkii* (Apocynaceae)	*L. amazonensis*	-	
Conodurine	*Peschiera vanheurkii* (Apocynaceae)	*L. amazonensis*	-	
Coreximine	*Annona muricata* (Apocynaceae)	*L. amazonensis*	25 μg/mL	
Coronaridine	*Peschiera australis* (Apocynaceae)	*L. amazonensis*	IC90: 22 μg/mL	93
Corydine	*Stephania dinklagei* (menispermaceae)	*L. donovani*		

TABLE 6-4 *(Continued)*

Active component	Occurrence	Parasite	IC_{50}/standard	Ref.
Corynantheidine	*Corynanthe pachyceras* (Rubiaceae)	*L. major*	IC50 3 μM	97
Corynanthine	*Corynanthe pachyceras (Rubiaceae)*	*L. major*	IC50 3 μM	97
Cusparine	*Cusparia trifoliate, Galipea officinalis* (Rutaceae)	*L. amazonensis*	-	
Daphnandrine	*Albertisia papuana* (Menispermaceae)	*L. donovani*	IC100 ~50 μg/mL	97
Dicentrinone	*Duguetia furfuracea* (Annonaceae)	*L. braziliensis* *L. donovani*	-	97
Dictyolamide A	*Dictyoloma peruviana (Rutaceae)*	*L. amazonensis*	100 μg/mL	97
Emetine	*Psychotria klugii* (Rubiaceae).	*L. donovani*	0.03 μg/mL	97
Formycin B	-	*L. donovani*	-	97
Gabunine	*Peschiera van heurkii* (Apocynaceae)	*L. amazonensis*	25 μg/mL	97
Isoguattouregidine	*Guatteria foliosa* (Annonaceae)	*L. amazonensis*	100 μg/mL	97
Gyrocarpine	*G. americanus* (Hernandiaceae)	*L. amazonensis*	IC100 ~50 μg/mL	97
Harmaline	*Peganum harmala* (Nitrariaceae)	*L. amazonensis*	1.16 μM	97
Harmine	*Peganum harmala* (Nitrariaceae)	*L. amazonensis*	-	
Harmicine	*Kopsia griffithii* (Apocynaceae)	*L. donovani*		
Liriodenine	*Annona foetida* (Annonaceae)	*L. braziliensis*	IC50 < 60 μM	
Julocrotine	*Croton pullei* (Euphorbiaceae)	*L. amazonensis*	19.8 μM	

TABLE 6-4 *(Continued)*

Active component	Occurrence	Parasite	IC_{50}/standard	Ref.
Limacine	*Caryomene olivasans* (Menispermaceae)	*L. donovani*	IC100 ~50 µg/mL	97
Liriodenine	*Annona foetida* (Annonaceae)	*L.braziliensis*	60 µM	
Lysicamine	*Guatteria amplifolia* (Annonaceae)	-	-	
Manzamines β-carboline	*Okinawan sponge* (Chalinidae)	-	0.9 µg/mL	
Moschatoline	*Atherosperma moschatum* (Atherospermataceae) *Annona foetida* (Annonaceae)	*L. braziliensis*	<60 µM	
N-Methyl-tetrahydroberberinium Iodide	*Enantia chlorantha* (Annonaceae)	*L. donovani* *L. braziliensis*	416 mg/kg caused 56% suppression	
N-hydroxy-annomontine	*Annona foetida* (Annonaceae)	*L. braziliensis*	34.8 µM	97
N-methylliriod endronine	*Stephania dinklagei* (Menispermaceae)	*L. braziliensis* *L. donovani*	36.1 µM	
Obaberine	*Pseudoxandra sclerocarpa* (Annonaceae)	*L. braziliensis*	IC100: ~50 µg/mL	97
Oxoisoaporphine derivatives	*Menispermum dauricum* (Menispermaceae)	*L. infantum*	-	
O-methylmo-schatoline	*Annona foetida* (Annonaceae)	*L. braziliensis*	-	
Piperine	*Piper auritum* (Piperaceae)	*L. donovani*	12.8 µg/mL	
Puertogaline A	*Guatteria boliviana* (Annonaceous)	*T. cruzi*	136.3 µg/mL	94
Puertogaline B	*Guatteria boliviana* (Annonaceous)	*T. cruzi*	43.9 µg/mL	94
Pyrimidine-β-carboline	*Annona foetida* (Annonaceae)	*L. braziliensis*	-	
Quinoline, 2-n-Propylquinoline	*Galipea longiflora* (Rutacea)	*L. amazonensis*	-	
Reserpine	*Rauwolfia serpentine* (Apocyanaceae)	*L. major*		

TABLE 6-4 *(Continued)*

Active component	Occurrence	Parasite	IC_{50}/standard	Ref.
Rhodesiacridone	*Thamnosma rhodesica* (Rutaceae)	*L. major*	10 µM	**
Sepeerine	*Chlorocardium rodiei* (Lauraceae)	*L. amazonensis*		
Simalikalactone D	*Quassia amara* (Simarubaceae)	*L. donovani*	NF	**
Skimmianine	*Spiranthera odoratíssima* (Rutaceae)	*L. amazonensis*	-	
Tetrandrine,Iso	*Stephania tetrandra* (Menispermaceae)	*L. amazonensis*	-	
Ushinsunine, nor	*Michelia alba* (Magnoliaceae) *Cananga odorata* (Annonaceae)	*L. amazonensis*	-	
Voacangine	*V.africana* (Apocynaceae)	*Leishmania* sp.	-	
Yohimbine	*Pausinystalia yohimbe* (Rubiaceae)	*L. major*		
	FLAVANOIDS			
Amentoflavone	*Celanodendron mexicanum*, (Alliaceae)	*L. donovani*	-	
Betuletol	*Ulicaria canariensis*,	*Leishmania* sp.	-	
	Betula ermanii (Betulaceae)			
Bractein	*Helichrysm buddleiodes* (Asteraceae)	*L. donovani*	-	
2′,6′-dihydroxy-4′-methoxychalcone	*Piper aduncum* (Piperaceae)	*L. amazonensis*	IC50 = 5.5 µM	95
Flavone, iso: 30,7-dihydroxy-40-methoxy		*L. amazonensis*	-	
Guaianolide	*Tanacetum parthenium* (Asteraceae)	*L. amazonensis*	IC45: 5µg/mL	
Luteolin	*Salvia tomentosa* (Lamiaceae)	*L. donovani*	IC70: 12.5 µM	

TABLE 6-4 *(Continued)*

Active component	Occurrence	Parasite	IC_{50}/standard	Ref.
Podocarpusflavone A	*Celanodendron mexicanum* (Alliaceae)	*L. donovani*	NF	97
Podocarpusflavone B	*Celanodendron mexicanum* (Alliaceae)	*L. donovani*	NF	97
Quercetin	*Fagopyrum esculentum,* Polygonaceae	*L. donovani*	IC70: 45.5 μM	
Sulfuretin	*Rhus verniciflua* (Anacardiaceae)	*L. donovani*	EC50: 1.24 μg/mL	97
Mammea A/B	*Calophyllum brasiliense* (Calophyllaceae)	*L. amazonensis*	3.0 μg/mL	
	DITERPENE			
15-monomethyl dehydropinifolic ester	*Polyalthia macropoda* (Annonaceae)	*L. donovani*	NF	97
Jatrogrossidione	*Jatropha grossidentata* (Euphorbiaceae)	*L. amazonensis*	IC100: 0.75 μg/mL	96
Jatrophone	*Jatropha isabelliin* (Euphorbiaceae)	*L. amazonensis*	<0.25 μg/mL	96
Labda-8-trans-13-dien		*L. donovani*	-	
Labda-9-14-diene,		*L. donovani*	-	
Rigidusine	*Haplopappus rigidus* (Asteraceae)	*L. donovani*	-	
Rollidesin B	Miscellaneous lactone	*L. amazonensis*		
Rosenolactone	*Holarrhena floribunda* (Apocynaceae)	*L. donovani*		97
Striatin A	*Acephalous molluscsa*, Cyclas *striatina* (Cycladae)	*L. amazonensis*	-	
Striatin B	*Acephalous molluscsa*, Cyclas *striatina* (Cycladae)	*L. amazonensis*	-	

TABLE 6-4 *(Continued)*

Active component	Occurrence	Parasite	IC_{50}/standard	Ref.
Taxol	*Taxus brevifolia* (Taxacae)	*L. major*	-	
Casearlucine A	*Laetia procera* (Flacourtiaceae)	*L. amazonensis*	11.1 µg/mL	
Caseamembrol A	*Laetia procera* (Flacourtiaceae)	*L. amazonensis*	11.0 µg/mL	
Laetiaprocerine A	*Laetia procera* (Flacourtiaceae)	*L. amazonensis*	10.9 µg/mL	
Laetiaprocerine D	*Laetia procera* (Flacourtiaceae)	*L. amazonensis*	50.9 µg/mL	
	MONOTERPENES			
Espintanol	*Oxandra espintana* (Annonaceae)	*L. amazonensis*	NF	97
Linalool	*Croton cajucara* (Euphorbiaceae)	*L. amazonensis*	8.7 ng/mL	
	TRITERPENE			
Bruceantin	*Brucea antidysenterica* (Simaroubaceae)	*L. donovani*	-	
Brucein A	*Brucea javanica* (Simaroubaceae)	*L. donovani*	-	
Brucein B,	*Brucea javanica* (Simaroubaceae)	*L. donovani*	-	
Chaparrinone	*Quassia undulata, Simaba multiflora* (Simaroubaceae)	*L. donovani*	-	
15-beta-heptyl Chaparrinone	*Quassia undulata, Simaba multiflora* (Simaroubaceae)	*L. donovani*	NF	97
Colchiside 4,7	*Hedera colchica* (Araliacea)	*L. infantum*	-	
Dihydrobetulinic acid	*Betula alba* (Betulaceae)	*L. donovani*	4.1 µM	
Glaucaruantine		*L. donovani*		

TABLE 6-4 *(Continued)*

Active component	Occurrence	Parasite	IC_{50}/standard	Ref.
Glaucarubin	*Simarouba glauca* (Simaroubaceae)	*L. donovani*	-	
Glaucarubinone	*Simarouba glauca* (Simaroubaceae)	*L. donovani*	-	
Glauacarubol, 15-beta-glucosyl	*Simarouba glauca* (Simaroubaceae)	*L. donovani*	-	
18β-glycyrrhetinic acid	*Glycyrrhizza glabra* (Leguminosae)	*L. donovani*	4.6 μg/mL	
Hederacolchiside	*Hedera colchica* (Araliaceae)	*L. infantum*	-	
Hederacolchiside A-1	*Hedera colchica* (Araliaceae)	*L. mexicana*	0.068 μM	
Hederagenin	*Ivy Hedera helix* (Araliaceae)	*L. infantum*		
Hederin (alpha, beta & delta)	*Hedera helix* (Araliaceae)	*L. tropica*		
16α- Hydroxycleroda-3,13 (14) Z-dien-15, 16-olide	*Polyalthia longifolia* (Annonaceae)	*L. donovani*	5.79±0.31 μg/mL	
Mimengoside A	*Buddleja madagascariensis* (Loganiaceae)	*L. infantum*	-	
Oleanolic acid,	*Pourouma guianensis* (Moraceae)	*L. amazonenesis*	11 μg/mL	
Sergeolide	*Picrolemma seudocoffea* (Simaroubaceae)	*L. donovani*	-	
Sergeolide, 15-deacetyl	*Picrolemma pseudocoffea* (Simaroubaceae)	*L. donovani*	-	
Simalikalactone D	*Quassia amara* (Simaroubaceae)	*L. donovani*	NF	97
Ursolic acid	*Baccharis dracunculifolia* (Asteraceae)	*L. donovani*	3.7 μg/mL	
	SESQUITERPENES			
Agarofuran	*Celastrus vulcanicola* (Celastraceae)	*L. tropica*		
Artemether	*Artemisia annua* (Asteraceae)	*L. major*	3 μM	

TABLE 6-4 *(Continued)*

Active component	Occurrence	Parasite	IC_{50}/standard	Ref.
Artemisinin	*Artemisia annua* (Asteraceae)	*L. major*	30 μM	
Anthecotulide	*Anthemisa uriculata* (Asteraceae)	*L. donovani*	8.18 μg/mL	
Brachycalyxolide,	*Vernonia brachycalyx* (Asteraceae)	*L. major*	17μg/mL	97
Eudesm	*Nardostachys chinensis* (Valerianaceae)	*L. donovani*	-	
Germacratien	Artemisia afra (Asteraceae) *Ballota africana* (Lamiaceae)	*L. major*	-	
Grifolin	*Peperomia galoides* (Piperaceae)	*L. amazonensis*	100 μg/mL	97
Incomptin B	*Decachaeta incompta* (Asteraceae)	*L. mexicana*	-	
Kudtriol	*Jasonia glutinosa* (Asteraceae)	*L. donovani*	250 μg/mL	97
Neurolenin B, C	*Neurolaena lobata* (Asteraceae)	*L. mexicana*	-	
Vernodalin Vernodalol Vernolide hydroxyl	*Vernonia amygdalina* (Asteraceae)	*L. infantum*	-	
	QUINOID			
Aloe emodin	*Stephania dinklagei* (Menispermaceae)	*L. donovani*	185.1μM	97
Alizarin, 3-methyl	*R.palmatum* (Polygonaceae) *Rubia cordifolia* (Rubiaceae)	*L. major*	-	
Anthraquinone-2-hydroxymethyl-3-hydroxy	*Rennellia elliptica* (Rubiaceae)	*L. major*	-	
Damnacanthal	*Morinda citrifolia* (Rubiaceae)	*L. major*	-	
Diospyrin	*Diospyros montana* (Ebenaceae)	*L. donovani*	10 μg/mL	

TABLE 6-4 *(Continued)*

Active component	Occurrence	Parasite	IC_{50}/standard	Ref.
Jacaranone	*Jacaranda copaia* (Bignoniaceae)	*L. amazonensis*	ED50: 0.02 mM	97
Plumbagin	*Plumbago zylenica* (Plumbaginaceae)	*L. amazonensis*	1.1 µg/mL	97
Parthenolide Guaianolide	*Tanacetum parthenium* (Asteraceae)	*L. amazonensis*	0.37 and 2.6 µg/mL (pro)	
Rubiadin-1-methyl ether	*C. australis* (Rubiaceae)	*L. major*	-	
	STEROID			
Holacurtine	*Holarrhena curtisii* (Apocynaceae)	*L. donovani*	(6.25>IC50>1.56 µg/mL)	97
Pregnan-20-one	*Cepaea nemoralis* (Helicidae)	*L. donovani*	-	
Sarachine		*L. chagasi*		
With-5-enolide	*Hibiscus abelmoschus* (Malvaceae)	*L. brasiliensis*	-	
	IRIDOID			
Amarogentin	*S. chirata* (Gentianaceae)	*L. donovani*	>60 µM	
Arbortristoside B, C	*Nyctanthes arbortristis* (Oleaceae)	*L. donovani*		97
Picroliv	*Picrorhiza kurroa* (Plantaginaceae)	*L. donovani*	NF	97
Picrosid I	*Picrorhiza kurroa* (Plantaginaceae)	*L. donovani*	NF	97
	COUMARIN			
Brachycoumarinone	*Vernonia brachycalyx* (Asteraceae)	*L. major*	NF	97
Epicycloisobrachycoumarinone	*Vernonia brachycalyx* (Asteraceae)	*L. major*	NF	97
	LIPID			
Decanoic acid	*E. maingayi* (Zingiberaceae)	*L. donovani*	-	

TABLE 6-4 *(Continued)*

Active component	Occurrence	Parasite	IC_{50}/standard	Ref.
Dodeca-tetra enoic acid	*E. purpurea* (Asteraceae)	*L. mexicana*	-	
Minquartynoic acid	*Minquartia guianensis* (Olacaceae)	*L. major*	-	
Tetradeca-7-11-dienoic acid	*Sarcotragus* sp.	*L. mexicana*	-	
	CHALCONES			
Licochalcone A	*G. uralensis* (Fabaceae)	*L. major*	IC95: 1 μg/mL	
2',6'-Dihydroxy-4'-methoxy chalcones	*Piper aduncum* (Piperaceae)	*L. amazonensis*	24 μg/mL	
2',4'-Dihydroxy-6'-methoxy-3',5'-dimethylchalcone	Psorothamnus polydenius (Fabaceae)	*L. donovani*	5.0 ± 1.3 to 25 μg/mL	
Chalconeflavokavain	*Piper rusbyi* (Piperaceae)	*L. amazonensis*	ND	
	SAPONINS			
Hederagenin	*Hedera helix* (Araliaceae)	*L. tropica*		
α-Hederin, β-Hederin	*Hedera colchica* (Araliaceae)	*L. infantum*	0.41 μM 0.35 μM	
Maesabalides III Maesabalides IV	*Maesa balansae* (Myrsinaceae)	*L. infantum*	7 ng/mL 14 ng/mL	
	LIGNANS			
Dyphillin	*Haplophyllum bucharicum* (Rutaceae)	*L. infantum*	0.2 μM	
	Tanins[98]			
Polyphenols, proanthocyanidins	*Diospyros kaki* (Ebenaceae)	*L. donovani*	0.8 nM	

TABLE 6-4 *(Continued)*

Active component	Occurrence	Parasite	IC_{50}/standard	Ref.
Flavan-3-olgallocatechin	*Camellia sinensis* (Theaceae)	*L. donovani*	-	
Proanthocyanidins (a hexamer)	*Camellia sinensis* (Theaceae) *Vitis vinifera* (Vitaceae)	*L. donovani*	-	
Ellagitannins	*Casuarina stricta* (Casuarinaceae)	*L. donovani*	$EC_{50} > 25$ µg/mL	
Oxylipin	*Tridax procumbens* (Asteraceae)	*L. mexicana*	0.48 µM	
Momordicartin	*Momordica charantia* (Cucurbitaceae)	*L. donovani*		
Glucantime	*Himatanthus sucuuba* (Apocynaceae)	L. amazonensis	IC80:20 µg/mL	
	LACTONE			
Sylvaticin	*Pythium sylvaticum* (Pythiaceae)	*L. amazonensis*		
Squamocin	*Annona squamosa* (Annonaceae)	*L. major*		97
Senegalene	*Annona squamosa* (Annonaceae)	*L. major*		97
Rollidesin B	Miscellaneous lactone	*L. amazonensis*		
Rolliniastatin 1,2	*Rollinia emarginata* (Annonaceae)	*L. amazonensis*	NF	
Pimaricin	*Streptomyces natalensis* (Streptomycetaceae)	*L. donovani*	-	
Nystatin	*Streptomyces noursei* (Streptomycetaceae)	*L. donovani*	-	
Mycophenolic acid	*Ginkgo biloba* (Ginkgoaceae)	*L. tropica*	-	
Molvizarin	*Annona senegalensis* (Annonaceae)	*L. major*		97

TABLE 6-4 *(Continued)*

Active component	Occurrence	Parasite	IC_{50}/standard	Ref.
Goniothalamicin	*Annona glauca* (Annonaceae)	*L.amazonensis*	NF	97
Glaucafilin	*Annona glauca* (Annonaceae)	*L.amazonensis*	-	
Glaucanisin	Annona glauca (Annonaceae)	*L. amazonensis*	-	
Cryptofolione	*Cryptocarya alba* (Lauraceae)	*L. amazonensis*	-	
Argentilactone	*Annona haernatantha* (Annonaceae)	*L. amazonensis*	-	
Annonacin A	*Annona glauca* (Annonaceae)	*L. amazonensis*	NF	97
Anonaine	*A. muricata* (Annonaceae)	*L. amazonensis*	-	
Amphotericin B	*Streptomyces nodosus* (Streptomycetaceae)	*L. braziliensis*	-	
Andrographolide	*Andrographis paniculata* (Acanthaceae)	*L. donovani*	-	
Quassin	*Quassia amara* (Simaroubaceae)	*L. donovani*	-	
4-Hydroxy-1-tetralone	Ampelocera edentula (Celtidoideae)	*L. amazonensis*	-	
Amarogentin	Swertia chirata (Gentianaceae)	*L. donovani*	-	97
Calceolarioside A	*N. arbortristis* (Oleaceae)	*L. donovani*	-	
Peganine HCL	*Peganum harmala* (Nitrariaceae)	*L. donovani*	-	
Physalins B	*Physalis angulata* (Solanaceae)	*L. amazonensis*	0.21 µM	
Gammapyrones	*Podolepsis hieraciodes* (Asteraceae)	*L. donovanii*	8.29–8.59 µg/mL	
Withaferin A	*Withania somnifera* (Solanaceae)	*L. donovani*	9.5±3.0 µg/ml	
Ajoene	*Allium sativum* (Amaryllidaceae)	*L. mexicana*	50 µM (IC90)	
Shikimic acid 3-5-O-gallate	*Pelargonium sidoides* (Geraniaceae) *Phyllanthusamarus* (Euphorbiacea)	*Leishmania parasite*	-	

KEYWORDS

- **natural products**
- **secondary metabolites**
- **antileishmania**
- ***Leishmania***

REFERENCES

1. Eltayeb, A.; Ibrahim, K. Potential Antileishmanial Effect of Three Medicinal Plants. *Indian J. Pharm. Sci.* **2012,** *74* (2), 171–174.
2. Zahir, A. A.; Abdul, R. A.; Pakrashi, S.; Ghosh, D.; Bagavan, A.; Kamaraj, C.; Elango, G.; Chatterjee, M. Evaluation of Antileishmanial Activity of South Indian Medicinal Plants against *Leishmania donovani. Experimental Parasitol.* **2012,** *132*, 180–184.
3. Shah, N.A.; Khan, M. R.; Nadhman.; A. Antileishmanial, Toxicity, and Phytochemical Evaluation of Medicinal Plants Collected from Pakistan. *Biomed. Res. Intern.* **2014,** *2014*, 7.
4. Filho V. C.; Meyre-Silva, C.; Niero, R.;Bolda Mariano, L. N.; Gomes do Nascimento, F.; Vicente Farias, I.; Gazoni, V. F.; Dos Santos Silva, B.; Giménez, A.; Gutierrez-Yapu, D.; Salamanca, E.; Malheiros, A. Evaluation of Antileishmanial Activity of Selected Brazilian Plants and Identification of the Active Principles. *Evid.-Based Complement. Alternat. Med.* **2013,** *2013*, 265025.
5. Colares, A. V.; Almeida-Souza, F.; Taniwaki, N. N.; Souza Cda, S.; da Costa, J. G.; Calabrese Kda, S.; Abreu-Silva, A. L. In Vitro Antileishmanial Activity of Essential Oil of *Vanillosmopsis arborea* (Asteraceae) Baker. *Evid. Based Complement. Alternat. Med.* **2013,** *2013*, 727042.
6. García, M.; Monzote, L.; Scull, R.; Herrera P. Activity of Cuban Plants Extracts against *Leishmania amazonensis. ISRN. Pharmacol.* 2012, *104540*, 7.
7. Muhammad I.; Midiwo, J.; Tekwani, B. L.; Samoylenko, V.; Sahu, R.; Machumi, F.; Rahman, A. A.; Walker, L. A.; Hester J. P. Antileishmanial Activity of Kenyan Medicinal Plants. *Planta Med.* **2011,** *77*, 47.
8. Al-Musayeib, N. M.; Mothana, R. A.; Matheeussen, A.; Cos, P.; Maes, L. *In vitro* Antiplasmodial, Antileishmanial and Antitrypanosomal Activities of Selected Medicinal Plants Used in the Traditional Arabian Peninsular Region. *BMC Complement Alternat. Med.* **2012,** *12*, 49.
9. Andrade, S. F.; da Silva Filho, A. A.; de O Resende, D.; Silva, M. L.; Cunha, W. R.; Nanayakkara, N. P. Antileishmanial, Antimalarial and Antimicrobial Activities of the Extract and Isolated Compounds from *Austroplenckia populnea* (Celastraceae). *Z. Naturforsch. C.* **2008,** *63*, 497–502.
10. Filho, A. A. D. S.; Resende, D. O.; Fukui, M. J.; Parreira, N. A.; Morais, D. R.; Santos, F. F.; Pauletti, P. M.; Cunha, W. R.; Silva, M. L. A.; Gregorio, L.; Bastos, J. K.; Nanayakkara, N. P. D. Constituents of *Baccharis dracunculifolia* DC (Asteraceae) with

in vitro Antileishmanial, Antiplasmodial and Cytotoxic Activities. *Planta Med.* **2009,** *75*, DOI: 10.1055/s-0029-1234499.

11. García, M.; Scull, R.; Osmany, C.; Boulet, G.; Maes, L.; Cos, P.; Monzote, L. Bioassay-guided in vitro Study of the Antileishmanial and Cytotoxic Properties of *Bixa orellana* Seed Extract. *J. Coastal Life Medicine* **2014,** *2* (6), 484–489
12. Al-Musayeib, N. M.; Mothana, R. A.; Al-Massarani, S.; Matheeussen, A.; Cos, P.; Maes, L. Study of the *in Vitro* Antiplasmodial, Antileishmanial and Antitrypanosomal Activities of Medicinal Plants from Saudi Arabia. *Molecules* **2012,** *17* (10), 11379–11390.
13. Oubada, García, M.; Bello-Alarcón, A.; Cuesta-Rubio, O.; Monzote, L. Antileishmanial Activity of Leaf Extract from *Calophyllum rivulare* against *Leishmania amazonensis. Emir. J. Food Agric.* **2014,** *26* (9), 807–812.
14. Ogeto, T. K.; Odhiambo R. A.; Shivairo, R. S.; Muleke, C. I.; Osero, B. O.; Anjili, C.; Ingonga, J. M.; Osuga, I. M. AntileishmanialAactivity of *Aloe secundiflora* Plant Extracts against *Leishmania major. Adv. Life Sci. Technol.* **2013,** *13*, 9–17.
15. Khan, I.; Yasinzai, M. M.; Mehmood, Z.; Ilahi, I.; Khan, J.; Khalil, A. T.; Saqib, M. S.; Rahman, W. U. Comparative Study of Green Fruit Extract of *Melia azedarach* Linn. with its Ripe Fruit Extract for Antileishmanial, Larvicidal, Antioxidant and Cytotoxic Activity. *Am. J. Phytomed. Clin. Therapeutics* **2014,** *2* (3), 442–454.
16. Sadeghi-Nejad, B.; Saki, J.; Khademvatan S.; Nanaei. S. *In vitro* Antileishmanial Activity of the Medicinal Plant - *Satureja khuzestanica* Jamzad. *J. Medicinal Plants Res.* **2011,** *5* (24), 5912–5915.
17. Adebayo, O. L.; Suleman, D.; Samson, A. A. Natural Products in Antileishmanial Drug Discovery: A Review. *J. Asian Scientific Res.* **2013,** *3* (2), 157–173.18. Singha, U. K.; Guru, P. Y.; Sen A. B.; Tandon J. S.. Antileishmanial Activity of Traditional Plants against *Leishmania donovani* in Golden Hamsters. *Int. J. Pharmacog.* **1992,** *30*, 289–295.
19. Beroa, J.; Hannaert, V.; Chataignéa, G.; Hérenta, M. F.; Quetin-Leclercq, J. *In vitro* Antitrypanosomal and Antileishmanial Activity of Plants Used in Benin in Traditional Medicine and Bio-guided Fractionation of the Most Active Extract. *J. Ethnopharmacol.* **2011,** *137*, 998–1002.
20. Falodun, A.; Imieje, V.; Erharuyi, O.; Joy, A.; Langer, P.; Jacob, M.; Khan, S.; Abaldry, M.; Hamann, M. Isolation of Antileishmanial, Antimalarial and Antimicrobial Metabolites from *Jatropha multifida. Asian Pac. J. Trop. Biomed.* **2014,** *4* (5), 374–378.
21 Fournet, A.; Barrios, A.; Muñoz', A. V.; Hocquemiller, R., Roblot, F.; Cavé, A. Antileishmanial Activity of a Tetralone Isolated from *Ampelocera edentula*, a Bolivian Plant Used as a Treatment for Cutaneous Leishmaniasis. *Planta Med.* **1994,** *60*, 8–12.
22. Soudia, S.; Hashemia, S. M.; Hosseinia, A. Z.; Ghaemib, A.; Jafarabadic, M. A. Antileishmanial Effect of *Echinacea purpurea* Root Extract Cultivated in Iran. *Iranian J. Pharmaceutical. Res.* **2007,** *6* (2), 147–149
23 Baloch, N.; Nabi, S.; Bashir, S.; AL-Kahraman, Y. M. S. A. *In vitro* Antileishmanial, Cytotoxic activity and Phytochemical Analysis of *Nepeta praetervisa* Leaves Extract and its Fractions. *Int. J. Pharm. Sci.* **2013,** *5* (4), 475–478 24. Yao, L.; Fiona, S.; Ten-Jin, K.; Christophe, W. Antileishmanial Assay and Antimicrobial Activity on Crude Extracts of *Melodinus eugeniifolus* Barks and Leaves from Malaysia. *Pharmacol. Pharm.* **2014,** *5*, 747–754.
25. Ngure, P. K.; Tonui, W. K.; Ingonga, J.; Mutai, C.; Kigondu, E.; Ng'ang'a, Z.; Rukunga, G.; Kimutai, A. *In vitro* Antileishmanial Activity of Extracts of *Warburgia*

ugandensis(Canellaceae), a Kenyan Medicinal Plant. *J. Medicinal Plants Res.* **2009,** *3* (2), 61–66.

26. Monzote, L.; García, M.; Montalvo, A. M.; Scull, R.; Miranda, M. Chemistry, Cytotoxicity and Antileishmanial Activity of the Essential Oil from *Piper auritum. Mem. Inst. Oswaldo. Cruz.* **2010,** *105* (2), 168–173.
27. Nabi, S.; Ahmed, N.; Javed Khan, M.; Bazai, Z. Yasinzai, M.; Al-Kahraman, Y. M. S. A. *In vitro* Antileishmanial, Antitumor Activities and Phytochemical Studies of Methanolic Extract and its Fractions of Juniperus Excelsa Berries. *World Appl. Sci. J.* **2012,** *19* (10), 1495–1500.
28. Hooshyar, H.; Talari, S.; Feyzi, F. Therapeutic Effect of *Hedera helix* Alcoholic Extract Against Cutaneous Leishmaniasis Caused by *Leishmania major* in Balb/c Mice. *Jundishapur J. Microbiol.* **2014,** *7* (4), e9432.
29. Mirzaie, M.; Nosratabadi, S. J. A.; Derakhshanfar; Sharif, I. Antileishmanial Activity of *Peganum harmala* Extract on the in vitro Growth of *Leishmania major* Promastigotes in Comparison to a Trivalent Antimony Drug. *Veterinarski arhi* **2007,** *77* (4), 365–375.
30. Naskar, M.; Bhattacharya, S.; Biswas, M.; Antileishmanial Effect of *Ixora coccinea* Leaf Extracts on the *in vitro* Growth of *Leishmania donovani* Promastigotes. *J. Adv. Pharmacy Edu. Res.* **2013,** *3* (4), 471–474.
31. Gopiesh, K. V.; Krishnan, K.; Giulia, G. Leishmanicidal Activity of Saponins Isolated from the Leaves of *Eclipta prostrata* and *Gymnema sylvestre. Indian J. Pharmacol.* **2009,** *41*, 32–35.
32. Iqbal, H.; Khattak, B.; Ayaz, S.; Rehman, A.; Ishfaq, M.; Naseer Abbas, M.; Rehman, H. U.; Waheed, S.; Wahab, A. Comparative Efficacy of *Aloe vera* and *Tamarix aphylla* against Cutaneous Leishmaniasis. *Int. J. Basic Med. Sci. Pharm.* **2012,** *2*, 2049–4963.
33. Singh, S. K.; Bimal, S.; Narayan, S.; Jee, C.; Bimal, D.; Das, P. *Leishmania donovani*: Assessment of Leishmanicidal Effects of Herbal Extracts Obtained from Plants in the Visceral Leishmaniasis Endemic Area of Bihar, India. *Raageeva Bimal Exp. Parasitol.* **2011,** *127*, 552–558.
34. Zahir, A. A.; Rahuman, A. A.; Pakrashi, S.; Ghosh, D.; Bagavan, A.; Kamaraj, C.; Elango, G.; Chatterjee, M. Evaluation of Antileishmanial activity of South Indian medicinal plants against *Leishmania donovani. Experimental. Parasitol.* **2012,** *132*, 180–184.
35. Corral-Caridad, M. J. Q.; Moreno, I.; Toraño, A.; Domínguez, M.; Alunda, J. M. Effect of Allicin on Promastigotes and Intracellular Amastigotes of *Leishmania donovani* and *L. infantum. Exp. Parasitol.* **2012,** *132*, 475–482.
36. Lenta, N.; Vonthron-S′en′echeau C.; Fongang Sohd, R.; Tantangmo F.; Ngouela, S.; Kaiser, M.; Tsamod, E.; Anton, R.; Weniger, B. *In vitro* Antiprotozoal Activities and Cytotoxicity of Some Selected Cameroonian Medicinal Plants B. *J. Ethnopharmacol.* **2007,** *111*, 8–12.
37. Patrício, F. J.; Costa, G. C.; Pereira, P. V.; Aragão-Filho, W. C.; Sousa, S. M.; Frazão, J. B.; Pereira, W. S.; Maciel, M. C.; Silva, L. A.; Amaral, F. M.; Rebêlo, J. M.; Guerra, R. N.; Ribeiro, M. N.; Nascimento, F. R. Efficacy of the Intralesional Treatment with *Chenopodium ambrosioides* in the Murine Infection by *Leishmania amazonensis. J. Ethnopharmacol.* **2008,** *115* (2), 313–319.
38. Santosa, A. O.; Ueda-Nakamurab, T.; Dias Filho, B. P.; Veiga Juniorc,V. F.; Pintod, A. C.; Nakamura, C. V.; Effect of Brazilian Copaiba Oils on *Leishmania amazonensis. J. Ethnopharmacol.* **2008,** *120*, 204–208.

39. Valadeau, C.; Pabon, A.; Deharo, E.; Albán-Castillo, J.; Estevez, Y.; Lores, F.A.; Rojas, R.;, Gamboa, D.; Sauvain, M.; Castillo, D.; Bourdy, G. Medicinal Plants from the Yanesha (Peru): Evaluation of the Leishmanicidal and Antimalarial Activity of Selected Extracts. *J. Ethnopharmacol.* **2009,** *123*, 413–422.
40. Moura-Costa, G. F.; Nocchi, S. R.; Ceole, L. F.; Carlos, P. M. J.; Vataru, N. C.; Dias Filho, B. P.; Temponi, L. G.; Ueda-Nakamura, T.; Parana, R. C. Antimicrobial Activity of Plants Used as Medicinal Sonan Indigenous Reserve in Brazil. *J. Ethnopharmacol.* **2012,** *143*, 631–638.
41. Muganza, D. M.; Fruth, B. I.; Lami, J. N.; Mesia, G. K.; Kambu,O. K.; Tona, G. L.; Kanyanga, C. R.; Cos, P.;, Maes, L.; Apers, S.; Pieters, L. In vitro Antiprotozoal and Cytotoxic Activity of 33 Ethonopharmacologically Selected Medicinal Plants from Democratic Republic of Congo. *J. Ethnopharmacol.* **2012,** *141*, 301–308.
42 Virendra K. D.; Vermaa, G.; Agarwalc, D. D.; Kaiserd, M.; Brund, R. Antiprotozoal Activities of Traditional Medicinal Plants from the Garhwal Region of North West Himalaya, India. *J. Ethnopharmacol.* **2011,** *136*, 123–128.
43. Shukla, A. K.; Patra, S.; Dubey V. K.; Deciphering Molecular Mechanism Underlying Antileishmanial Activity of *Nyctanthes arbortristis*, an Indian Medicinal Plant. J. Ethnopharmacol. **2011,** *134*, 996–998.
44. de Toledoa, C. E.; Britta, E. A.; Ceole, L. F.; Silva, E. R.; de Mello, J. C.; Dias Filho, B. P.; Nakamuraa, C. V.; Ueda-Nakamura, T. J. Antimicrobial and Cytotoxic Activities of Medicinal Plants of the Brazilian Cerrado, Using Brazilian Cachac, a as Extractor Liquid. *J. Ethnopharmacol.* **2011,** *133*, 420–425.
45. Odonnea, G.; Bourdyb, G.; Castillo, D.; Estevez, Y.; Lancha-Tangoad, A.; Alban-Castillo, J.; Deharob, E.; Rojasf, R.; Stiena, D.; Sauvainb, M. *Ta'ta Huayani*: Perception of Leishmaniasis and Evaluation of Medicinal Plants Used by the Chayahuita in Peru. Part II. *J. Ethnopharmacol.* **2009,** *126*, 149–158.
46. Oskuee, R. K.; Jafari, M. R.; Amel Farzad, S.; Ramezani, M. *In vitro* LeishmanicidalAactivity of *Calotropis gigantea* and its Fractions against *Leishmania major*. *J. Med. Plants Res.* **2012,** *6* (23), 3977–3983.
47. García, M.; Perera, W. H.; Scull, R.; Monzote, L. Antileishmanial Assessment of Leaf Extracts from *Pluchea carolinensis, Pluchea odorata* and *Pluchea rosea. Asian Pac. J. Trop. Med.* **2011,** *4*, 836–840
48. Zhang, J.; Rahman, A. A.; Jain, S.; Jacob, M. R.; Khan, S. I.; Tekwani, B. L.; Ilias, M. Antimicrobial and Antiparasitic Abietane Diterpenoids from *Cupressus sempervirens. Res. Rep. Medicinal Chem.* **2012,** *2*, 1–6.
49. Monzote, L.; García, M.; Scull, R.; Cuellar, A.; Setzer, W. N. Antileishmanial Activity of the Essential Oil from *Bixa orellana. Phytother. Res.* 2014, *28* (5), 753–758.
50. Carneiro, S. M.; Carvalho, F. A.; Santana, L. C.; Sousa, A. P.; Neto, J. M.; Chaves, M. H. The Cytotoxic and Antileishmanial Activity of Extracts and Fractions of Leaves and Fruits of *Azadirachta indica* (A Juss.). *Biol Res.* **2012,** *45* (2), 111–116.
51. Tiuman Tatiana, S.; Santos Adriana, O.; Ueda-Nakamura, T.; Dias Filho, B. P.; Nakamura, C .V. Recent Advances in Leishmaniasis Treatment. *Int. J. Infectious Diseases* **2011,** *5*, e525–e532.
52. Rochaa, L. G.; Almeidab, J. R. G. S.; Mace^dob, R. O.; Barbosa-Filhob, J. M. A Review of Natural Products with Antileishmanial Activity. *Phytomedicine* **2005,** *12*, 514–535.
53. González-Coloma, A.; Reina, M.; Sáenz, C.; Lacret, R.; Ruiz-Mesia, L.; Arán, V. J.; Sanz, J.; Martínez-Díaz, R. A. Antileishmanial, Antitrypanosomal, and Cytotoxic

Screening of Ethnopharmacologically Selected Peruvian Plants. *Parasitol. Res.* **2012,** *110*, 1381–1392.

54. Dutta, A.; Ghoshal, A.; Mandal, D.; Mondal, N. B.; Banerjee, S.; Sahu, N. P.; Mandal, C. Racemoside A, an Anti-leishmanial, Water-soluble, Natural Steroidal Saponin, Induces Programmed Cell Death in *Leishmania donovani*. *J. Med. Microbiol.* **2007,** *56* (9), 1196–1204.
55. Monzote, L.; García, M.; Pastor, J.; Gil, L.; Scull, R.; Maes, L.;Cos, P.; Gille, L. Essential Oil from *Chenopodium ambrosioides* and Main Components: Activity against *Leishmania*, their Mitochondria and Other Microorganisms. *Exp. Parasitol.* 2014, *136*, 20–6.
56. Ozer, L.; El-On, J.; Golan-Goldhirsh, A.; Gopas, J. *Leishmania major*: Anti-leishmanial Activity of *Nuphar lutea* Extract Mediated by the Activation of Transcription Factor NF-jB. *Experimental Parasitol.* **2010,** *126*, 510–516.
57. dos Santos, A. O.; Aparecida Britta, E.; Bianco,E. M.; Ueda-Nakamura, T.; Dias Filho, B. P.; Crespo Pereira, R.; Vataru Nakamura, C. 4-Acetoxydolastane Diterpene from the Brazilian Brown Alga *Canistrocarpus cervicornis* as Antileishmanial Agent. *Mar. Drugs.* **2011,** *9* (11), 2369–2383.
58. Sabina, H.; Tasneem, S.; Kausar, S. Y.; Choudhary, M. I.; Aliya, R. Antileishmanial Activity in the Crude Extract of Various Seaweed from the Coast of Karachi, Pakistan. *Pak. J. Bot.* **2005,** *37* (1), 163–168.
59. Spavieri, J.; Kaiser, M.; Casey, R.; Hingley-Wilson, S.; Lalvani, A.; Blunden, G.; Tasdemir, D. Antiprotozoal, Antimycobacterial and Cytotoxic Potential of Some British Green Algae. *Phytother. Res.* 2010, *24* (7), 1095–1098.
60. Parra, M. G.; Monzote Fidalgo, C. L.; Castañeda Pasarón, C. O.; García Delgado, N.; Pérez Hernández, A. Antileishmanial Activity of Six Extracts from Marine Organisms. *Rev. Cubana Med. Trop.* **2012,** *64* (1), 61–64.
61. Ben Kahla-Nakbi, A.; Haouas, N.; El Ouaer, A.; Guerbej, H.; Ben Mustapha, K.; Babba, H. Screening of Antileishmanial Activity from Marine Sponge Extracts Collected off the Tunisian Coast. *Parasitol. Res.* **2010,** *106* (6), 1281–1286.
62. Carballeira Néstor, M.; Montano, N.; Cintrón, G. A.; Márquez, C.; Fernández Rubio, C.; Prada, C. F.; Balaña-Fouce, R. First Total Synthesis and Antileishmanial Activity of (*Z*)-16-methyl-11-Heptadecenoic Acid, a New Marine Fatty Acid from the Sponge *Dragmaxia undata*. *Chem. Phy. Lipids* 2011, *164* (2), 113–117.
63. Márquez Diana, F.; Robledo, S. M. R.; Alejandro Martínez, M. Antileishmanial Epidioxysterols from Extracted Sterols of the Colombian Marine Sponge *Ircinia campana*. Porifera Research: Biodiversity, Innovation and Sustainability **2007,** *14*, 433–437.
64. Yoichi, N.; Shiroiwa, T.; Murayama, S.; Matsunaga, S.; Goto, Y.; Matsumoto, Y.; Fusetani, N. Identification of Renieramycin A as an Antileishmanial Substance in a Marine Sponge *Neopetrosia* sp. *Mar. Drugs* **2004,** *2*, 55–62.
65. Parra, M. G.; Fidalgo, L. M.; Martinez, J. M.; Alvarez, A. M; Iglesias, O. V. Leishmanicidal Activity of *Echinaster (Othilia) echinophorus* Crude Extract. *Rev. Inst. Med. Trop. Sao Paulo* **2010,** *52*, 89–93.
66. Sabina, H.; Aliya, R. Bioactive Assessment of Selected Marine Red Algae against *Leishmania major* and Chemical Constituents of *Osmundea pinnatifida*. *Pak. J. Bot.* **2011,** *43* (6), 3053–3056.
67. Vonthron-Sénécheau, C.; Devambez, I.; Vastel, A.; Mussio, I.; Rusig, A. Antiprotozoal Activities of Organic Extracts from French Marine Seaweeds. *Mar. Drugs* **2011,** *9*, 922–933.

68. Fouladvand, M.; Barazesh, A.; Farokhzad, F.; Malekizadeh, H.; Sartavi K. Evaluation of in vitro Anti-leishmanial Activity of Some Brown, Green and Red Algae from the Persian Gulf. *Eur. Rev. Med. Pharmacol. Sci.* **2011**, *15*, 597–600.
69. Freile-Pelegrin ,Y.; Robledo, D.; Chan-Bacab, M. J.; Ortega-Morales B. O. Antileishmanial Properties of Tropical Marine Algae Extracts. *Fitoterapia* **2008,** *79*, 374–377.
70. Lehnhardt Pires, C.; Rodrigues, S. D.; Bristot, D.; Gaeta, H. H; de Oliveira Toyama, D.; Farias, W. R. L.; Toyama, M. H. Evaluation of Macroalgae Sulfated Polysaccharides on the *Leishmania (L.) amazonensis* Promastigote. *Mar Drugs.* **2013,** *11* (3), 934–943.
71. Dube, A.; Singh, N.; Saxena, A.; Lakshmi, V. Antileishmanial Potential of a Marine Sponge, *Haliclona exigua* (Kirkpatrick) against Experimental Visceral Leishmaniasis. *Parasitol. Res.* **2007,** *101* (2), 317–324.
72. Rosa, L. H.; Machado, K. M.; Rabello, A. L.; Souza-Fagundes, E. M.; Correa-Oliveira, R.; Rosa, C. A.; Zani, C. L. Cytotoxic, Immunosuppressive, Trypanocidal and Antileishmanial Activities of Basidiomycota Fungi Present in Atlantic Rainforest in Brazil. *Antonie Van Leeuwenhoek* **2009,** *95* (3), 227–237.
73. AM Metwaly. A. M.; Kadry, H. A.; El-Hela, A. A.; Mohammad, A. I.; Ma, G.; Cutler, S. J.; Ross, S. A. Antileukemic, Antileishmanial and Antifungal Activities of Secondary Metabolites from the Endophytic Fungus *Nigrospora sphaerica. Planta Med.* **2013,** *79*, P52.
74. Rodrigues, A. P. D.; Farias, L. H. S.; Carvalho, A. S. C.; Santos, A.S.; do Nascimento, J. L. M.; Silva, E. O. A Novel Function for Kojic Acid, a Secondary Metabolite from *Aspergillus* Fungi, as Antileishmanial Agent. *Plos One* **2014,** *9*, e91259.
75. Ma, G.; Khan, S. I.; Jacob, M. R.; Tekwani, B. L.; Li, Z.; Pascol, D. S.; Walker,L. A.; Khan, I. A. Antimicrobial and Antileishmanial Activities of Hypocrellins A and B. *Antimicrob. Agents Chemother.* **2004,** *48*, 114450–114452.
76. Martínez-Luis, S.; Della-Togna, G.; Coley, P. D.; Kursar, T. A;. Gerwick William, H.; Cubilla-Rios, L. Antileishmanial Constituents of the Panamanian Endophytic Fungus *Edenia* sp. *J. Nat. Prod.* **2008**, *71* (12), 2011–2014.
77. Awaad, A. S.; Al-Zaylaee, H. M.; Alqasoumi, S. I.; Zain, M. E.; Aloyan, E. M.; Alafeefy, A. M.; Awad, E. S. H.; El-Meligy R. M. Anti-leishmanial Activities of Extracts and Isolated Compounds from *Drechslera rostrata* and *Eurotium tonpholium. Phytotherapy Res.* **2014,** *28* (5), 774–780.
78. Kumar, M.; Tripathi, M. K.; Srivastava, A.; Kumar Gour, J.; Kumar Singh, R.; Tilak, R.; Asthana, R. K. Cyanobacteria, *Lyngbya aestuarii* and *Aphanothece bullosa* as Antifungal and Antileishmanial Drug Resource. *Asian Pac. J. Trop. Biomed.* **2013,** *3* (6), 458–463.
79. Dragonamide, E.; Balunas, M. J.; Linington, R. G.; Tidgewell, K.; Fenner, A. M.; Ureña, L. D.; Togna, G. D.; Kyle, D. E.; Gerwick, W. H. A Modified Linear Lipopeptide from *Lyngbya majuscula* with Antileishmanial Activity. *J. Nat. Prod.* 2010, *73* (1), 60–66.
80. Balunas, M. J.; Grosso, M. F.; Villa, F. A.; Engene, N.; McPhail, K. L.; Tidgewell, K.; Pineda, L. M.; Gerwick, L.; Spadafora, C.; Kyle, D. E.; Gerwick, W. H. Coibacins A-D, Antileishmanial Marine Cyanobacterial Polyketides with Intriguing Biosynthetic Origins. *Organic Lett.* **2012,** *14*, 3878–3881.
81. Simmons, T. L.; Engene, N.; Urena, L. D.; Romero, L. I.; Ortega-Barrı, E.; Gerwick, L.; Gerwick, W. H. Viridamides A and B, Lipodepsipeptides with Antiprotozoal Activity

from the Marine Cyanobacterium *Oscillatoria nigro-viridis*. *J. Nat. Prod.* **2008,** *7*, 1544–1550.

82. Valadares, D. G.; Duarte, M. C.; Oliveira, J. S.; Chávez-Fumagalli, M. A.; Martins, V. T.; Costa, L. E.; Leite, J. P.; Santoro, M. M.; Régis, W. C.; Tavares, C. A.; Coelho, E. A. Leishmanicidal Activity of the *Agaricus blazei* Murill in Different *Leishmania* Species. *Parasitol. Int.* **2011,** *60*, 357–363.
83. Martínez-Luis, S.; Cherigo, L.; Higginbotham, S.; Arnold, E.; Spadafora, C.; Ibañez, A.; Gerwick, W. H.; Cubilla-Rios, L. Screening and Evaluation of Antiparasiticand in vitro Anticancer Activitiesof Panamanian Endophytic Fungi. *Int. Microbiol.* **2011,** *14*, 95–102
84. Pierre, G.; Salah, R.; Gardarin, C.; Traikia, M.; Petit, E.; Delort, A. M.; Mameri, N.; Moulti-Mati, F.; Michaud, P. Enzymatic Degradation and Bioactivity Evaluation of C-6 OxidizedC. *Int. J. Biol. Macromol.* **2013,** *60*, 383–392.
85. Mukherjee, T.; Roy, K.; Bhaduri, A. Acivicin: A Highly Active Potential Chemotherapeutic Agent against Visceral Leishmaniasis. *Biochem. Biophys. Res. Commun.* **1990,** *170* (2), 426–432.
86. Staerk, D.; Lemmich, E.; Christensen, J.; Kharazmi, A.; Erik Olsen, C.; Jaroszewski, J. W. Leishmanicidal, Antiplasmodial and Cytotoxic Activity of Indole Alkaloids from *Corynanthe pachyceras*. *Planta Med.* **2000,** *66*, 531–536.
87. Ashok, P.; Lathiya, H.; Murugesan, S. Manzamine Alkaloids as Antileishmanial Agents: A Review. *Eur. J. Med. Chem.* **2014,** *97*, 928–936.
88. Costa, E. V.; Pinheiro, M. L.; Xavier, C. M.; Silva, J. R.; Amaral, A. C.; Souza, A. D.; Barison, A.; Campos, F. R.; Ferreira, A. G.; Machado, G. M.; Leo, L. L. A Pyrimidine-beta-Carboline and Other Alkaloids from *Annona foetida* with Antileishmanial Activity. *J. Nat. Prod.* **2006,** *69*, 292–294.
89. da Silva, F. M. A.; Koolen, H. H. F.; de Lima, J. P. S.; Santos, D. M. F.;Jardim, I. S.; Souza, A. D. L.; Belém Pinheiro, M. L. Leishmanicidal activity of fractions rich in aporphine alkaloids from Amazonian Unonopsis species. *Brazilian J. Pharmacogn.* **2012,** *22* (6), 1368–1371.
90. Bodley, A. L.; Shapiro T. A. Molecular and Cytotoxic Effects of Camptothecin, a Topoisomerase I Inhibitor, on Trypanosomes and *Leishmania*. *Proc. Natl. Acad. Sci. USA*. **1995,** *92* (9), 3726–3730.
92. Fournet, A.; Angelo Barrios, A.; Muñoz, V.; Hocquemiller, R.; Roblot, F.; Cavé, A.; Richomme, P.; Bruneton, J. Antiprotozoal Activity of Quinoline Alkaloids Isolated from *Galìpea longijlora,* a Bolivian Plant Used as a Treatment for Cutaneous Leishmaniasis. *Phytotherapy Res.* **1994,** *8*, 174–178.
93. Delorenzi, J. C.; Freire-de-Lima, L.; Gattass, C. R.; Andrade Costa, D.; He, L.; Kuehne, M. E.; Saraiva, E. M. B. In *vitro* Activities of Iboga Alkaloid Congeners Coronaridine and 18-Methoxycoronaridine against *Leishmania amazonensis*. *Antimicrob. Agents Chemother.* **2002,** *46* (7), 2111–2115.
94. Mahioua, V.; Roblot, F.; Fournet, A.; Hocquemiller, R. Bisbenzylisoquinoline Alkaloids from *Guatteria boliviana* (Annonaceae). *Phytochemistry* **2000,** *54*, 709–716.
95. Torres-Santos, E. C.; Sampaio-Santos, M.; Buckner, I. F. S., Yokoyama, K.; Gelb, M.; Urbina J. A.; Rossi-Bergmann, B. Altered Sterol Profile Induced in *Leishmania amazonensis* by a Natural Dihydroxymethoxylated Chalcone. *J. Antimicrob. Chemother.* **2009,** *63*, 469–472.
96. Schmeda-Hirschrnann, G.; Razmilic, I.; Sauvain, M.; Moretti, C.; Muiioz, V.; Ruiz, E.; Balanza, E.; Fournet, A. Antiprotozoal Activity of Jatrogrossidione from *Jatropha*

grossidentata and Jatrophone from *Jatropha isabellii. Phytotherapy Res.* **1996,** *10*, 375–378.

97. Mishra, B. B.; Kale, R. R.; Prasad, V.; Tiwari, V. K.; Singh, R. K. Scope of natural products in fighting against leishmaniasis In *Opportunity, Challenge and Scope of Natural Products in Medicinal Chemistry*, Research Signpost: Varanasi, India, 2011; pp 121–154.
98. Kolodziej, H.; Burmeister, A.; Trun, W.; Radtke, O. A.; Kiderlen, A. F.; Ito, H.; Hatano, T.; Yoshidac, T.; Foo, L. Y. Tannins and Related Compounds Induce Nitric Oxide Synthase and Cytokines Gene Expressions in *Leishmania major*-infected Macrophage-like RAW 264.7 Cells. *Bioorg. Med. Chem.* **2005,** *13*, 6470–6476.

CHAPTER 7

ELEMENTS SUPPLEMENTATION IN LEISHMANIASIS

CONTENTS

7.1 INTRODUCTION

Macro and micronutrient deficiencies are a significant problem among people in rural areas in developing countries. Deficiencies may lead to an impaired immune system making the organism vulnerable to infections and diseases. Leishmaniasis is an infectious disease, endemic in 21 countries in America, and 39 million people in America are at risk for acquiring the disease. Malnutrition and micronutrient deficiencies are likely to interfere with several important functions of the immune system resulting in an impaired capability to overcome the leishmaniasis infection; nutritional status of the host is a key factor for the outcome of infection. Supplementation of macro and micronutrients under traditional medicine prescription may be a better strategy to heal immune-compromised aliments like *Leishmania.* Role of different elements in leishmaniasis is described in Table 7-1.

7.2 IRON *(LAUHA KALPAS)*

Infection with the protozoan parasite *Leishmania* impairs the health of millions of people throughout the world. Amastigotes are the most important *Leishmania* life cycle forms in the context of human disease. Iron (Fe) transport is a major factor regulating the transition of promastigotes to amastigotes. A report suggested that Fe supplementation whether used prophylactically or therapeutically, promoted parasite (*Leishmania donovani*) multiplication.[1] It has been reported that that low Fe in the environment is a potent trigger for the differentiation of noninfective promastigotes into infective amastigotes.[2]This report clearly indicate that Fe depletion from the culture medium triggered expression of the ferrous Fe transporter LIT1 (*Leishmania* Fe transporter 1), an increase in Fe content of the parasites, growth arrest, and differentiation of wild-type (WT) promastigotes into infective amastigotes. In contrast, development of mutant, *LIT1*-null promastigotes showed reduced intracellular Fe content and sustained growth in Fe-poor media, followed by cell death.[2] Vale-Costa et al. (2013) recently reported that supplementation of Fe improves the host's capacity to eliminate *Leishmania infantum.*[3] Furthermore, Fe levels were found to be lower in patients with acute and chronic cutaneous leishmaniasis than in the control group (Faryadi and Mohebali, 2003).[4] These reports demonstrated that the direct toxicity of Fe against *Leishmania* advises a potential use of this metal as a therapeutic tool or the further exploration of Fe anti-parasitic mechanisms for the design

TABLE 7-1 Role of different elements in leishmaniasis

Element name	Ayurvedic	Current reported work	Ref.
Iron	*Lauha Kalpas*	Iron supplementation improves the host's capacity to eliminate *L. infantum* parasites through interaction with reactive oxygen and nitrogen species	2, 3
Cu	*Munivreehi, Sharkara, Dhanyaka, Panchamrut-Parpati, Kutaj-Parpati, Triphala, Sukshma-Triphala, Patol, Patha, Kutki and Rohitak like Panchamrut-Parpati*	Wilson disease (copper is deposited in the brain and liver) is susceptible to those patients that are suffering from visceral leishmaniasis (Pandey et al., 2007).	9
Zn	*Chintamoni rasa, Mrutasanijivani rasa, Pratapa tapana rasa, Yasadamruta ointment, Visweswara rasa, Pitalla rasayana*	Zinc deficiency possibly increases vulnerability and endemicity of visceral leishmaniasis	9, 19
K	Panchakarma therapy, *Aarogya vardhini* ras, *Vasadi ghan, Anchamrut loh*	Hypokalaemia (muscular weakness and associated tiredness, cardiac ventricular arrhythmias, polydipsia) during the treatment of *Leishmania* may sometime lead to rhabdomyolysis. Potassium supplementation should prevent this side effect.	17, 16
Vit A,B, C, and E	Alma (for vitamin c)	Prophylactic administration of vitamin C significantly reduced the intake of *Leishmania donovani* in hamsters but had no therapeutic effect. In contrast, vitamins A, B complex, and E, whether used prophylactically or therapeutically, promoted parasite multiplication.	1
Mg		Serum Mg was increased in chronic VL as compared to acute cases.	19

TABLE 7-1 *(Continued)*

Element name	Ayurvedic	Current reported work	Ref.
Ca		Tetany is usually caused by low ionized serum calcium concentration which causes increased excitability of peripheral nerves resulting in carpo-pedal spasm, convulsion and stridor.	15, 29, 30
Aresnic and antimony	*Pravala bhsasma, Tamra bhasma*, *Yakrit pleehodarari loha*	Arsenicals and antimonials are first line drugs for the treatment of trypanosomal and leishmanial diseases. Because arsenic and antimony are related metalloids, and arsenical resistant *Leishmania* strains are frequently cross-resistant to antimonials.	31
Mercury	*Mahkardhawja mercury, Parad, Hingwastika, Trifla, Guggulu, Praval pishti, Ekangvir ras, Yograj guggul, Agnitundi bunti, Arogya vardhini banti*	HgCl2 treatment enhances the susceptibility to L. major in SJL mice consistent with the induction of host Th2 parameters. These findings have implications for the role of mercury contamination in areas of endemic leishmaniasis.	32
Selenium	Food sources such as garlic, onion, wheat germs and red grapes contain selenium in sufficient amount	Selenium (Se) is an essential trace element for *Leishmania* organisms and is present in proteins as selenocysteine (Sec or U), an amino acid that is chemically distinct from serine and cysteine by a single atom (Se instead of O or S, respectively). Sec is incorporated into selenoproteins. Plasma selenium, zinc, and iron concentrations were significantly lower and copper concentrations was significantly higher in patients with CL than those of healthy controls. Some reports related with anti-leishmanial properties selenium NPs have more and less cytotoxic effects than SeO_2 against *L. infantum*	25–27

of new drugs. Therefore, this may justify importance of Fe against intracellular infections.

Contemporary medicine advises Fe supplements in Fe deficiency anemia. Several reports already proven that the *Leishmania* parasite induces *anemia* in by differentially altering erythropoiesis in bone marrow and spleen. In folk medicine, there are various types of prescriptions recommended for Fe supplementation. Ayurvedic classics also quote significant information about administration of Fe. *Lauha Kalpas* are the unique compound herbo-mineral formulations where Fe (*Lauha*) is used as a major ingredient. Various prepeartions of *Lauha Kalpas* that are mentioned in *Bhaishajya Ratnavali, Charaka Samhita, Rasendra Sara* Samgraha, and so forth were known for their profound effect in various ailment. Critical analysis of these *Lauha Kalpas* reveals that ancient seers administered Fe in a better acceptable form. In Ayurveda, *Lauha Kalpas* are present in form of Khalviya preparations (medicine is prepared grinding the ingredients in a *Khalva Yantra* i.e., with mortar and pestle), *Churna* (powders), *Avaleha* (confectionaries), *Rasakriya* (solidified decoctions), and *Putapaka* (incinerated) preparations. Apart from solid dosage forms, semisolid dosage forms mentioned in classics are very much useful.[5]

7.3 ZINC *(YASADA, RASAKA, OR KHARPARA)*

Zinc (Zn) is essential trace elements of great importance for many enzymes and biological processes and their deficits or excesses may lead to different health problems. It has been introduced as a drug in the prevention and treatments of diseases since past two decades. Zn deficiency in particular has a great impact on the defense mechanisms of the body and the immune response to infections. Zn plays an important role in *Leishmania.* In a few studies, patients with cutaneous leishmaniasis were injected with Zn sulfate under the skin. One previous report demonstrated the role of oral Zn sulphate in both treatment and prophylaxis for cutaneous leishmaniasis.[6] Mishra et al. (2009) reported the low serum Zn levels, in healthy subjects from Bihar and more significantly in visceral leishmaniasis (VL) patients of this region, are possibly associated with vulnerability and endemicity of VL in the region. Mishra et al. (2009) also suggested role of oral Zn supplementation in better management and prevention of VL, particularly in endemic areas.[7] Zn and Fe levels were found to be lower in patients with acute and chronic cutaneous leishmaniasis than in the control group.[3] Zn deficiency in VL indicates possible therapeutic administration of Zn in these severe forms of leishmaniasis. The process of elimination of intracellular pathogens, such as *Leishmania*, requires a Th1 type immune response, whereas a dominant Th2 response leads to exacerbated disease. Experimental human Zn deficiency decreases Th1 but not Th2 immune response. A recent report suggested the Serum Zn levels were much decreased were increased in chronic VL as compared to acute cases.[8] Weyenbergh et al. (2004) demonstrated the Zn deficiency in VL and mucocutaneous leishmaniasis (MCL) and its possible therapeutic administration in these severe forms of leishmaniasis.[9] These reports suggest that the Zn supplementation may prevent or decrease the severity of infection. The Ayurvedic physicians have practiced both oral and topical applications of Zn after *sodhana* (purification) and *marana* (calcification) before 14th century A.D. *Rasaka* or *Kharpara* (Zn ore or Zn carbonate), *Yasada* (Zn metal), *Puspanjana* (Zn oxide), and *Pittala* (brass) are Zn-containing minerals used as therapeutic agents in Ayurveda. *Rasaka* or *Kharpara* are found in most (20 i.e., 66.66%) of the formulations, *Yasada* (Zn metal) in 5 (16.66%), *Pittala* (brass) in 4 (13.33%) and *Puspanjana* (Zn oxide) is used in one formulation.[10] *B. Chintamoni rasa* (spleen and liver growth, fever), *Mrutasanijivani rasa* (fever, anemia, edema), *Pratapa tapana rasa* (Intermittent fever), *Yasadamruta ointment* (all types of skin diseases, fistula); *Visweswara rasa* (all types fever, night fever, irregular fever), *Pitalla rasayana* (vigor and vitality) and many others are known to Zn-based Ayurvedic formulations that are extensively utilized for various ailments.[10] A report also suggested that the *Zn bhasma* appears safe for human use.[11]

Serum Zn levels were much decreased in chronic VL as compared to acute cases. Zn deficiency in VL indicates possible therapeutic administration of Zn in these severe forms of leishmaniasis. The process of elimination of intracellular pathogens, such as *Leishmania,* requires a Th1 type immune response, whereas a dominant Th2 response leads to exacerbated disease. Experimental human Zn deficiency decreases Th1 but not Th2 immune response.

7.4 COPPER

Copper (Cu) is also an essential trace elements of great importance for many enzymes and biological processes. It was founded that serum Cu concentration was found to be significantly higher in the patients with acute and chronic cutaneous leishmaniasis than those of control group.[9] Environmentally or genetically determined increases in Cu levels might augment susceptibility to infection with intracellular pathogens, by causing a decrease in interferon-γ production.[9] *Furthermore,* no statistically significant differences founded in serum Cu level in patients with acute and chronic cutaneous leishmaniasis.[4] Wilson disease (Cu is deposited in the brain and liver) is susceptible to those patients that are suffering from VL.[12]

Recent report also demonstrated the high antileishmanial activity of various Cu complexes. Thiosemicarbazones and their metallic complexes are an important class of compounds that have been extensively studied in recent years, mainly because of their broad profile of pharmacological activity. Benzaldehyde thiosemicarbazone derived from limonene complexed with Cu induced lipoperoxidation and the production of mitochondrial superoxide anion radicals in promastigotes and axenic amastigotes of *Leishmania amazonensis*.[13]

In Ayurveda, Cu poisoning or its related ailments can be healed by administration of *Munivreehi*, *Sharkara*, and *Dhanyaka* for 3 days (*Rasaratna samucchaya* and *Arogya prakasha*). Most individuals need a lifelong chelating therapy to reduce Cu deposition. Ayurvedic treatment is aimed at improving the excretion of Cu through the liver and from the intestines with the help of specific herbal medicines that promote excretion of harmful and toxic substances from the body. The basic pathology of Wilson disease is treated by using medicines like *Panchamrut-Parpati, Kutaj-Parpati, Triphala* (Three fruits), *Sukshma-Triphala*, *Patol* (*Tricosanthe dioica*), *Patha* (*Cissampelos pareira*), *Kutki*, and *Rohitak*. These medicines reduce the absorption of Cu from the intestines and increase Cu excretion from the liver, and need to be given long term in order to reduce the effects resulting from excessive Cu deposition in the body. Consuming spirulina has been found to reduce the toxicity due to Cu. It also increases the blood circulation and promotes growth. Regular intake of Spirulina causes the excess Cu to get expelled from the body. Most of the wastes get expelled through feces from the body.

7.5 POTASSIUM

Physiological saline with potassium chloride (KCl) supplementation plays an important role in *Leishmania*. It has been suggested that salt loading protects against amphotericin B (AmB)-induced nephrotoxicity. It is very important to study the influence of saline loading on the nephrotoxic response to AmB in patients who were diagnosed with MCL. Llanos et al. (1991) reported that serum potassium (K) levels fell during supplementation of saline on AmB nephrotoxicity.[14] The saline group required significantly greater amounts of K supplementation to maintain a normal serum K. Oral K supplementation to maintain a normal serum K. Further report suggested that supplementation of AmB physiologic saline and KCl during treatment could help to prevent an increase in serum creatinine levels and severe rigor and would make the treatment of kala-azar with AmB easier.[15] Post-kala-azar dermal leishmaniasis (PKDL) is a neglected complication of VL—a deadly, infectious disease that claims approximately 20,000 to 40,000 lives every year. PKDL is thought to be a reservoir for transmission of VL, thus, adequate control of PKDL plays a key role in the ongoing effort to eliminate VL. Treatment of PKDL suffering patients with AmB formulation causes hypokalemia, which may lead to rhabdomyolysis. Many patients probably have mild or moderate hypokalemia during treatment, and only a few progresses to rhabdomyolysis. K supplementation should prevent this side effect.[16,17] Ayurveda and herbal medicine could be a hope for correcting the rhabdomyolysis. According to Ayurveda, *Panchakarma* is cleansing of the body. These is a set of five (*panch* = five in Sanskrit) procedures. They are *Vamana, Virechana, Nirooha, Nasya*, and *Anuvasana. Nirooha, Anuvasana*, and *Uttaravasthi* form the basic types of *Vasthi* purification technique in Ayurveda called *Panchakarma* which is very effective for correcting this type of disorder. These procedures include whole body massage with medicated oils, streaming of medicinal oil on forehead, herbalized stream treatment, nasal administration of medicinal oils, emesis, purgation, and enemas. *Aarogya vardhini* ras (2 tablets twice a day), *Vasadi ghan* (2 tablets twice day), or *Anchamrut loh* (guggle 2 tablets) twice a day are the general prescriptions that are frequently used to treat hypokalemia. Some herbs are also responsible hypokalemic-induced rhabdomyolysis. Toyohara et al. (2008) reported the hypokalemic rhabdomyolysis induced by the low dose daily intake of licorice (2.0 g/day).[18] Similar report is also available on *Ginkgo biloba*. Administration of such herbal medicine and its related products can aggravate the condition. Thus prior consultation from herbalist or Ayurvedic expert is required for starting the suitable medication.

7.6 MAGNESIUM

Magnesium (Mg) deficiency aggravates hypokalemia, which often becomes refractory to treatment. Serum Mg could be a potential prognosis factor for chronic VL patients. AmB, also in liposomal form, induces Mg wasting further worsening a possible deficiency. It has been suggested that the high prevalence of eclampsia among young Bangladeshi women is explained by high rates of Mg deficiency.[16] But there are some strong evidences depicting the role of Mg^{2+} in increasing parasite proliferation. Lal et al. (2012) serum Mg was increased in chronic VL as compared to acute cases.[19] Hypermagnesemia is a rare electrolyte abnormality because the kidney is very effective in excreting excess Mg.

7.7 CALCIUM

There are only few reports that indicate that *Leishmania* parasite may often cause hypercalcemia.[20] A report also suggested that a leishmaniasis patient who suffers from liver problems often becomes hypercalcemic.[21] In contrast, there are some reports available on hypercalcemia induced by few anti-leishmanial drugs such as paromomycin, and AmB.[22] According to a report AmB-induced hypomagnesemia caused hypoparathyroidism and hypocalcemia in thalassemia patient and all three abnormalities resolved after the drug was withdrawn. Similarly drugs, for example, paromomycin, that are used in the treatment of *Leishmania* may cause tetany (low ionized serum calcium concentration). Drugs, for example, paromomycin, that are used in the treatment of *Leishmania* may cause tetany. Prompt detection of symptoms and intravenous calcium gluconate treatment promptly reverse the situation. To get the herbal treatment, some leishmaniasis patients of Indian origin applies curcumin extract on the skin wounds caused by *Leishmania* parasite. However, treatment with curcumin leads to the elevation of cytosolic calcium. Therefore, proper consultation with Ayurvedic expert is required to get the proper Ayurvedic treatment against this disease.

7.8 ANTIMONY AND ARSENIC

Antimony and arsenic are elements that have a long history of use as poisons, therapeutic agents, or cosmetics. For over a century, compounds containing pentavalent antimony (antimonials) have formed the basis of treatment of the leishmaniases worldwide. Antimonial preparations remain first-line drugs for VL. In modern science, antimony preparations are used. Probably it may have been influenced by Ayurveda because even in Ayurveda antimony is used as *Shuddha neelanjana* in the dose of 100 mg with *Pravala bhsasma*, *Tamra bhasma* each 100 mg along with *Yakrit pleehodarari loha* (100 mg).[23] Treatment with antimony has been started in 1925.[24] Clarke in his prescriber says that antimony is the antidote to kala-azar. Calcutta Medical Club (1962) reported the use of antimony in the treatment of kala-azar (Calcutta Medical Journal, Volume 59). Homeopathic remedies for kala-azar (related to antimony and arsenic compounds) are *Antimonium crudrum, Antim metallicum or Antim tart*, and *Ferrum arsenicosum*.

Recent research in India explored that arsenic contamination may have played a significant role in the development of *Leishmania* antimonial resistance in Bihar because inadequate treatment with antimonial drugs is not exclusive to India, whereas widespread antimonial resistance is.

Arsenicals and antimonials are first-line drugs for the treatment of trypanosomal and leishmanial diseases.

To create the active form of the drug, Sb(V) must be reduced to Sb(III). Because arsenic and antimony are related metalloids, and arsenical-resistant *Leishmania* strains are frequently cross-resistant to antimonials.

Arsenic treatment resulted in an elevation of intracellular Ca^{2+} levels that did not occur with antimony exposure. Cellular glutathione level was reduced after antimony treatment but arsenic did not affect glutathione. Inhibition of Ca^{2+} influx during arsenic treatment reduced cell death, whereas supplementation of glutathione during antimony treatment rescued cell loss. Under Fe-depleted conditions, the cytotoxic effects of arsenic and antimony did not occur and cell survival increased; in contrast, the presence of excess Fe resulted in higher cell death. Therefore, Fe can potentiate parasite death.

In United States, Ayurvedic medicines are sold under the dietary supplement act of 1994 and are considered as dietary supplements. As such they are not required to meet rigorous standard for conventional medicines. In some cases, metals are a part of the formulation. *Bhasmas* are an example of such medicinal preparations that are combinations of metals, herbal juices, and fruits. It is believed that, as used metals exists as nanoparticles and are rendered nontoxic effects when they complex with the components of medicinal plants. Some of the Ayurvedic formulations that are contaminated with arsenic are *Trifla guggulu* and *Yograj guggulu.*

7.9 MERCURY

Leshmania is a life-threatening disease. The severity of disease is dependent on the *Leishmania* strain as well as the immune status of the infected host. Because of the strong immunomodulatory properties of mercury in promoting Th2-type responses, it is worth worthy to discuss its role in *Leishmania.* It has been found that mercury treatment enhances the susceptibility against the *Leishmania* parasite, possibly via an upregulation of Th2 responses. Mercury-treated mice exhibit a dramatic activation of Th2 cells, marked by production of IL-4 and IL-4-mediated increases in serum IgE and IgG, which may probably lead to the enhancement of susceptibility to *Leishmania major*. These reports may have potential implications for human leishmaniasis in endemic areas, which often have high environmental levels of mercury pollution.

In *siddha mahkardhawja,* mercury is present as sulfide as a component. *Bhasma* called as *parad* also contain mercury as a cative principal. Products such as *hingwastika, trifla guggulu, praval pishti, ekangvir ras, yograj guggul, agnitundi bunti,* and *arogyavardhini banti (badyanath)* contain mercury were present in Indian market as Ayurvedic medicine. Precaution should be taken while administering any mercury-based Ayurvedic formulations to the *Leishmania* patient.

7.10 SELENIUM

Selenium (Se) is an essential trace element for *Leishmania* organisms and is present in proteins as selenocysteine (Sec or U), an amino acid that is chemically distinct from serine and cysteine by a single atom (Se instead of O or S, respectively). Se is incorporated into selenoproteins. Plasma Se, Zn, and Fe concentrations were significantly lower and Cu concentrations were significantly higher in patients with cutaneous leishmaniasis than those of healthy controls. Some reports related with antileishmanial properties Selenium nanoparticles (NPs) have more and less cytotoxic effects than SeO_2 against *L. infantum.*[25–27]

According to Ayurveda, glutathione which is required for healthy immune function contains four atoms of Se atoms. Thus, it is a main component of glutathione peroxide. This trace mineral is therefore a crucial component of the glutathione system. The body obtains Se from food and water and tissue level tends to match Se levels in the surrounding environment. Deficiency of Se leads to cardiomyopathy of keshan. Se toxicity causes loss of hairs, nails, dermatitis, and so forth. Food sources such as garlic, onion, wheat germs, and red grapes contain Se in sufficient amount.[28]

7.11 VITAMIN C

Prophylactic administration of vitamin C significantly reduced the intake of *L. donovani* in hamsters but had no therapeutic effect. In contrast, vitamins

A, B complex, and E if used prophylactically or therapeutically, promoted parasite multiplication. Amla contains high amount of vitamin C that is every 100 g of fresh fruit contains 460 to 685 mg of vitamin C.

KEYWORDS

- **Ayurved**
- **elements**
- **kala azar**
- **leishmaniasis**
- **supplementation**

REFERENCES

1. Garg, R.; Singh, N.; Dube, A. Intake of Nutrient Supplements Affects Multiplication of *Leishmania donovani* in Hamsters. *Parasitology* **2004,** *129*, 685–691.
2. Mittra, B.; Cortez, M.; Haydock, A.; Ramasamy, G.; Myler, P. J.; Andrews, N. W. Iron Uptake Controls the Generation of *Leishmania* Infective Forms through Regulation of ROS Levels. *J. Exp. Med.* **2013,** *210* (2), 401–416.
3. Vale-Costa, S.; Gomes-Pereira, S.; Teixeira, C. M.; Rosa, G.; Rodrigues, P. N, Appelberg, A. T. R.; Gomes, M. S. Iron Overload Favors the Elimination of *Leishmania infantum* from Mouse Tissues through Interaction with Reactive Oxygen and Nitrogen Species. *PLoS Negl. Trop. Dis.* 2013, *7* (2), e2061.
4. Faryadi, M.; Mohebali, M. Alterations of Serum Zinc, Copper and Iron Concentrations in Patients with Acute and Chronic Cutaneous Leishmaniasis. *Iranian J. Publ. Health* **2003,** *32* (4), 53–58.
5. Gupta, K. L. V.; Pallavi, G.; Patgiri, B. J.; Galib, Prajapati, P. K. Critical Review on the Pharmaceutical Vistas of Lauha Kalpas (Iron Formulations). *J. Ayurveda Integr. Med.*. **2012,** *3*, 21–28.
6. Najim, R. A.; Sharquie, K. E.; Farjou, I. B. Zinc Sulphate in the Treatment of Cutaneous Leishmaniasis: An in Vitro and Animal Study. *Mem. Inst. Oswaldo Cruz*. **1998,** *93* (6), 831–837.
7. Mishra J.; Carpenter S.; Singh S. Low Serum Zinc Levels in an Endemic Area of Visceral Leishmaniasis in Bihar, India. *Indian J. Med. Res.* **2010,** *131*, 793–798.
8. Lal, C. S.; Kumar, S.; Ranjan, A.; Rabidas, V. N.; Verma, N.; Pandey, K.; Verma, R. B.; Das, S.; Singh, D.; Das, P. Comparative Analysis of Serum Zinc, Copper, Magnesium, Calcium and Iron Level in Acute and Chronic Patients of Visceral Leishmaniasis. *J. Trace Elem. Med. Biol.* **2013,** *27* (2), 98–102.
9. Weyenbergh, J. V.; Santana, G.; D'Oliveira, A.; Santos, A. F.; Costa, C. H.; Carvalho, E. M.; Barral, A.; Barral-Netto, M. Zinc/Copper Imbalance Reflects Immune

Dysfunction in Human Leishmaniasis: An ex vivo and in vitro Study. *BMC. Infectious Dis.* **2004,** *4*, 50.

10. Panda, A. K.; Rout, S. Zinc in Ayurvedic Herbo-mineral Products. *Natural Product Radiance* **2006,** *5* (4), 284–288.
11. Umrani, R. D.; Paknikar, K. M. Ayurvedic Medicine Zinc Bhasma: Physicochemical Evaluation, Anti-diabetic Activity and Safety Assessment. *J. Biomed. Nanotechnol.* **2011,** *7* (1), 148–149.
12. Pandey, K.; Sinha, P. K.; Das, V. N. R.; Kumar, N.; Verma, N.; Bimal, S.; Lal, C. S.; Topno, R. K.; Singh, D.; Verma, R. B.; Bhattacharya, S. K.; Das, P. Wilson Disease with Visceral Leishmaniasis: An Extremely Uncommon Presentation. *Am. J. Trop. Med. Hyg.* **2007,** *77* (3), 560–561.
13. Britta, E. A.; Barbosa Silva, A. P.; Ueda-Nakamura, T.; Dias-Filho, B. P.; Silva, C. C.; Sernaglia, R. L.; Nakamura, C. V. Benzaldehyde Thiosemicarbazone Derived from Limonene Complexed with Copper Induced Mitochondrial Dysfunction in *Leishmania amazonensis. PLoS One* **2012,** *7* (8).
14. Llanos, A.; Cieza, J.; Bernardo, J.; Echevarria, J.; Biaggioni, I.; Sabra, R.; Branch, R. A. Effect of Salt Supplementation on Amphotericin B Nephrotoxicity. *Kidney Int.* **1991,** *40*, 302–308.
15. Thakur, C. P.; Kumar, A.; Mitra, D. K.; Roy, A.; Sinha, A. K.; Ranjan, A. Improving Outcome of Treatment of Kala-azar by Supplementation of Amphotericin B with Physiologic Saline and Potassium Chloride. *Am. J. Trop. Med. Hyg.* **2010,** *83* (5), 1040–1043.
16. Marking, U.; Boer, M. D.; Das, A. K.; Ahmed, E. M.; Rollason, V.; Ahmed, B.; Davidson, R. N.; Ritmeijer, K. Hypokalaemia-Induced Rhabdomyolysis after Treatment of Post-Kala-azar Dermal Leishmaniasis (PKDL) with High-Dose AmBisome in Bangladesh-A Case Report. *PLoS Negl. Trop. Dis.* **2014,** *8* (6), e2864.
17. Desjeux, P.; Ghosh, R. S.; Dhalaria, P.; Strub-Wourgaft, N.; Zijlstra, E. E. *Report of the Post Kala-Azar Dermal* Leishmaniasis *(PKDL), Consortium Meeting, New Delhi, India, 27–29, June 2012. Parasit. Vectors* 2013, 6, 196.
18. Toyohara, T.; Tanemoto, M.; Uruno, A.; Abe, M.; Abe, T.; Ito, S. Case of Rhabdomyolysis Induced by the Approved Daily Dose of a Traditional Chinese Medicine. *Nihon Jinzo Gakkai Shi.* **2008,** *50* (2), 135–139.
19. Lal, C. S.; Kumar, S.; Ranjan, A.; Rabidas, V. N.; Verma, N.; Pandey, K.; Verma, R. B.; Das, S.; Singh, D.; Das, P. Comparative Analysis of Serum Zinc, Copper, Magnesium, Calcium and Iron Level in Acute and Chronic Patients of Visceral Leishmaniasis. *J. Trace Elem. Med. Biol.* **2013,** *27* (2), 98–102.
20. Freeman, K. S.; Miller, M. D.; Breitschwerdt, E. B.; Lappin, M. R. Leishmaniasis in a Dog Native to Colorado. *J. Am. Vet. Med. Assoc.* **2010,** *237* (11), 1288–1291.
21. Aladesanmi, O.; Jin, X. W.; Nielsen, C. *A 56-Year-old Man with Hypercalcemia. Cleve. Clin. J. Med.* 2005, 72, 707–712
22. Marcus, N.; Garty, B. Z. Transient Hypoparathyroidism due to Amphotericin B-induced Hypomagnesemia in a Patient with Beta-thalassemia. *Ann Pharmacother.* **2001,** *35* (9), 1042–1044.
23. Devaraj, T. L. Speaking of ayurvedic remedies. In *Speaking of Ayurvedic Remedies*; New Dawn Press, New Delhi, India, 2005.
24. Ghose, R. C. *The Homoeopathic Director*; Arya Chemical Works, Ltd.: Calcutta, India, 1925; pp 5–6.

25. Kocyigit, A.; Gur, S.; Erel, O.; Gurel, M. S. Associations among Plasma Selenium, Zinc, Copper, and Iron Concentrations and Immunoregulatory Cytokine Levels in Patients with Cutaneous Leishmaniasis. *Biol. Trace Elem. Res.* **2002,** *90* (1-3), 47–55.
26. da Silva, M. T.; Silva-Jardim, I.; Thiemann, O. H. Biological Implications of Selenium and its Role in Trypanosomiasis Treatment. *Curr. Med. Chem.* **2014,** *21* (15), 1772–1780.
27. Soflaei, S.; Dalimi, A.; Abdoli, A,; Kamali, M.; Nasiri, V.; Shakibaie, M.; Tat, M. Anti-leishmanial Activities of Selenium Nanoparticles and Selenium Dioxide on *Leishmania infantum. Comp. Clinical Pathol.* 2014, 23, 15–20.
28. Sharma, H.; Clark, C. Ayurvedic healing: Contemporary Maharishi Ayurveda. In *Medicine and Science*; Singing Dragon: London, United Kingdom, 2011; p 120.
29. Das, R.; Roy, A.; Data, N.; Majumde H. K. Reactive Oxygen Species and Imbalance of Calcium Homeostasis Contributes to Curcumin Induced Programmed Cell Death in *L. donovani. Apoptosis* **2008,** *13*, 867–882.
30. Thakur, C. P. Tetany in Kala Azar Patients Treated with Paromomycin. *Indian J. Med. Res.* **2008,** *127*, 489–493.
31. Ashish M.; Chandrima, S. Mechanism of Metalloid-induced Death in *Leishmania* spp.: Role of Iron, Reactive Oxygen Species, Ca^{2+}, and Glutathione. *Free Radical Biol. Med.* **2006,** *40* (10), 1857–1868.
32. Bagenstose, L. M.; Mentink-Kane, M. M.; Brittingham, A.; Mosser, D. M.; Monestier, M. Mercury Enhances Susceptibility to Murine Leishmaniasis. *Parasite Immunol.* **2001,** *23* (12), 633–640.

CHAPTER 8

ALTERNATIVE THERAPIES FOR LEISHMANIASIS

CONTENTS

PART VIII ALTERNATIVE THERAPIES FOR LEISHMANIASIS

ABSTRACT

There are several alternative therapies available for leishmaniasis. Among these therapies, we are chiefly focusing on oil, chelation, and acupuncture therapies. Plant essential oils used traditionally in folk medicine are emerging as alternative sources for chemotherapeutic compounds. Recently various antileishmanian plants are identified. Antileishmanian activities of these plants are based on their essential oils. These essential oils can be used in form of combined therapy for monotherapeutic regimen. Acupuncture is a well-known form of Asian medical treatment and it is used not only as an effective curative method but also to prevent illness and maintain health. In recent years, intensive studies have been carried out to explain the underlying mechanisms of the efficacy of acupuncture in leishmaniasis. Chelation is also one of the most effective treatments and is a safe alternative to various diseases.

8.1 INTRODUCTION

Leishmaniasis is a neglected tropical disease caused by *Leishmania* parasite. Leishmaniasis is one of the most important parasitic infections, but current treatments are unsatisfactory due to their toxicity, cost, and resistance. Therefore, the development of new antileishmanial compounds is imperative. Many people who live in endemic areas use plants as an alternative to treat the disease. The search for new immunopharmacological chemical agents to treat various diseases caused by bacteria, fungi, and protozoa, such as leishmaniasis, for example, has led to the exploration of potential products from plant species and their main active ingredients. Antimonial drugs are the current treatment for leishmaniasis. There is currently no vaccine against leishmaniasis, and chemotherapy remains the only effective control. These drugs cause major side effects and frequent discontinuation of treatment. Recent research on plants has shown a successful approach to obtain new antileishmanial alternatives. Medicinal and aromatic plants constitute a major source of natural organic compounds. Plant essential oils (EOs) used traditionally in folk medicine are emerging as alternative sources for chemotherapeutic compounds. Several plant EOs exert their independent antileishmanial activity. In most of the cases, it was observed that isolated components of EO exert lesser antileishmanial potential then whole oil fraction. After increased unresponsiveness to most of the monotherapeutic regimens, the combination therapy has found new scope in the treatment of both cutaneous and visceral leishmaniasis. In addition, the combination of antileishmanial drugs could reduce the potential toxic side effects and prevent drug resistance. There are various reports that demonstrated the role of various EOs in combined therapy for monotherapeutic regimen. For those reasons, it is important to critically evaluate the role of combination therapy as new data.

Chelation therapy has also been proven effective in the removal of heavy toxic metals and other harmful substances that have entered the body through food, water, and environmental pollution. Once these damaging metals are removed, the body has greater access to the vital nutrients obtained through diet and supplements. The most common form of intravenous chelation therapy is with ethylenediaminetetraacetic acid (EDTA), and when properly used, it has been found to be nontoxic. This therapy is administered by intravenous infusion which is significantly different from the oral chelation therapy for general measures. Interfering in ion-dependent processes in *Leishmania* may be an interesting approach to defeat these microorganisms.

Acupuncture is a well-known form of Asian medical treatment and it is used not only as an effective curative method but also to prevent illness and maintain health. In China, acupuncture has been used in the treatment of several diseases for at least 5200 years. Acupuncture has a beneficial effect when treating many diseases and painful conditions, and therefore it is thought to be useful as a complementary therapy or to replace generally accepted pharmacological intervention. The basic health concept in traditional Chinese medicine consists of the body's vital energy, circulating unidirectionally through a complex network of channels (meridians) just beneath the skin, but also moving within blood vessels. It permeates organs and tissues, and is behind all physiological processes. Health is the harmonious, uninterrupted flow of body's vital energy, and disease ensues when there is disruption of body's vital energy flow. Large randomized trials demonstrating the immediate and sustained effect of acupuncture are missing. It is used for the production of analgesic effect, stress-related physical-mental disorders and homeostasis. The attributive effect of acupuncture has been investigated in inflammatory diseases, including asthma, rhinitis, inflammatory bowel disease, rheumatoid arthritis, epicondylitis, complex regional pain syndrome type 1, and vasculitis. Factors that can affect body's vital energy flow include emotional states such as anxiety, stress, anger, fear or grief, poor nutrition, weather conditions, hereditary factors, infections, and trauma. A number of observations on the anti-inflammatory actions of acupuncture have been published for various acupoints, acupuncture frequencies, and additional application of electrostimulation. Electroacupuncture (EA) stimulation, an application of electrical current on acupuncture needles, is one of the most popular types of this traditional therapy. By inserting needles, the acupuncturist tries to recover the equilibrium between physical, emotional, and spiritual aspects of the individual, and to improve energy flow and energy quality. Additional activation can be obtained through manipulation of the needle or electrostimulation at different frequencies. The insertion of a needle into an acupoint induces the release of pro-inflammatory mediators such as substance P, calcitonin gene-related peptide, histamine, bradykinin, serotonin, proteases, pro-inflammatory cytokines, and others, thereby causing vasodilatation and producing danger signals that are transmitted *via* the afferent vagus nerve. Mechanisms underlying the ascribed immunosuppressive actions of acupuncture is essential to understand the huge gap between specific skin point applications and immune responses. An increase in the release of endogen opioid peptides is generally accepted to be a keystone pathway that affects the immune system after the acupuncture application. The acupuncture-controlled release of neuropeptides from nerve endings and subsequent vasodilative and anti-inflammatory effects through calcitonine gene-related peptide is hypothesized. The complex interactions with substance P, the analgesic contribution of b-endorphin and the balance between cell-specific pro-inflammatory and anti-inflammatory cytokines tumor necrosis factor-α (TNF) and interleukin (IL)-10 are discussed. In response to these stimuli, the hypothalamus secretes corticotropin-releasing hormone (CRH), which leads to a decrease in pro-inflammatory cytokines and an increase in anti-inflammatory cytokines such as IL-10. Leukocytes also respond to CRH and secrete anti-inflammatory cytokines.

8.2 OIL-BASED THERAPY

8.2.1 EUGENIA UNIFLORA

Eugenia uniflora L. is a member of the Myrtaceae family and is commonly known as Brazilian cherry tree contains EO of 32 compounds, which constituted 92.65% of the total oil composition. The most abundant components were sesquiterpenes (91.92%), with curzerene (47.3%), γ-elemene (14.25%), and trans-β-elemenone (10.4%) being the major constituents. In addition, potential antileishmanial activity of its EO fraction was explored by increases in both the phagocytic capacity and the lysosomal activity.[1]

8.2.2 SYZYGIUM AROMATICUM

Researchers have been examining whether clove oil could be used to treat visceral leishmaniasis. Researchers in India found that the EO of clove possesses significant activity against this parasite when tested with mice. The parasites attack the macrophages of the immune system. Clove oil did not have cytotoxic effects against healthy macrophage cells. The study authenticated the promising antileishmanial activity of clove oil, which could be useful for the treatment of this disease in humans. Potential of oil from *Syzygium aromaticum* flower buds (clove) was demonstrated by Islamuddin et al. (2014). He has shown that eugenol-rich EO from *S. aromaticum* possesses significant activity against *Leishmania donovani*, with 50 % inhibitory concentration against promastigotes and intracellular amastigotes. Reported leishmanicidal effect was mediated via apoptosis as confirmed by externalization of phosphatidylserine, DNA nicking, dyskinetoplastidy, cell cycle arrest at sub-G_0-G_1 phase, loss of mitochondrial membrane potential, and reactive oxygen species generation with no adverse cytotoxic effects against murine macrophages.[2]

8.2.3 THYMUS CAPITELLATUS

In one report, *Thymus capitellatus* Hoffmanns. & Link (family Lamiaceae) volatile extract and its major compounds, 1,8-cineole and borneol, were evaluated against *Leishmania infantum*, *Leishmania tropica*, and *Leishmania major*. It was found that *T. capitellatus* volatile extract without having any cytotoxic effect, exhibited anti-parasite activity on *Leishmania* species, with IC50 values ranging from 35 to 62 μg/mL. However, major compounds 1,8-cineole and borneol did not show biological activity suggesting that these monoterpenes are not responsible for the antileishmanial activity of *T. capitellatus* EO.[3]

8.2.4 CYMBOPOGON CITRATUS

Cymbopogon citratus EO and major compounds, mrycene and citral. *C. citratus* and citral were found to be the most active inhibiting *L. infantum*,

L. tropica, and *L. major* growth at IC(50) concentrations ranging from 25 to 52 μg/mL and from 34 to 42 μg/mL, respectively. In addition, it was also reported that citral was responsible for antileishmania activity of the *C. citratus* and both may represent a valuable source for therapeutic control of leishmaniasis.[3]

8.2.5 OCIMUM

There are various reports available on leishmanicidal activity of *Ocimum bascilicum, Ocimum gratissimum, Origanum vulgare*, and *Ocimum sanctum*. The eugenol-rich EO of *O. gratissimum* progressively inhibited *Leishmania amazonensis* growth at concentrations ranging from 100 to 1000 μg/mL.[4] The EO of *O. basilicum* was found to be active against promastigotes of *Leishmania* and innocuous to J774 macrophages at concentrations up to 1600 μg/mL.[5] In one report, a relative antileishmanian study was studied on major oil of *O. basilicum* L. [(-)-linalool (30–40%) and eugenol (8–30%)] and *O. sanctum* [eugenol (8–43%) and methylchavicol (15–27%)]. EOs from both species were found to be in vitro activity against *L. donovani* (IC50 = 37.3–49.6 μg/mL), which was comparable to the activity of commercial oil (IC50 = 40–50 μg/mL). Minor basil oil constituents (+)-delta-cadinene, 3-carene, alpha-humulene, citral, and (-)-trans-caryophyllene had antileishmanial activity, whereas other constituents were ineffective. Suzuki et al. (2009) isolated and identified 16 neolignan derivatives from the ethyl acetate soluble fraction of the plant *O. sanctum*. It was found that some of these compounds show leishmanicidal activity. It was also discovered that none of the EO obtained from *Ocimum* sp. was cytotoxic to mammalian cells.[4–7] These reports suggested that *O. sanctum*-derived EO and its compounds could be used as sources for new antileishmanial drugs.

8.2.6 ACHILLEA MILLEFOLIUM

Achillea L. (Compositae or Asteraceae) is a widely distributed medicinal plant throughout the world and has been used since ancient time. There are many reports on the mentioned folk and traditional effects. Recently, *Achillea millefolium* is explored for its EO-based medicinal properties. The oil *content of A. millefolium* differed greatly between the vegetative state (0.13%). The predominant constituents were sabinene (17.58%), 1,8-cineole (13.04%), borneol (12.41%), bornyl acetate (7.98%), -pinene(6.28%),-pinene (6.26%), terpinine-4-ol (6.17%), and chamazulene (5.28%). An EO of *A. millefolium* was recently extracted from the leaves and flowers and tested for in vitro activity against *L. amazonensis* and murine macrophages (i.e., the J774G8 cell line). It was suggested that the EO obtained from *A. millefolium* significantly inhibited *L. amazonensis* promastigotes at 7.8 μg/mL and amastigotes at 6.5 μg/mL.[8]

8.2.7 LIPPIA SP.

Lippia gracilis, popularly known in Brazil as "alecrim-de-tabuleiro," is used for many purposes, especially antimicrobial and antiseptic activities. Previous reports suggested the variation of thymol and carvacrol concenteration in the EO, obtained from *L. gracilis* plants (obtained from various germ plasms) by hydrodistillation. Regarding leishmanicidal activity, the IC50, for LGRA-106 and LGRA-110, was found to be 86.32 and 77.26 μg/mL, respectively. It is also reported that EO, rich in thymol and thymol itself presented best antidermatophytic activity, whereas the best leishmanicidal activity was obtained with EO from genotype rich in carvacrol and carvacrol itself.[9]

Similarly in vitro leishmanicidal effects of a thymol- and a carvacrol-rich EO from leaves of *Lippia sidoides* Cham. It was studied in another report that *Lippia sidoides* EOs showed significant activity against promastigote forms of *Leishmania chagasi*.[10]

The EOs were obtained from different species of *Lippia*, also a widely distributed genus of Colombian plants. Colombian *Lippia* EO contains geranial, neral, limonene, nerol, carvacrol, p-cymene, gamma-terpinene, carvone, and thymol. *Lippia* were reported against free and intracellular forms of *L. chagasi*. *Lippia alba* and *Lippia origanoides* are the well-known species of this genus. Thymol and S-carvone are the two major components of the active EOs. The EO of *L. alba* exhibited the highest activity against *Trypanosoma cruzi* epimastigotes and intracellular amastigotes and EO of *L. origanoides* was active against *L. chagasi* promastigotes but none of the EOs or major components tested in this study was active on amastigotes of *L. chagasi*-infected THP-1 cells.[11]

8.2.8 COPAIBA OIL

In addition, the American flora is one of the world's wealthiest sources of material with pharmacological activity, due to its biodiversity. Copaiba oil has been used in folk medicine since the 19th century. The use of copaiba oils to treat leishmaniasis is cited in several ethnopharmacological studies. Nevertheless, the potential antileishmania of copaiba oils had not been studied. Recent literatures revealed a significant activity profile of copaiba oils against the parasite *L. amazonensis*. Santos et al. (2008) investigated eight different kinds of Brazilian copaiba oils for antileishmanial activity. In his study, he suggested that copaiba oils showed variable levels of activity against promastigote forms with IC(50) values in the range between 5 and 22 μg/mL. The most active oil was that from *Copaifera reticulata* with IC(50) values of 5, 15, and 20 μg/mL for promastigote, axenic amastigote, and intracellular amastigote forms, respectively. In addition, he has also suggested the low cytotoxicity profile of *C. reticulata* against J774G8 macrophages.[12] In 2011, it was discovered that the oral treatment of copaiba oil (Group IV) caused a significant reduction in the average lesion size against *L. amazonensis* lesions compared with untreated mice. There were no toxic and genotoxic effects. Morphological and ultrastructural changes such as mitochondrial swelling, increase in plasma membrane permeability, and depolarization in the mitochondrial membrane potential in parasite cells was reported in the groups treated with this oleoresin.[13] Dos Santos et al. (2012) demonstrated the role of copaiba oil in inducing morphological and ultrastructural changes in *L. amazonensis.*[14] It was also reported that copaiba oil caused notable morphological and ultrastructural changes in the promastigote and axenic amastigote forms, including extensive mitochondrial damage and denaturation of the plasma membrane. Copaiba oil treatment also induced a decrease in Rh123 fluorescence, suggesting interference with the mitochondrial membrane potential and loss of cell viability with an increase in plasma membrane permeability.[14] In 2012 and 2013, Diterpene (Hydroxycopalic acid, methyl copalate, pinifolic acid, and kaurenoic acid) and sesquiterpenoidal compounds (β –caryophyllene), those are responsible for the leishmanicidal activity, were explored from various commercial varieties of copaiba oil. Hydroxycopalic acid and methyl copalate were found to be the most active against promastigotes. However, pinifolic acid and kaurenoic acid was reported most active against axenic amastigotes. In addition, it was also observed that the compounds such as agathic acid, kaurenoic acid, and pinifolic acid yielded significant increases in plasma membrane permeability and mitochondrial membrane depolarization.[15] Soares et al. (2013) reported that diterpenes-rich oils showed antipromastigote activity whereas sesquiterpenes-rich oil presented a dose-dependent activity against intracellular amastigotes.[16] These sesquiterpenoidal and diterpenoidal compounds were found to be less active against *L. amazonensis* and more toxic for the macrophages than the whole commercial oil. The leishmanicidal activity of these compounds appears to be independent of nitric oxide (NO) production by macrophages.[16] In conclusion; copaiba oil could be exploited for the development of new antileishmanial drugs.[17]

8.2.9 PIPER SP.

Piper species are widely used in folk medicine in Latin America and the West Indies, to heal wounds, reduce swelling and skin irritations, and treat the symptoms of cutaneous leishmaniasis (CL). Several studies emphasize the importance of *Piper* species in the treatment of this disease. In fact, various classes of antiparasitic active compounds have been identified in *Piper* species, such as chalcones and dihydrochalcones, benzoic acid derivatives, and neolignans. The chemical composition of EOs of *Piper* is mainly composed of phenylpropanoids such as safrole, dillapiol and myristicin, or terpenes such as limonene, β-caryophyllene, spathulenol, (*E*)-nerolidol, α-bicyclogermacrene, and cadinol. Insecticidal, fungicidal, bactericidal, larvicidal, and molluscicidal properties are attributed to these species.[18] EO from *Piper auritum* oil was found to be active against the promastigotes of *L. major, Leishmania mexicana, Leishmania braziliensis*, and *L. donovani* with a favorable selectivity index against peritoneal macrophages from BALB/c mice.[19] Monzote et al. (2010) also reported the safrole as abundant compound, comprising 87% of the oil of *P. auritum.*[19] Guerrini and collaborators carried out extensive pharmacological evaluation of EOs obtained from *Piper aduncum* and *Piper obliquum*, with interesting results. The EOs obtained from leaves of *Piper duckei* and *Piper demeraranum* exhibited potent biological activity against two *Leishmania* species and *P. duckei* oil was found to the most active. IC50 values of main mono- and sesquiterpene, limonene, and caryophyllene compounds were found to be lower than those found for the EOs of the *Piper* species.[18] In one report, the nerolidol-rich EO from *Piper claussenianum,* Piperaceae, was assayed on arginase activity of *L. amazonensis.* The effect of this EO on arginase activity levels showed an enzyme inhibition of 62.2%.[20] Garcia et al. reported the antileishmanial activity of eupomatenoid-5, a neolignan obtained from leaves of *Piper regnellii var. pallescens*. He has also clarified the mode of action of eupomatenoid-5 against *L. amazonensis.*[21] By using biochemical and morphological techniques, he has demonstrated that eupomatenoid-5-induced cell death in *L. amazonensis* promastigotes, sharing some phenotypic features observed in metazoan apoptosis, including increased reactive oxygen species production, hypopolarization of mitochondrial potential, phosphatidylserine exposure, decreased cell volume, and G_0/G_1 phase cell cycle arrest.[21] These reports demonstrated the usefulness of the EOs as a promising alternative to treat leishmaniasis.

8.2.10 *CHENOPODIUM AMBROSIOIDES*

Natural products are often overlooked in antiprotozoal chemotherapy. Plants have been used traditionally in the treatment of leishmaniases, in particular against cutaneous disease. *Chenopodium ambrosioides* is an aromatic herb used by native people to treat parasitic diseases. Monzote et al. (2007) reported the significant in vitro antileishmanial effect of the EO from *C. ambrosioides* against *L. donovani* without affecting the phagocytic activity of the macrophages at a concentration toxic to the parasite.[22] Monzote et al. (2007) demonstrated the role of *C. ambrosioides* EO in the combination therapy of various antileishmanial drugs on promastigotes of *L. amazonensis*. In his study, he has reported the synergic effect of EO from *C. ambrosioides* with pentamidine against promastigotes of *L. amazonensis.*[22] However, an indifferent effect has been found for combinations of meglumine antimoniate or amphotericin B and the EO.[22] Monzote and his coworkers (2014) demonstrated the relative antileishmanial activity of the EO from *C. ambrosioides* and its major components (alpha-terpinene, p-cymene, ascaridole, carvacrol, and caryophyllene oxide) with their mechanism of action and activity against a panel of microorganism.[23] In his report, he has also demonstrated that all chemical components were active against promastigote and amastigote forms of *Leishmania*; however, ascaridole exhibited the better antileishmanial activity and the EO was having highest selectivity index. He has suggested that the breakdown of mitochondrial membrane potential and a modification of redox indexes is the mechanism followed by these components to exert antileishmanian activity.[23] He and his coworkers also demonstrated the drug delivery-mediated activity of the EO from *C. ambrosioides* in BALB/c mice infected with *L. amazonensis*. Findings of reports suggested that the intraperitoneal administration of the EO prevented lesion development and decrease the parasite burden whereas oral administration also retarded the infection although it was less effective than the intraperitoneal route. Furthermore, administration by intralesional route did not show activity. In his report, he examined the signs of toxicity those were evident only in the animals treated by intraperitoneal route and no resistance was detected in *L. amazonensis* isolates obtained from treated mice.

Intraperitoneal and oral treatment of EO at 30 mg/kg was found to better antileishmanial effect than treatment with the reference drug, amphotericin B at 1 mg/kg.

8.2.11 CROTON CAJUCARA

Croton cajucara Benth. (family Euphorbiaceae), locally known as "sacaca," is a plant found in the Amazon region that has been used in folk medicine against gastrointestinal and liver disorders, diabetes, and for cholesterol reduction. The leaves of *C. cajucara* are used as an infusion in popular medicine to combat several diseases. In earlier reports, two morphotypes were identified, namely white sacaca and red sacaca. The EOs of white sacaca and red sacaca were classified in two groups: one rich (up to 45%) in linalool, and other containing up to 44% of an aromatic sesquiterpene, 7-hydroxycalamenene. Previous studies have demonstrated that the linalool-rich EO from *C. cajucara* (white sacaca) is extremely efficient against the tegumentary specie *L. amazonensis*. Rodrigues et al. (2013) reported the minimum inhibitory concentrations of the EO from the leaves of *C. cajucara* (red sacaca) and its purified component 7-hydroxycalamenene against *L. chagasi* were 250 and 15.6 μg/mL, respectively.[1] He and his coworkers also demonstrated nuclear and kinetoplastic alterations in *L. chagasi* promastigotes.[1] In the same work, he has demonstrated the potential of EO in reducing parasite/macrophage interaction after the pretreatment of macrophage with EO whereas NO production is increased by *L. chagasi*-infected macrophages. The extreme toxicity of *C. cajucara* leaf extracts for *L. amazonensis* was reported with no effect upon mammalian cells, enables linalool-rich EO to be a source of a new lead compound for novel antileishmanial drugs.[24] Morphological changes such as leishmanial nuclear, kinetoplast chromatin destruction, followed by cell lysis in *L. amazonensis* promastigotes was reported in EO-treated group. In addition, pretreatment of mouse peritoneal macrophages with EO reduced 50% percent interaction between these macrophages and *L. amazonensis*, with a concomitant increase in the level of NO production by the infected macrophages.[24]

8.2.12 MITRACARPUS FRIGIDUS

Mitracarpus frigidus was found to be having significant antibacterial, antifungal, and leishmanicidal activities. It was reported that the EO obtained by hydrodistillation of the aerial parts of *M. frigidus* composed of 11 compounds, in which linalool and eugenol acetate are the major components. EO was proved to be active against *L. major* and *L. amazonensis* promastigote forms. The cytotoxicity of EO against *Artemia salina* was found to be moderate.[25]

8.2.13 SATUREJA BAKHTIARICA

The chemical composition and the anti-*L. major* activity of the EOs obtained from *Satureja bakhtiarica* were reported under in vitro conditions against *L. major*. A total of 13 compounds were identified in earlier studies out of which major components were found to be phenolic compounds, thymol and p-cymene. It was reported that EO of *S. bakhtiarica* showed higher activity against *L. major* than the standard antileishmanial drug, glucantime. Perhaps because of the high concentration of phenolic compounds in the EO, all the parasites were killed after 24 hours. The EO from *S. bakhtiarica* is a potential plant drug against leishmaniasis.[26]

8.2.14 BACCHARIS DRACUNCULIFOLIA

Baccharis dracunculifolia DC. (Asteraceae), popularly known as "alecrim do campo," is a native plant from Brazil used in folk medicine as febrifuge, anti-inflammatory, antiseptic, and to treat skin sores. Parreira et al. (2010) isolated and identified 14 compounds mainly oxygenated sesquiterpenes, such as (E)-nerolidol and spathulenol.[27] He has also demonstrated the activity of EO from the leaves of *B. dracunculifolia* against promastigote forms of *L. donovani*. da Silva Filho et al. (2009) demonstrated the potential role of ursolic acid, hautriwaic acid, uvaol, acacetin, and ermanin against *Leishmania*.[28] It was later found that components such as ursolic acid, methyl linolenate, caryophyllene oxide, and trans-nerolidol are also active against amastigote forms of *Leishmania, L. amazonensis*. It was also demonstrated that during this process, caryophyllene oxide interacts with ergosterol, hence increases the effectiveness if antileshmanian drug against the parasite.[28] The in vitro antileishmanial activity of the EO and eight extracts obtained from *Xylopia* discrete was studied in one report. The leaf methanol extract and the EO induced a differential production of monocyte chemoattractant protein-1, a chemokine associated with a *Leishmania*-resistant phenotype (Th1).[29]

8.2.15 CYMBOPOGON CITRATUS

Cymbopogon citratus (DC) Stapf, Family Poaceae, is a widely used herb in tropical countries and is also known as a source of ethnomedicines. In 2009, *C. citrates* along with two more oils proved to be active against *L. chagasi* promastigotes growth in a dose-dependent way. It was reported that the EO from *C. citrates* caused the drastic morphological alterations in all EO-treated parasites, including cell swelling, accumulation of lipid droplets in the cytoplasm, and increase of acidocalcisome volume. Furthermore, aberrant-shaped cells with multi-septate body were also reported. Taken together, our data show that these EOs affect the parasite viability being the *C. citratus* EO the most effective against *L. chagasi*.[30] In an antileishmnail reports on *C. citrates*, the antiproliferative activity of its EO on promastigotes and axenic amastigotes, and intracellular amastigote forms of *L. amazonensis* was found to be significantly better than citral, indicated a dose-dependent effect. Furthermore, this report also suggested that EO has no cytotoxic effect on macrophage strain J774G8.[31] Machado et al. (2010) suggested the relative antileishmanian potential of EO obtained from *C. citratus, Juniperus oxycedrus* berries, and *Thymus capitelatus* oils. Machado and his coworkers (2012) also reported the susceptibility of *L. infantum, L. tropica*, and *L. major* to *C. citratus* EO and major compounds, mrycene and citral.[32] *C. citratus* and citral were the most active inhibiting *L. infantum, L. tropica,* and *L. major* growth. In his study, he has also demonstrated the effects of citral and EO-mediated considerable ultrastructural alterations, namely mitochondrial and kinetoplast swelling, autophagosomal structures, disruption of nuclear membrane, and nuclear chromatin condensation of *L. infantum* promastigotes. His findings suggested leishmanicidal effect of *C. citratus* EO and citral promoted by triggering a programmed cell death by the externalization of phosphatidylserine, loss of mitochondrial membrane potential, and cell-cycle arrest at the G_0/G_1 phase.[32]

8.2.16 SYZYGIUM CUMINI

Dias et al. (2013) reported the relative compositional and whole EO significant potential of *Syzygium cumini* leaves against *L. amazonensis*. EO contained high abundance of monoterpenes (87.12%) with the major components α-pinene (31.85%), (Z)-β-ocimene (28.98%), and (E)-β-ocimene (11.71%).[33]

8.2.17 VANILLOSMOPSIS ARBOREA

Colares et al. (2013) reported in vitro leishmanicidal activity of EO of *Vanillosmopsis arborea* (VAEO) and its major compound α-bisabolol against *L. amazonensis.* He has suggested the potential role of EO and α-bisabolol against promastigotes and intracellular amastigotes without having any toxicity on treated macrophages. It was also reported that promastigotes when incubated with EO or α-bisabolol showed morphological changes with the accumulation of vesicles electrodense lipid.[34]

8.2.18 BIXIA ORELLANA

Monzote et al. (2014) reported the in vitro and in vivo effects of the EO from *Bixa orellana* seeds against *L. amazonensis*. A total of 73 compounds were explored from EO of *B. orellana* seeds out of which ishwarane and geranylgeraniol were the major components. It was proved that oil showed potential activity against intracellular amastigote, whereas the cytotoxic concentration was seven-fold higher for the host cells. Intraperitoneal administration of Bixa oil to control disease progression of established CL in BALB/c mice was also demonstrated in the same study.[23] Lopes et al. (2012) demonstrated the activity of geranylgeraniol, the major bioactive constituent from seeds of *B. orellana*, against *L. amazonensis*. Geranylgeraniol inhibited the promastigote and intracellular amastigote forms. It was reported that this compound was more toxic to parasites than to macrophages and did not cause lysis in human blood cells. In addition, geranylgeraniol-induced morphological changes in parasite such as mitochondria alterations and an abnormal chromatin condensation in the nucleus with increased production of superoxide anion production in mitochondaria.[35]

8.2.19 KEETIA LEUCANTHA

Keetia leucantha is a West African tree used in traditional medicine to treat several diseases such as parasitic infections. The dichloromethane extract of leaves was previously shown to possess growth-inhibitory activities on *Plasmodium falciparum, T. brucei,* and *L. mexicana* with low or no cytotoxicity (>100 μg/mL on human normal fibroblasts). Twenty-seven compounds were reported in the oil out of which seven constituents and the three triterpenic acids are the major components of this oil. Three triterpenic acids present in the dichloromethane leaves extract were reported for their higher antitrypanosomal activity on bloodstream forms. β-ionone, ursolic acid, oleanolic acid, and betulinic acid from the EO of *Keetia leucantha* were proven for their potential in the inhibition of trypanosomal glyceraldehyde 3-phosphate dehydrogenase, which may in part explain these antitrypanosomal activities.[36]

8.2.20 *ECHINOPS KEBERICHO AND ARTEMISIA ABSINTHIUM*

To justify the significance in *Leishmania* strains (*Leishmania aethiopica and L. donovani*), and toxicity on the human monocytic leukemia (THP-1) cell line and red blood cells in vitro, 65 compounds from *Artemisia absinthium* and 43 compounds from *Echinops kebericho* were reported from their EOs. Oxygenated monoterpene camphor and the sesquiterpene lactone dehydrocostus lactone were found to be the major constituents of these oils. Both oils showed potential activity against promastigote and axenic amastigote forms of both *Leishmania* species with weak hemolytic effect against the human monocytic leukemia cell line. It was suggested that among the two oils tested, *E. kebericho* exerted strong antileishmanial activity that was even higher than that of amphotericin B with significant cytotoxicity.[37]

8.2.21 *ARTEMISIA HERBA-ALBA*

Hatimi et al. (2001) reported the EO of Artemisia herba-alba Asso was tested for their antileshmanial activity against *L. tropica* and *L. major*. The strongest leishmanicidal activity was observed with the EO at 2 μg/mL as versus the other two strains tested.[38]

8.2.22 *ARTEMISIA ABYSSINICA* AND *SATUREJA PUNCTATA*

In 2010, the oils of *Artemisia abyssinica* and *Satureja punctata* were reported for leishmanicidal activity against promastigote and axenic amastigotes of *L. donovani* and *L. aethiopica*, including toxicity studies on human monocytic leukemia cells (THP-1) and erythrocytes in vitro. A total of 67 compounds were reported from *A. abyssinica* oil including yomogi alcohol, artemisyl acetate, and artemisia alcohol, and many oxygenated monoterpenes as the major constituents. In addition, 67 compounds were also reported from

S. punctata containing main constituents geranial, neral, alpha-bisabolol, and (E)-nerolidol, of which oxygenated mono- and sesquiterpenes showed highest abundance. Both oils were active against promastigotes and amastigotes with varying toxicities in human monocytic leukemia cells were found. It was also suggested that *S. punctata* oil exerted highest activity against both *Leishmania* sp. and toxicity.[39]

8.2.23 CROTON MACROSTACHYUS

The main chemical composition of the volatile oil from berries of *Croton macrostachyus* was found to be benzyl benzoate, linalool, gamma-muurolene, (E,E)-alpha-farnesene, delta-cadinene, and alpha- urcumene. The oil was found to be effective against *L. donovani* and *L. aethiopica* promastigotes and axenic amastigote stages. Thus, the observed high efficacy and moderate toxicity of the volatile oil from *C. macrostachyus* makes the plant a promising source of new lead compounds in the search for safe and effective antileishmanial drugs.[40]

8.2.24 CHAMOMILLA RECUTITA

Many of the drugs used to treat leishmaniasis are associated with numerous adverse effects. Agents of natural origin have shown activity against different parasites. Morales-Yuste et al. (2010) reported the potential in vitro antileishmanian effects on the activity of (-)alpha-bisabolol, the principal component of *Chamomilla recutita* EO, against *L. infantum* promastigotes, the main species responsible for human leishmaniasis in Spain. At the two highest concentrations tested (1000 and 500 μg/mL), (-)alpha-bisabolol and pentamidine (control agent) achieved 100% inhibition of *L. infantum* promastigote.[41]

8.2.25 DIETARY FISH OIL

Dietary fish oil (FO) supplementation has been shown to inhibit inflammation in various clinical disease states and to be beneficial in the experimental models of inflammation and bacterial and plasmodial infection. In mice, Dietary FO increases macrophage production of TNF-α. Production of TNF has been reported to be important in the resistance of mice against various *Leishmania* spp. Blok et al. (2002) reported dietary supplementation with FO protects susceptible BALB/c mice against infection with *L. amazonensis*. No influence of the FO diet on the course of infection was reported whereas lipopolysaccharide (LPS)-induced TNF production of peritoneal cells was significantly increased in FO-fed mice. Thus, it was concluded that dietary supplementation with FO is of no benefit in leishmaniasis in susceptible BALB/c mice.[42]

8.2.26 MELALEUCA ALTERNIFOLIA (TEA TREE) OIL

Complementary and alternative medicines such as tea tree (melaleuca) oil have become increasingly popular in recent decades. This EO has been used for almost 100 years in Australia but is now available worldwide both as neat oil and as an active component in an array of products. The primary uses of tea tree oil (TTO) have historically capitalized on the antiseptic and anti-inflammatory actions of the oil. This review summarizes recent developments in our understanding of the antimicrobial and anti-inflammatory activities of the oil and its components, as well as clinical efficacy. Specific mechanisms of antimicrobial and anti-inflammatory action are reviewed, and the toxicity of the oil is briefly discussed. Two publications show that TTO has antiprotozoal activity. TTO caused a 50% reduction in growth (compared to controls) of the protozoa *L. major* and *T. brucei* at concentrations of 403 mg/mL and 0.5 mg/mL, respectively (109). Further investigation showed that terpinen-4-ol contributed significantly to this activity.[43]

8.3 ROLE OF CHELATION THERAPY IN *LEISHMANIA*

Chelation is one of the most effective treatments and is a safe alternative to vascular surgery. Most patients of chelation IV therapy are treated for vascular disease.

Chelation therapy has also been proven effective in the removal of heavy toxic metals and other harmful substances that have entered the body through food, water, and environmental pollution. Once these damaging metals are removed, the body has greater access to the vital nutrients obtained through diet and supplements. The most common form of intravenous chelation therapy is with EDTA, and when properly used, it has been found to be nontoxic. This therapy is administered by intravenous infusion which is significantly different from the oral chelation therapy for general measures. Interfering in ion-dependent processes in *Leishmania* may be an interesting approach to defeat these microorganisms.

Iron is crucial for all living organisms since it is involved in a wide variety of important metabolic processes and pathogenesis. It is an essential element for the survival of microorganisms in vitro and in vivo, acting as a cofactor of several enzymes and playing a critical role in host–parasite relationships. *L. (Viannia) braziliensis* is a parasite that is widespread in the new world and considered the major etiological agent of American tegumentary leishmaniasis. Although iron depletion leads to promastigote and amastigote growth inhibition, little is known about the role of iron in the biology of *Leishmania*. Iron is vital for all trypanosomatid parasites and plays a significant role in pathogenesis and immune control of these organisms. Iron chelation leads to a multifactorial response that results in cellular collapse, starting with the interruption of cell proliferation and culminating in marked mitochondrial impairment in some parasites and their subsequent cell death, whereas others may survive and resume proliferating. In this sense, the depletion of this essential nutrient in trypanosomatids rapidly decreases the rate of DNA synthesis, increases the oxidative stress levels via loss of superoxide dismutase and ascorbate-dependent peroxidase activity, blocks the J-base synthesis, and stops electron transfer to the alternative oxidase, leading inexorably to the death of the protozoan.[44]

To understand the basic mechanism involved in chelation therapy against *Leishmania*, it is important to highlight leucyl aminopeptidase (LAP) gene. Just in the case of malaria, the activity of *P. falciparum*, in fact its whole life cycle is much dependent on the LAP activity to complete its whole life cycle. Some chelating agents are very efficient in inhibiting in aminopeptidases activity. However, when this pathogen superexpresses LAP gene, it becomes more resistant to chelating agent (bestatine). Similarly, Intron-less genes encoding a LAP were cloned in 2002 from *L. amazonensis, L. donovani, and L. major*. It was reported that *Leishmania* LAP activity was inhibited by metal ion chelators and enhanced by divalent manganese, cobalt, and nickel cations; although only zinc was detected in the purified LAP, indicating that zinc is the natural LAP cofactor.[45,46] Calcium chelator also plays an important role in NO production by *Leishmania* sp.[47] Zinc-dependent metalloproteases or zinc-dependent glycoproteins can also considered as good targets for zinc chelating agents. Most vegetables, however, are not good sources of zinc owing to the presence of phytate, a component of plants that chelates zinc and prevents its absorption.

8.4 ROLE OF ACUPUNCTURE THERAPY IN *LEISHMANIA*

8.4.1 ELECTROACUPUNCTURE

In recent years, intensive studies have been carried out to explain the underlying mechanisms of the efficacy of acupuncture. EA has been used to treat inflammatory diseases. It has been shown that electrical stimulation of the ST36 acupoint significantly reduces both the serum and tissue levels of the pro-inflammatory cytokines such as TNF in rats with ulcerative colitis, chronic inflammation induced by Freund's complete adjuvant, experimental arthritis, inflammation induced by carrageenan injection, and other conditions. Furthermore, alternatively activated macrophages (AAMos) are associated with the improvement of several inflammatory diseases, such as experimental arthritis and colitis.

8.4.1.1 ELECTROACUPUNCTURE AND MACROPHAGES

Macrophages have well established roles in the primary responses to pathogens, and can be activated in different ways, giving rise to classically activated macrophages or AAMo. AAMo stimulated by cytokines such as IL-4, IL-10, and IL-13 are anti-inflammatory and mildly microbicidal. Corticoids and IL-10 can also act on macrophages and increased the generation of AAMo. AAMo are mainly induced after stimulation with IL-4 and IL-13, and produces cytokines and enzymes for the inflammation modulation and initiation of wound healing. The properties of AAMo depend on their arginase activity, which increases ornithine and urea production. Ornithine can be metabolized to collagen or purine, which are both fundamental for wound healing. Arginase is the prototypic marker for AAMo. This enzyme increases in murine macrophages involved in helminthic infection, tumors and tissue repair, converting L-arginine to ornithine and urea, whereas induced NO synthase (iNOS) present in cMO converts L-arginine to citrulline and NO. Arginase and iNOS share the same substrate, leading to an inverse correlation between these two enzymes in helminthic infection, tumors, and tissue-repair environments. In addition, AAMo are more susceptible to intracellular pathogens such as *L. major.*

Classically activated macrophages (cMO) are induced by interferon-γ (IFNγ) and produce NO (NO) through iNOS to enhance the resistance to intracellular pathogens such as *L. major.* Therefore, cMO are able to control the growth of intracellular pathogens, whereas AAMo are susceptible to infection with such pathogens, both in vitro and in vivo.

8.4.1.2 ELECTROACUPUNCTURE AND NO PRODUCTION

Earlier report suggested that EA suppressed the NO production induced by LPS or LPS and IFNγ in peritoneal macrophages. Although the arginase activity in cells after EA treatment or cultured in the absence of IL-4 does not change, the activity was increased in macrophages from EA-treated mice in the presence of IL-4. It was not clarified how EA increases the IL-4 responsiveness of macrophages, although EA and IL-4 could synergistically potentiate the responsiveness or interfere with some signal transduction from the IL-4 receptor. However, the mechanism is unlikely due to an increase in IL-4 receptor expression, because the IL-4 receptor expression was similar between macrophages from sham- and EA-treated mice. There are some reports available on the role of EA at the *Zusanli* acupoint (ST36) to change the profile of healthy murine macrophages, particularly the generation of AAMos and susceptibility to *L. major* infection.

The generation of AAMo with high arginase activity is associated with a decreased ability to control intracellular parasites such as *L. major*, whereas NO production by cMO is associated with better control of these parasites. Experiments have been performed using IFNγ-stimulated macrophages to observe the killing of *L. major* in vitro. In addition, IL-4 can prevent NO production and decrease the killing of the parasites. These findings are in agreement with our results, showing an increase in the percentage of cells infected by *L. major* after IL-4 treatment. Macrophages from EA-treated mice were more responsive to IL-4 and enhanced the growth of the parasite inside the cells. An ability of IFNγ-stimulated macrophages to kill parasites was not observed in our experiments, possibly because the combination of LPS and IFNγ is required to produce the optimal stimulation for NO production to kill parasites, and only IFNγ was used in some of our experiments.

In a recent report, it was suggested that infection of BALB/c mice with *L. major* induces early production of IL-4 by $CD4^+$ T cells. This early production of IL-4 and the presence of AAMo are associated with the susceptibility of this mouse strain to *L. major* infection. Because macrophages from EA-treated mice were more responsive to IL-4, the outcome of infecting mice with *L. major* was examined. The lesion size in EA-treated mice was more pronounced than that in sham-treated mice, suggested that EA increases

IL-4 responsiveness in vivo and interferes with the outcome of infection by intracellular pathogens such as *L. major*.[48]

Aguiar and his coworkers (2012) demonstrated the peritoneal cells freshly obtained from EA-treated mice had similar arginase and microbicidal activities to cells from sham-treated mice. It was reported that cells from EA-treated mice exhibited significant increases in the arginase activity and decreases the NO production when cultured in the presence of a combination of IFNγ and LPS. In addition, the lesion size in mice infected with *L. major* promastigotes was larger in EA-treated mice.[49]

CL is an endemic parasitic disease in Iran. Current treatments for the disease are not satisfying, have many side effects and are expensive. The healing effect of T-helper 1 (Th1) immune response, especially IFN-Î³ secretion in CL has been previously documented. It has been shown that acupuncture, a traditional Chinese medicine, also might activate Th1 immune response. Shakibapour et al. (2013) studied the effect of acupuncture on serum level of IFN-Î³ in experimental CL of BALB/c mice. It was proven that the mean serum level of IFN-Î³ was not significantly different between and within the groups at the beginning and at the sessions 5 and 10 of the therapy. This report suggested that acupuncture may not affect the serum level of IFN-Î³ in BALB/c model of CL. Moreover, diazepam does not interfere with the serum level of IFN-Î³ in such a study. Analysis of other immune factors and early measurement of IFN-Î³ in the course of treatment possibly may display the activated protective immune response against leishmaniasis by acupuncture.[50]

KEYWORDS

- ***Leishmania***
- **therapy**
- **essential oil**
- **chelation**
- **acupuncture**

REFERENCES

1. Rodrigues, K. A.; Amorim, L. V.; de Oliveira, J. M.; Dias, C. N.; Moraes, D. F.; Andrade, E. H.; Maia, J. G.; Carneiro, S. M.; Carvalho, F. A. *Eugenia uniflora* L. Essential Oil as a Potential Anti-*Leishmania* Agent: Effects on *Leishmania amazonensis* and Possible Mechanisms of Action. *Evid. Based Complement. Alternat. Med.* **2013**, 2013, 279726.
2. Mohammad, J.; Mohammad, I.; Abuzer, A.; Farhat A.; Mohammed, A. Isolation, characterization and antimicrobial evaluation of a novel compound N-octacosan 7*β* ol, from *Fumaria parviflora Lam. BMC Complement. Altern. Med.* **2014,** 14, 98.
3. Machado M.; Dinis, A. M.; Santos-Rosa, M.; Alves, V.; Salgueiro, L.; Cavaleiro, C.; Sousa, M. C. Activity of *Thymus capitellatus* Volatile Extract, 1,8-Cineole and Borneol against *Leishmania* sp. *Vet. Parasitol.* **2014,** *200* (1-2), 39–49.
4. Ueda-Nakamura, T.; Mendonça-Filho, R. R.; Morgado-Díaz, J. A.; Korehisa Maza, P.; Prado Dias Filho, B.; Aparício Garcia Cortez, D.; Alviano, D. S.; Rosa Mdo, S.; Lopes, A. H.; Alviano, C. S.; Nakamura, C. V. Antileishmanial Activity of Eugenol-rich Essential Oil from *Ocimum gratissimum Parasitol. Int.* **2006,** *55* (2), 99–105.
5. Sanchez-Suarez, J.; Riveros, I.; Delgado, G. Evaluation of the Leishmanicidal and Cytotoxic Potential of Essential Oils Derived from Ten Colombian Plants. *Iran J. Parasitol.* **2013,** *8* (1), 129–136.
6. Zheljazkov, V. D.; Cantrell, C. L.; Tekwani, B.; Khan, S. I. Content, Composition, and Bioactivity of the Essential Oils of Three Basil Genotypes as a Function of Harvesting. *J. Agric. Food Chem.* **2008,** *56* (2), 380–385.
7. Suzuki, A.; Shirota, O.; Mori, K.; Sekita, S.; Fuchino, H.; Takano, A.; Kuroyanagi, M. Leishmanicidal Active Constituents from Nepalese Medicinal Plant Tulsi (*Ocimum sanctum* L.). *Chem. Pharm. Bull.* **2009,** *57* (3), 245–251.
8. Santos, A. O.; Santin, A. C.; Yamaguchi, M. U.; Cortez, L. E.; Ueda-Nakamura, T.; Dias-Filho, B. P.; Nakamura, C. V. Antileishmanial Activity of an Essential Oil from the Leaves and Flowers of *Achillea millefolium*. *Ann. Trop. Med. Parasitol.* **2010,** *104* (6), 475–483.
9. de Melo J. O.; Bitencourt, T. A.; Fachin, A. L.; Cruz, E. M.; de Jesus, H. C.; Alves, P.B.; de Fátima Arrigoni-Blank, M.; de Castro Franca, S.; Beleboni, R. O.; Fernandes, R. P.; Blank, A. F.; Scher, R. Antidermatophytic and Antileishmanial Activities of Essential Oils from *Lippia gracilis* Schauer Genotypes. *Acta. Trop.* **2013,** *128* (1), 110–115.
10. Farias-Junior, P. A.; Rios, M. C.; Moura, T. A.; Almeida, R. P.; Alves, P. B.; Blank, A. F.; Fernandes, R. P.; Scher, R. Leishmanicidal Activity of Carvacrol-rich Essential Oil from *Lippia sidoides* Cham. *Biol. Res.* **2012,** *45*, 399–402.
11. Escobar, P.; Milena L. S.; Herrera, L. V.; Martinez, J. R.; Stashenko, E. Chemical Composition and Antiprotozoal Activities of Colombian Lippia spp Essential Oils and Their Major Components. *Mem. Inst. Oswaldo Cruz.* **2010,** *105* (2), 184–190.
12. Santos, A. O.; Ueda-Nakamura, T.; Dias Filho, B. P.; Veiga Junior, V. F.; Pinto, A. C.; Nakamura, C.V. Effect of Brazilian Copaiba Oils on *Leishmania amazonensis*. *J. Ethnopharmacol.* **2008,** *120* (2), 204–208.
13. dos Santos, A. O.; Costa, M. A.; Ueda-Nakamura, T.; Dias-Filho, B. P.; da Veiga-Júnior, V. F.; de Souza Lima, M. M.; Nakamura, C. V. *Leishmania amazonensis*: Effects of Oral Treatment with Copaiba Oil in Mice. *Exp. Parasitol.* **2011,** *129* (2), 145–151.
14. Dos Santos, A. O.; Ueda-Nakamura, T.; Dias Filho, B. P.; da Veiga Junior, V. F.; Nakamura, C. V. Copaiba Oil: An Alternative to Development of New Drugs against Leishmaniasis. *Evid. Based Complement. Alternat. Med.* 2012, 2012, 898419.

15. Santos, D.; Izumi, E.; Ueda-Nakamura, T.; Dias-Filho, B. P.; Veiga-Júnior, V. F.; Nakamura, C. V. Antileishmanial Activity of Diterpene Acids in Copaiba Oil. *Mem Inst Oswaldo Cruz* **2013,** *108* (1), 59–64.
16. Soares, D. C.; Portella, N. A.; Ramos, M. F.; Siani, A. C.; Saraiva, E. M. Trans-β-Caryophyllene: An Effective Antileishmanial Compound Found in Commercial Copaiba Oil (*Copaifera spp.*). *Evid. Based Complement. Alternat. Med.* **2013,** *2013*, 761323. 17. Johann S.; Oliveira F. B.; Siqueira, E. P.; Cisalpino, P. S.; Rosa, C. A.; Alves, T. M.; Zani, C. L.; Cota, B. B. Activity of Compounds Isolated from *Baccharis dracunculifolia* D.C. (Asteraceae) against *Paracoccidioides brasiliensis. Med. Mycol.* **2012,** *50* (8), 843–851.
18. Moura do Carmo, D. F.; Amaral A. C.; Machado, G. M.; Leon, L. L.; Silva, J. R. Chemical and Biological Analyses of the Essential Oils and Main Constituents of *Piper* Species. *Molecules* **2012,** *17*,1819–1829.
19. Monzote, L.; García, M.; Montalvo, A. M.; Scull, R.; Miranda, M. Chemistry, Cytotoxicity and Antileishmanial Activity of the Essential Oil from *Piper auritum. Mem. Inst. Oswaldo Cruz.* **2010,** *105* (2), 168–173.
20. Marques, A. M.; Bareto, A. L. S.; Curvelo, J. A. R.; Romanos, M. T. V.; Soares, R. M. A.; Kaplan, M. A. C. Antileishmanial Activity of Nerolidol-rich Essential oil from *Piper claussenianum. Braz. J. Pharmacognosy* **2011,** *21* (5), 908–914.
21. Garcia, F. P.; Lazarin-Bidóia, D.; Ueda-Nakamura, T.; Oliveira Silva, S. D.; Nakamura, C. V. Eupomatenoid-5 Isolated from Leaves of *Piper regnellii* Induces Apoptosis in *Leishmania amazonensis. Evid. Based Complement. Alternat.Med.* 2013, 2013, 940531.
22. Monzote, L.; García, M.; Montalvo, A. M.; Scull, R.; Miranda, M.; Abreu, J. *In vitro* Activity of an Essential Oil against *Leishmania donovani. Phytother. Res.* **2007,** *21* (11), 1055–1058.
23. Monzote, L.; García, M.; Scull, R.; Cuellar, A.; Setzer, W. N. Antileishmanial Activity of the Essential Oil from *Bixa orellana. Phytother. Res.* **2014,** *28* (5), 753–758.
24. do Socorro S Rosa Mdo, S.; Mendonça-Filho, R. R.; Bizzo, H. R.; de Almeida Rodrigues, I.; Soares, R. M.; Souto-Padrón, T.; Alviano, C. S.; Lopes, A. H. Antileishmanial Activity of a Linalool-rich Essential Oil from *Croton cajucara. Antimicrob. Agents Chemother.* **2003,** *47* (6), 1895–1901.
25. Fabri, R. L.; Coimbra, E. S.; Almeida, A. C.; Siqueira, E. P.; Alves, T. M.; Zani, C. L.; Scio, E. Essential Oil of *Mitracarpus frigidus* as a Potent Source of Bioactive Compounds. *An. Acad. Bras. Cienc.* **2012,** *84* (4), 1073–1080.
26. Mohammadpour, G.; Marzony, E. T.; Farahmand, M. Evaluation of the Anti-*Leishmania major* Activity of *Satureja bakhtiarica* Essential Oil in vitro. *Nat. Prod. Commun.* **2012,** *7* (1), 133–136.
27. Parreira, N. A,; Magalhães, L. G.; Morais, D. R.; Caixeta, S. C.; de Sousa, J. P.; Bastos, J. K.; Cunha, W. R.; Silva, M. L.; Nanayakkara, N. P.; Rodrigues, V.; da Silva Filho, A. A. Antiprotozoal, Schistosomicidal, and Antimicrobial Activities of the Essential Oil from the Leaves of *Baccharis dracunculifolia. Chem. Biodivers.* **2010,** *7* (4), 993–1001.
28. da Silva, Filho A. A.; Resende, D. O.; Fukui, M. J.; Santos, F. F.; Pauletti, P. M.; Cunha, W. R.; Silva, M. L.; Gregório, L. E.; Bastos, J. K.; Nanayakkara, N. P. *In vitro* Antileishmanial, Antiplasmodial and Cytotoxic Activities of Phenolics and Triterpenoids from *Baccharis dracunculifolia* D. C. (Asteraceae). *Fitoterapia.* **2009,** ***80*** (8), 478–482.
29. López, R.; Cuca, L. E.; Delgado, G. Antileishmanial and Immunomodulatory Activity of *Xylopia discreta. Parasite Immunol.* **2009,** *31* (10), 623–630.

30. Oliveira, V. C.; Moura, D. M.; Lopes, J. A.; de Andrade, P. P.; da Silva, N. H.; Figueiredo, R. C. Effects of Essential Oils from *Cymbopogon citratus* (DC) Stapf., *Lippia sidoides Cham.,* and *Ocimum gratissimum* L. on Growth and Ultrastructure of *Leishmania chagasi* Promastigotes. *Parasitol. Res.* **2009,** *104* (5), 1053–1059.
31. Santin, M. R.; dos Santos, A. O.; Nakamura, C. V.; Dias Filho, B. P.; Ferreira, I. C.; Ueda-Nakamura, T. In vitro Activity of the Essential Oil of *Cymbopogon citratus* and its Major Component (citral) on *Leishmania amazonensis. Parasitol. Res.* **2009,** *105* (6), 1489–1496.
32. Machado, M.; Pires, P.; Dinis, A. M.; Santos-Rosa, M.; Alves, V.; Salgueiro, L.; Cavaleiro, C.; Sousa, M. C. Monoterpenic Aldehydes as Potential Anti-*Leishmania* Agents: Activity of *Cymbopogon citratus* and Citral on *L. infantum, L. tropica* and *L. major. Exp. Parasitol.* **2012,** *130* (3), 223–231.
33. Dias, C. N.; Rodrigues, K. A.; Carvalho, F. A.; Carneiro, S. M.; Maia, J. G.; Andrade, E. H.; Moraes, D. F. Molluscicidal and Leishmanicidal Activity of the Leaf Essential Oil of *Syzygium cumini* (L.) SKEELS from Brazil. *Chem. Biodivers.* **2013,** *10* (6), 1133–1141.
34. Colares, A.V.; Almeida-Souza, F.; Taniwaki, N. N.; Souza Cda, S.; da Costa, J. G.; Calabrese Kda, S.; Abreu-Silva, A. L. In Vitro Antileishmanial Activity of Essential Oil of *Vanillosmopsis arborea* (Asteraceae) Baker. *Evid. Based Complement. Alternat. Med.* **2013,** *2013*, 727042.
35. Lopes, M. V.; Desoti, V. C.; Caleare Ade, O.; Ueda-Nakamura, T.; Silva, S. O.; Nakamura, C. V. Mitochondria Superoxide Anion Production Contributes to Geranylgeraniol-Induced Death in *Leishmania amazonensis. Evid. Based Complement. Alternat. Med.* **2012,** *2012*, 298320.
36. Bero, J.; Beaufay, C.; Hannaert, V.; Hérent, M. F.; Michels, P. A.; Quetin-Leclercq, J. Antitrypanosomal Compounds from the Essential Oil and Extracts of *Keetia leucantha* Leaves with Inhibitor Activity on *Trypanosoma brucei* Glyceraldehyde-3-phosphate Dehydrogenase. *Phytomedicine* **2013,** *20* (3-4), 270–274.
37. Tariku,Y.; Hymete, A.; Hailu, A.; Rohloff, J. In vitro Evaluation of Antileishmanial Activity and Toxicity of Essential Oils of *Artemisia absinthium* and *Echinops kebericho. Chem. Biodivers.* **2011,** *8* (4), 614–623.
38. Hatimi, S.; Boudouma, M.; Bichichi, M.; Chaib, N.; Idrissi, N. G. *In vitro* Evaluation of Antileishmania Activity of *Artemisia herba* Alba Asso. *Bull. Soc. Pathol. Exot.* **2001,** *94* (1), 29–31.
39. Tariku Y.; Hymete, A.; Hailu, A.; Rohloff, J. Essential-oil Composition, Aantileishmanial, and Toxicity Study of *Artemisia abyssinica* and *Satureja punctata* ssp. Punctata from Ethiopia. *Chem. Biodivers.* **2010,** *7* (4), 1009–1018.
40. Tariku, Y.; Hymete, A.; Hailu, A.; Rohloff, J. Constituents, Antileishmanial Activity and Toxicity Profile of Volatile Oil from Berries of *Croton macrostachyus. Nat. Prod. Commun.* **2010,** *5* (6), 975–980.
41. Morales-Yuste, M.; Morillas-Márquez, F.; Martín-Sánchez, J.; Valero-López, A.; Navarro-Moll, M. C. Activity of (-)alpha-bisabolol against *Leishmania infantum* Promastigotes. *Phytomed.* **2010,** *17* (3-4), 279–281.
42. Blok, W. L.; Rabinovitch, M.; Zilberfarb, V.; Netea, M. G.; Buurman, W. A.; van der Meer, J. W. The Influence of Dietary Fish-oil Supplementation on Cutaneous *L. amazonensis* Infection in Mice. *Cytokine.* **2002,** *19* (5), 213–217.
43. Carson, C. F.; Hammer, K. A.; Riley, T. V. *Melaleuca alternifolia* (Tea Tree) Oil: A Review of Antimicrobial and Other Medicinal Properties. *Clin. Microbiol. Rev.* **2006,** *19* (1), 50–62.

44. Marques A. M.; Barreto, A. L. S.; Curvelo, J. A. D. R.; Romanos, M. T. V; Soares, R. M. D. A.; Kaplan, M. A. C. Antileishmanial Activity of Nerolidol-rich Essential Oil from *Piper claussenianum. Rev. Bras. Farmacogn.* **2011,** 21.
45. Morty, R. E.; Morehead J. Cloning and Characterization of a Leucyl Aminopeptidase from Three Pathogenic *Leishmania* Species. *J. Biol. Chem.* **2002,** *277*, 26057–26065.
46. Teixeira, A.; Vinaud, M.; Castro, A. M. *Emerging Chagas Disease*; Bentham Science Publishers: Sharjah, UAE, 2011; p 149.
47. Genestra, M.; Cysne-Finkelstein, L.; Guedes-Silva, D.; Leon, L. L. Effect of L-arginine Analogs and a Calcium Chelator on Nitric Oxide (NO) Production by *Leishmania sp. J. Enzyme Inhib. Med. Chem.* **2003,** *18* (5), 445–452.
48. Cabioğlu, M. T.; Cetin, B. E. Acupuncture and Immunomodulation. *Am. J. Chin. Med.* **2008,** *36*, 25.
49. Danillo, N. A., Mayara, M. S., Parreira W. V., Tome, F. D., Batista, L. F.; Gomes, C. M.; Oliveira, M. A. P. Electroacupuncture at the ST36 Acupoint Increases Interleukin-4 Responsiveness in Macrophages, Generation of Alternatively Activated Macrophages and Susceptibility to *Leishmania major* Infection. *Chinese Medicine* **2012,** *7*, 17.
50. Shakibapour, M; Hoseini, S, G.; Mahmoodi, M.; Rostami, F.; Hejazi, S. Effect of Acupuncture Treatment on Level of Serum Interferon (IFN)-Î³ in BALB/c Model of *Leishmania* Major Infection. *Hossein J. Isfahan Med. School* **2013,** *31*, 1077.

CHAPTER 9

INFLAMMATION AND LEISHMANIASIS

CONTENTS

PART XI ROLE OF ANTI-INFLAMMATORY AND ANALGESIC PLANTS IN LEISHMANIA

ABSTRACT

Inflammatory and pain conditions are common in clinical practice. Inflammatory and pain related diseases are widespread in the aging society of developed and developing countries, nevertheless the drugs used to combat pain and inflammatory diseases often have serious side effects. Botanical remedies have been used for centuries to treat such conditions. Our database covers updated information of 216 traditional and their Ayurvedic formulations that are widely used to treat inflammatory and pain conditions. Efforts were also being made to describe the general anti-inflammatory mechanism followed by plants and their extracts. Role of anti-inflammatory plants in leishmania is also described. This database will help the common people for their primary health care and researchers in their research work as they could select the anti-inflammatory medicinal plants from which they can isolate active constituents by using various separation techniques. These types of research works may unveil some new molecules that help us to fight against inflammatory disorders.

9.1 INTRODUCTION

Plants are vital for the existence of life in the universe. About 200,000 plant species known, 300 species were cultivated for food production. The universal role of plants in the treatment of disease is exemplified by their employment in all the major systems of medicine irrespective of the underlying philosophical premise.[1] The use of medicinal plants for health reason started thousands of years ago and it is still a part of medicinal practice in China, Egypt, India, and other developing countries.[2] Over the centuries, the use of medicinal herbs has become an important part of daily life despite significant progress made in modern medical and pharmaceutical research.[3]

Medicinal plants not only play an important role in the public health services, but also offer an established basis of searching for new drugs by means of modern scientific methods.[4]

The earliest mention of the medicinal use of the plants has been found in "Rig Veda," which was written between 4000 and 1600 B.C. In the "Atharva Veda," we find still more varied use of drugs. It is in the "Ayurveda" which is considered as an "Upa Veda" that definite properties of drugs and their use have been given in great detail. "Charaka Samhita" is another earliest treatise on "Ayurveda" (600 B.C) which list a total of 341 plants and plant products for use in health management. "*Susruta Samhita*" also deals with plant related to medicines.

Millions of people in the Third World still use herbal medicines because of their faith and belief in the traditional system of medicine and because of the general awareness of the widespread toxicity and harmful aftereffects associated with the long use of synthetic drugs and antibiotics.[5] During the past two decades considerable changes have taken place in the medicinal system all over the World. Today people prefer the drugs from natural sources rather than the synthetics. In United States and United Kingdom, the plant-based drugs are being used substantially. Russia and China have adopted an integrated system of allopathic, traditional, and folk system of medicine. Plants appear to have involved the chemical pathways to produce compounds capable of curing many diseases.[5]

Medicinal plants have curative properties due to the presence of various complex phytoconstituents that are found as secondary plant metabolites in one or more parts of plants. These plant metabolites, according to their composition, are grouped as alkaloids, glycosides, corticosteroids, essential oils, and so forth.[6]

There are various plants that are used in various system of medicine in the treatment of different disorders such as aconite root (*Aconitum napellus*, family Ranuculaceae) used as topically to skin numbness, acorus (*Acorus calamus*, family Araceae) as a carminative and spasmolytic, adiantum (*Adiantum capillus-vernis*, family Ferns) as a antitussive and expectorant, alertis (*Alertis farinosa*, family Liliaceae) as a mild sedative, allium (*Allium sativum*, family Liliaceae) as an expectorant and hypolipidemic, apium (*Apium graveolens*, family Umblliferae) as a antirheumatic and sedative, hawthorn berries (*Crataegus oxycantoides*, family Rosaceae) as a cardioactive and hypotensive, and mistletoe (*Viscum album*, family Loranthaceae) as a hypotensive and cardiac depressant.[7]

Inflammatory diseases including different types of rheumatic diseases are a major cause of morbidity of the working force throughout world. Inflammation involves changes in blood flow, increased vascular permeability, tissue destruction through the activation and migration of reactive oxygen species and the production of local mediators such as platelet activating factors induced by phospholipase A2, cycloxygenases, lipoxygenases. During this process, this key biological intermediate known as arachidonic is converted in to large number of eicosanoids with biological activities.[67]

This has been called the "King of Human Miseries." Although rheumatism is one of the oldest known diseases of the mankind and affects a large percentage of population of the World, no substantial progress was seen till the synthesis of aspirin in 1899 by the German Company Bayer, the hint of which also was obtained from a plant, the Willow bark (*Salix alba*, family Salicaceae) used worldwide in folk medicine for the relief of aches, fever, and rheumatic pain. Since then many compounds were introduced as a result of laboratory search for drugs with anti-inflammatory activity (AIA); though many of them produced a dramatic symptomatic improvement in rheumatic processes, but did not arrest the progress of the diseases process and all of them shared the common side effect, that is, gastrointestinal irritations.[8]

Nonsteroidal anti-inflammatory drugs ($NSAID_s$) are most commonly used drugs to treat inflammatory conditions but the long-term usage of NSAIDs cause gastric erosions, which can become stomach ulcers and in extreme cases result in death. The risk of death as a result of use of NSAIDs is 1 in 10,000 for young adults aged 16–45. The risk increases 10-fold for those over 75. Patients who take these drugs are at increased risk of clinically important injury to the gastrointestinal mucosa. Estimates suggest that NSAIDs lead to ulcer complications (bleeding or perforation) in 1–4% of chronic users each year, and NSAIDs use is associated with up to 2,500 deaths each year in the U.K. population, which may be attributed to inhibition of COX-1.[9]

In view of these side effects, many plants have been screened for anti-inflammatory/analgesic activity (Table 9-1) based on the traditional reports (Table 9-2) in search of a new entity with least side effects.

TABLE 9-1 Plants reported as analgesics and anti-inflammatory agents

Sr. No.	Plant name	Extracts	Ref.
1.	*Abutilon indicum*	Ethanol extract of root	10
2.	*Achillea santolina*	80% methanol extract of leaves	11
3.	*Ageratum conyzoides*	Hydroalcoholic extract of leaves	12
4.	*Alnus hirsuta*	80% aqueous extract of bark	13
5.	*Anacardium occidentale*	Aqueous extract of stem-bark	14
6.	*Angelica dahurica*	Aqueous extract of root	15
7.	*Angelica pubescens*	Aqueous extract of root	15
8.	*Anthemis nobilis*	Aqueous extracts of whole plant	16
9.	*Apium graveolens*	80% methanol extract of stem	11
10.	*Araucaria bidwillii*	Alcoholic extracts of leaf	17

TABLE 9-1 *(Continued)*

Sr. No.	Plant name	Extracts	Ref.
11.	*Artemisia absinthium*	Methanol extract of stem	18
12.	*Astragalus membranaceus*	Ethanol extract of whole plant	15
13.	*Barleria lupulina Lindl.*	Methanol extract of aerial parts	19
14.	*Calendula officinalis*	Ethanol extract of petals	20
15.	*Cardiospermum halicabum*	Alcoholic fraction of leaves	21
16.	*Cardiosperum helicacabum*	Alcoholic extract of leaves	21
17.	*Commiphora mukul*	Ethyl acetate-soluble potion	21
18.	*Curcuma xanthorrhiza*	Methanol extract of the dried rhizomes	22
19.	*Desmodium gangeticum*	Hexane extract of root	21
20.	*Erigeron floribundus*	Aqueous extract of whole plant	23
21.	*Erythrina crista-galli.*	Ethanol extract of dead twig	24
22.	*Forsythia suspensa*	Ethanol extract of whole plant	15
23.	*Gynura procumbens*	Ethanol extract of whole plant	25
24.	*Hedychium spicatum*	Ethyl acetate extract of rhizomes	26
25.	*Hygrophila auriculata*	Aqueous extract of aerial parts	27
26.	*Imperata cylindrica*	Chloroform and aqueous extract of whole plant	28
27.	*Inula viscosa*	Dichloromethane extract	21
28.	*Jacaranda mimosifolia*	Methanol extract of stembark	29
29.	*Lactuca scariola*	Methanol extract of seeds	18
30.	*Lagenaria siceraria*	The fresh, rind fruit juice extract.	30
31.	*Matricaria chamomilla*	80% methanol extract of root	11
32.	*Matricaria recutita*	Aqueous extracts of whole plant	16
33.	*Mikania cordifolia.*	Leaf decoction of	21
34.	*Morinda morindoides*	80% MeOH extract of leaves	21
35.	*Myrsine australis.*	Methanol extract of the leaves	21
36.	*Myrtus communis*	80% methanol extract of root	11
37.	*Nothospondias staudtii*	Aqueous, methanol and chloroform extracts of leaves	31
38.	*Nyctanthes arbertritis*	Water soluble fraction of ethanol extract of leaves	21
39.	*Paeonia daurica*	Ethanolic extract of the roots	32
40.	*Pedilanthus tithymaloides*	Tincture	33
41.	*Perilla frutescens* var *acuta*	Dichloromethane extract of the stems	21
42.	*Plumeria acuminata*	Methanol extract of leaves	20
43.	*Poria cocos*	Ethanol extract of whole plant	15
44.	*Protium kleinii*	Ether extract of whole plant	34

TABLE 9-1 *(Continued)*

Sr. No.	Plant name	Extracts	Ref.
45.	*Ruta graveolens*	Aqueous, ethanolic and methanolic extracts of aerial parts	35
46.	*Salvia apiana*	Diluted tincture	36
47.	*Salvia officinalis*	*n*-hexane and the chloroform extract of leaves	36
48.	*Santolina oblongifolia* Boiss.	Ethyl acetate extract of the flower tops	21
49.	*Securidaca longipedunculata*	Methanol and petroleum ether extract of root bark	37
50.	*Stachytarpheta cayennensis*	Freeze-dried aqueous extracts of whole plant	38
51.	*Symplocos spicata*	Methanol extract of stem-bark	21
52.	*Tanacetum microphyllum*	Dichloromethane extract of the aerial parts	21
53.	*Tessaria integrifolia*	Leaf decoction of	21
54.	*Trichodesma indicum*	Chloroform extract of root	39
55.	*Turnera ulmifolia*	Lyophilized infusion of the aerial parts	40
56.	*Vitex negundo*	Suspension of dried powered leaves	21
57.	*Withania somnifera*	80% methanol extract of bark	11
58.	*yucca schidigera*	Aqueous extract of whole plant	41
59.	*Zanha Africana*	Methanol extract of root bark	21

TABLE 9-2 Plants used traditionally as anti-inflammatory/analgesics agents

Sr. No.	Plant name	Family	Part used	Ref.
1.	*Abrus precatorius*	Leguminosae	Root and seeds	44
2.	*Acacia catechu* (Katha)	Leguminosae	Bark and stem	42
3.	*Acalypha indica*	Euphorbiaceae	Whole plant	43
4.	*Acorus calamus*	Araceae	Rhizomes	44
5.	*Adenanthera pavonina*	Fabaceae	Barks	45
6.	*Albizia lebbeck*	Fabaceae	Bark	46
7.	*Alhagi camelorume*	Leguminosae	Seeds	44
8.	*Allium sativum*	Liliaceae	Bulb	44
9.	*Allium stracheyi* (Pharna)	Liliaeceae	Leaves	63
10.	*Alocasia indica*	Araceae	Rhizomes	61
11.	*Alpinia officinarum*	Zingiberaceae	Dried rhizome	44
12.	*Amaranthus spinosus* (Prickly amaranth)	Amaranthaceae	Whole plant	63
13.	*Amaranthus Viridis* (Green amaranth)	Amaranthaceae	Whole plant	63
14.	*Amomum subulatum*	Zingiberaceae	Fruit	44
15.	*Amoora cucullata*	Meliaceae	Leaves	47

TABLE 9-2 *(Continued)*

Sr. No.	Plant name	Family	Part used	Ref.
16.	*Ananas comosus*	Bromeliaceae	Fruit juice	44
17.	*Anarcadium occidentale*	Anarcardiaceae	Seed coat	44
18.	*Andrographis peniculata*	Acanthaceae	Leaves	44
19.	*Apium graveolens*	Umbelliferae	Fruit	11
20.	*Apuleia Leiocarpa* (Grapia)	Leg-ceae	Bark and duramen	48
21.	*Argyreia argentea*	Convolvulaceae	Leaves	49
22.	*Asphadeline lutea* (Jacob's rod)	Asphodelaccae	Aerial	62
23.	*Asystasia dalzelliana* (Lavana-valli)	Acanthaceae	Whole plant	63
24.	*Atropa belladonna*	Solanaceae	Fruits	44
25.	*Azadirachta indica*	Meliaceae	Leaves	50
26.	*Baliospormum Montanum* (Danti)	Euphorbiaceae	Roots	63
27.	*Banda tessellate*	Orchidaceae	Roots	44
28.	*Baugainvilla spectabillis* (Booganbel)	Nyctaginaceae	Leaves	51
29.	*Bauhinia racemosa* (Asoda)	Caesalpiniaceae	Stem bark	64
30.	*Boswellia serrata*	Burseraceae	Oleogum	44
31.	*Brassica nigra*	Brassicaceae	Leaves	52
32.	*Brunfelsia uniflora* (Manaca)	Solanaceae	Leaves	48
33.	*Bryonia laciniosa* (Gargumar)	Cucurbitaceae	Whole plant, fruits	63
34.	*Butea monosperma* (Palash)	Fabaceae	Leaves	63
35.	*Calophyllum inophyllum*	Clusiaceae	Nuts	44
36.	*Calophyllum inophyllum*	Hypericaceae	Seeds	44
37.	*Calotropis gigantea* (Crown flower)	Asclepiadaeceae	Leaves	63
38.	*Cannabis sativa*	Cannabaceae	Leaves	44
39.	*Canscora decussatta*	Gentianaceae	Whole plant	44
40.	*Carpolobia lutea* (cattle stick)	Polygalaceae	Roots	63
41.	*Casearia sylvestris* Swartz. (wild coffee)	Flacurteaceae	Leaves and bark	48
42.	*Cassia absus*	Leguminosae	Seeds	44
43.	*Cassia sophera* (Kasunda)	Caesalpiniaceae	leaves	53
44.	*Celosia argentia* (Lalmurga)	Amaranthaceae	Leaves	54
45.	*Chococca brachiata*	Rubiaceae	Root	48
46.	*Cissampelos pareira* (Akanadi)	Menispermaceae	Aerial parts	63
47.	*Cissus quadrangularis* (Hadjod)	Vitaceae	whole plant	63
48.	*Cissus rependa* (Pani bel)	Vitaceae	Root, Stem	55
49.	*Clausena suffruticosa*	Rutaceae	Root	56
50.	*Clerodendron viscosum*	Verbanaceae	Aerial parts	57
51.	*Clerodendrum phlomidis* (Arni)	Verbanaceae	Stem bark	63

TABLE 9-2 *(Continued)*

Sr. No.	Plant name	Family	Part used	Ref.
52.	*Colchicum autumnale*	Liliaceae	Seeds and corns	44
53.	*Colchicum luteum*	Liliaceae	Seeds and corns	44
54.	*Commiphora mukul*	Burseraceae	Balsam	44
55.	*Curcuma longa*	Zingiberaceae	Rhizomes	44
56.	*Cuscuta reflexa*	Convolvulaceae	Whole plant	44
57.	*Cymbidium aloifolium*	Orchidaceae	Leaves	58
58.	*Cynara scolymus* (Globe artichoke)	Asteraceae	Leaves	48
59.	*Cyperus rotendus*	Cyperaceae	Root and seeds	44
60.	*Dalbergia volubilis*	Leguminaceae	Bark	44
61.	*Dendranthema indica*	Compositae	Seeds	44
62.	*Desmodium triflorum*	Fabeceae	Whole plant	59
63.	*Dorstonia brasiliensis* (Carapia)	Moraceae	Root	48
64.	*Echinaceae purpurea*	Compositae	Root	44
65.	*Elephantopus scaber* (Elephant foot)	Asteraceae	Leaves	48
66.	*Eucalyptus citriodora* (lemon eucalyptus)	Myrtaceae	Essential oil	63
67.	*Ficus bengalensis* (Bar)	Moraceae	Leaves	51
68.	*Ficus glomerata* (Cluster Fig Tree)	Moraceae	Bark and leaves	44
69.	*Ficus racemosa* (Udumbar)	Moraceae	fruits	63
70.	*Garcinia mangostana*	Guttiferae	Gum	44
71.	*Glinus oppositifolius*	Molluginaceae	Whole plants	60
72.	*Harpagophytum procumbens*	Pedaliaceae	Dried root	44
73.	*Hedera nepalense*	Araliaceae	Fruit	44
74.	*Hedychium coronarium*	Zingiberaceae	Rhizome	61
75.	*Hedyotis puberula* (Surbuli)	Rubiaceae	Whole plant	63
76.	*Hemidesmus indicus*	Asclepiadaceae	Root, flower and latex	44
77.	*Hibiscus rosa sinensis* (China rose)	Malvaceae	leaves	63
78.	*Hibiscus sabdariffa*	Malvaceae	Calyx	61
79.	*Hibiscus tiliaceus* (Beach Hibiscus)	Malvaceae	Leaves	63
80.	*Holarrhena antidysenterica* (Indrajao)	Apoynaceae	Bark	63
81.	*Hygrophila auriculata*	Acanthaceae	Seed	44
82.	*Hyoscyamus niger*	Solanaceae	Seeds	44
83.	*Juglans regia*	Juglandiaceae	Seeds	44
84.	*Kaempferia galangal* (Aromatic ginger)	Zingiberaceae	Fresh rhizome	63
85.	*Kigelia pinnata*	Bignoniaceae	Leaves	61
86.	*Kyllinga monocephala* (Nirbishi)	Cyperaceae	Leaves	63
87.	*Leonurus sibiricus*	Lamiaceae	Aerial part	61

TABLE 9-2 *(Continued)*

Sr. No.	Plant name	Family	Part used	Ref.
88.	*Leucas cephalotes* (dronpushpi)	Labiatae	Leaves	63
89.	*Linum usitatissimum*	Linaceae	Oil & leaves	44
90.	*Lippia nodiflora*	Verbenaceae	Leaves	61
91.	*Mangifera indica*	Anacardiaceae	Leaves	61
92.	*Manihot esculenta* (Simal alu)	Euphorbiaceae	Whole plant	63
93.	*Manilkara zapota* (Chickoo)	Sapotaceae	Leaves	63
94.	*Marsilea trifolia* (Goldthread)	Marsilea-ceae	Fresh leaf	63
95.	*Marsypianthes chanaedrys* (Konmonmi mawon)	Lamiaceae	Leaves	48
96.	*Melaleuca leucadandron*	Myrtaceae	Leaves and oil	44
97.	*Mentha arvensis*	Labiatae	Leaves	44
98.	*Mesua ferrea*	Guttiferae	Whole plant	44
99.	*Mesua nagassarium*	Clusiaceae	Leaves	61
100.	*Mikania glomerata* (sprengel)	Asteraceae	Leaves	48
101.	*Mimosa pudica*	Leguminosae	Leaves and roots	44
102.	*Mitragyna parvifolia* (kadam)	Rubiaceae	fruits	63
103.	*Mucuna pruriens*	Fabaceae	Aerial parts	61
104.	*Murraya paniculata* (Orange Jessamine)	Rutaceae	Bark	63
105.	*Myristica fragrans*	Myristicaceae	Seeds and ariallus	44
106.	*Myrsine australis*	Myricaceae	Leaves	44
107.	*Nelumbo nucifera* (Kamal)	Nelumbonaceae	Seeds	63
108.	*Nyctanthes arbor-tristis* (Shefali)	Oleaceae	Bark	63
109.	*Oxalis corniculata* (Creeping oxalis)	Oxalidaceae	Whole plant	63
110.	*Papaver somniferum*	Papaveraceae	Latex	44
111.	*Peganum harmalla* (Harmal)	Zygophylaceae	Whole plant	62
112.	*Peltophorum pterocarpum*	Peltophoreaceae	Pods	44
113.	*Pergularia daemia* (Utaran)	Asclepiadaceae	Roots	63
114.	*Persicaria stagnina*	Polygonaceae	Whole plant	61
115.	*Phyllanthus emblica*	Euphorbiaceae	Flowers	63
116.	*Phyllanthus niruri* (Gulf-leaf flower)	Phyllanthaceae	whole plant	63
117.	*Phyllanthus reticulatus*	Euphorbiaceae	Aerial parts	61
118.	*Pimpinella anisum* (Saunf)	Umbellifera	Seeds	62
119.	*Piper chaba*	Piperaceae	Stem	61
120.	*Pletranthus amboinicus* (Maxican mint)	Lamiaceae	Leaves	63
121.	*Plumbago zeylanica* (Chitrak)	Plumbaginaceae	Roots	63
122.	*Polyalthia longifolia* (Devadaru)	Annonaceae	Leaves	63
123.	*Polygonum lanatum*	Polygonaceae	Whole plant	28

TABLE 9-2 *(Continued)*

Sr. No.	Plant name	Family	Part used	Ref.
124.	*Polygonum stagninum*	Polygonaceae	Aerial parts	61
125.	*Polygonum viscosum*	Polygonaceae	Aerial parts	61
126.	*Psila spartioides*	Asteraceae	Whole plant	44
127.	*Randia dumetornm* (Mainphal)	Rubiaceae	Seeds	63
128.	*Rubia cordifolia* (Indian Madder)	Rubiaceae	Root	63
129.	*Sacropthyte piriei*	Balanophoraceae	Rhizomes	44
130.	*Santolina oblongifolia*	Compositae	Flower tops	21
131.	*Saraca indica* (Asok)	Leguminosae	Leaves	63
132.	*Scoparia dulcis*	Scrophulariaceae	Leaves	61
133.	*Scoparia dulcis* (Mithi patti)	Scrophulariacae	Whole herb	61
134.	*Sida acuta* (Bariara)	Malvaceae	Whole plant	51
135.	*Sida cordifolia*	Malvaceae	Aerial parts	61
136.	*Sinapis arvensis* (Field mustard)	Solanaceae	Aerial	62
137.	*Solanum surattense*	Solanaceae	Fruiting plant	44
138.	*Solanum trilobatum* (Alarka)	Solanaceae	Root	63
139.	*Sphaeranthus indicus* (Mundi)	Compositae	Whole plants	63
140.	*Spilanthus oleraceae*	Compositae	Whole plant	44
141.	*Sterculia foetida* (Jangli badam)	Sterculiaceae	Seeds	63
142.	*Stylosanthes fruitcosa* (Saillekampa)	Papilionaceae	Whole plant	51
143.	*Swertia decussata*	Gentianaceae	Leaves & seeds	44
144.	*Tamarix indica*	Tamaricaceae	Root	61
145.	*Tanacetum artemisioides* (Paloyo Zoon)	Asteraceae	Whole plant	30
146.	*Tectona grandis* (Sagwan)	Vervenaceae	Leaves	63
147.	*Thesium chinense* (bai rui cao)	Santalaceae	Leaves	63
148.	*Toona celiata* (Tun)	Meliaceae	Heart wood	51
149.	*Trianosperma tayaya* (Mart)	Curcurbitaceae	Root	48
150.	*Tribulus terrestris* (Bindii)	Zygophyllaceae	Aerial	62
151.	*Trichosanthes dioica*	Cucurbitaceae	Fruit	61
152.	*Tridax procumbens* (Tridax daisy)	Compositae	Leaves	63
153.	*Tridex procumbens* (Ghamra)	Asteraceae	Leaves	63
154.	*Xanthium indicum* (Banokra)	Compositae	Leaves	63
155.	*Xeromphis spinosa*	Rubiaceae	Bark	61
156.	*Zanha Africana*	Sapindaceae	Root bark	21
157.	*Zingiber officinale*	Zingiberaceae	Rhizomes	44

9.2 EVIDENCE ACQUISITION

The plant kingdom is undoubtedly valuable as a source of new medicinal agents. The present work constitutes a review of the literature on plant and their extracts showing analgesics and AIA. The review refers to 216 plants with their families, and biological source, the parts utilized, the type of extract tested. With this objective of contributing to these studies, a literature search on the use of natural products, crude plant extracts, which have already been evaluated particularly for inflammation and pain, has been carried out using biological abstracts, chemical abstracts, and the data bank of the Jadavpur University and updated to December 2013. The references found in the search were then studied in detail.

9.3 DESCRIPTION OF THE DATABASE OF ANTI-INFLAMMATORY PLANTS

In spite of the development in present medicine, it has been accounted that more than 70% of the developing world's population still depends on traditional system of medicine. This database explores various herbs that possess anti-inflammatory properties and have the potential to reduce pain and inflammation. Day by day herbal remedies and its related drugs are gaining more popularity. Safety, efficacy and cost-effectiveness are the most considerable reasons for their wide usage. In India, there are several indigenous medicinal plants available that have anti-inflammatory capabilities. Lists of these medicinal plants are given in Tables 9-1 and 9-2.

9.4 MECHANISM OF ACTION OF NATURAL DRUGS

Though a number of plants have been investigated for anti-inflammatory and analgesic activity, but there still remain a number of plants which are traditionally used for this ailment and need scientific investigations for their anti-inflammatory and analgesic activity. One such plant identified is *Tephrosia purpurea* Pers. For the treatment of inflammation and pain, currently most of the population is moving toward herbal remedies. We have highlighted a database on various medicinal plants (Tables 9-1 and 9-2) that are having strong potential in reducing pain and inflammation. These plants were already screened against pain and inflammation but their utilization will be more advisable after finding out the mechanism of action at molecular level. In response to the external or other stimuli, the activation of transcription factor nuclear factor-kappaB (NF-κB) occurs. For the development of novel anti-inflammatory agent, one of the recent focused mechanisms is the inhibition of transcription factor, activation inflammation that controls over 500 different gene products. The agents that can inhibit NF-κB and diminish chronic inflammation have potential to prevent or delay the onset of the chronic diseases and further even treat them. Various other reported mechanisms followed by anti-inflammatory components of these plants are illustrated in Figures 9-1 and 9-2.

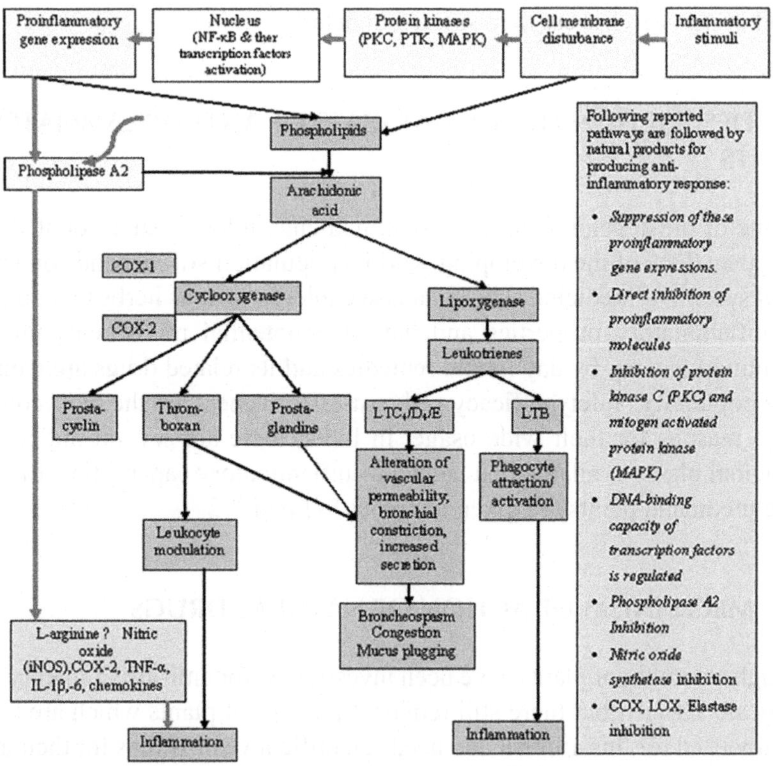

FIGURE 9-1 Illustration of several mechanisms of natural products and their respective pathways for producing anti-inflammatory response.

Dark red boxes with light arrows indicates eicosanoid pathway whereas light red boxes with dark arrows indicates the direct production of iNOS, COX-2, TNF-α, and IL-β, -6 for inflammation. Blue arrow indicates the direct production of phospholipase-2. Green box explores the pathways adopted by various natural substances to inhibit or reduce the inflammatory response. Yellow box represents transcription factors activation in response to the various stimuli that lead to the activation of various genes that may further cause inflammation.[65,66,68]

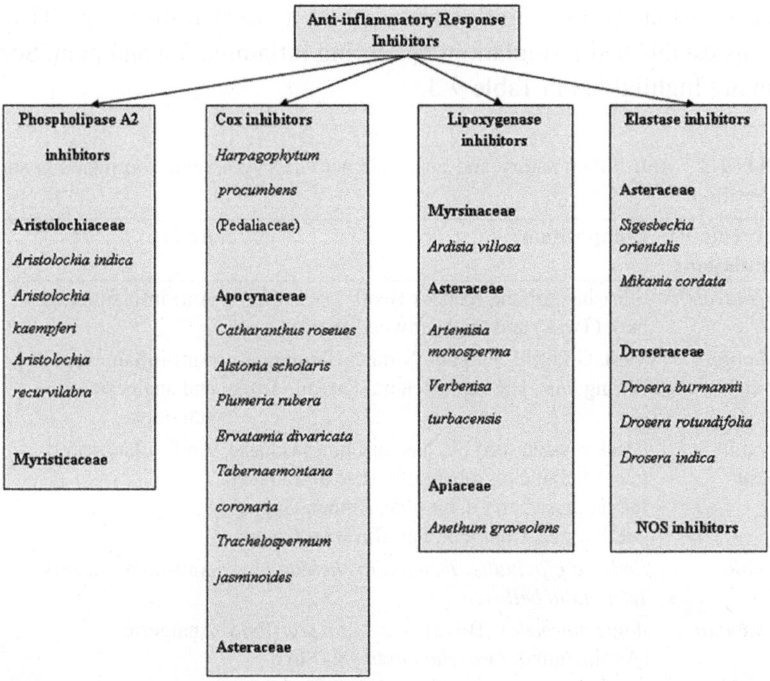

FIGURE 9-2 Illustration of the various classes of anti-inflammatory plants according to their mechanism of inhibition.

9.5 AYURVEDA FOR PAIN AND INFLAMMATION MANAGEMENT

Inflammation in Ayurveda is known by different names in different contexts namely *Shotha*, *Shopha*, *Svayatu*, *Utsedha*, and *Samhata*; whereas arthritic pain is known as *Sandhi vata* (*sandhi* means joint in Sanskrrit), caused by vitiation of *Vata dosha* in the human body. Ayurveda believes that *sandhi vata* can be caused due to various reasons such as rheumatism, gout, infections, digestive problems, and so forth, which results in a buildup of ama (toxins in the body). Ayurveda treats the concept of pain and inflammation as (1) symptom of a disease, (2) an independent disease, and (3) a complication of diseases. Ayurveda can serve as a "goldmine" for novel anti-inflammatory and analgesic agents used for centuries to treat chronic diseases. In this work, almost 200 Ayurvedic plants have been identified that exhibit analgesic and AIA (Table 9-1–9.3). Nowadays, transcription factor, NF-κB is a key target for all the anti-inflammatory agents. Plants those are efficiently inhibit the NF-κB are highlighted in Figure 9-3. For the development of polyherbal formulations, the combination of these plants can be utilized against various types of inflammation and its related disorders. There are various established formulations for curing inflammation and pain. Some of them are highlighted in Table 9-3.

TABLE 9-3 Anti-inflammatory and analgesic activities Ayurvedic formulations and their composition

Ayurvedic formulations	Composition	Action	Ref.
Shirishavaleha	Shirisha (Albizia lebbeck Benth.), viz. the bark (Twak) and the heartwood (Sara).	Anti-inflammatory	69
Dashanga ghana	Vasa, Guduchi, Parpata, Nimba, Bhunimba, Bhringaraja, Haritaki, Behera, Parwal, Amla	Anti-inflammatory and analgesic activities	70
Nimbadi thailam	Black sesame seed oil, Neem, Chinese chaste tree, Chebulic myrobalan, Beleric myrobalan, Indian gooseberry, Chir pine, Amber, Guggul, Sal tree, Camphor, Paraffin wax, water.	Anti-inflammatory	71
Triphala	*Emblica officinalis*, *Terminalia chebula*, *Terminalia bellirica*	Anti-inflammatory	72
Dashamula	*Aegle marmelos* (Bilva), *Premnain tegrifolia* (Agnimantha), *Oroxylum indicum* (Shyonaka), *Stereospermum suaveolens* (Patla), *Gmelina arborea* (Kashmiri), *Desmodium indicum* (Shaliparni), *Urari alagopoides* (Prishniparni), *Solanum indicum* (Brahati), *Solanum xanthocarpum* (Kantkari) and *Tribulus terrestris* (Gokshura).	Analgesic	73
Draksharishta	Dry grapes, Cinnamon, Cardamom, *Cinnamomum tamala*, *Mesua ferrea*, *Callicarpa macrophylla*, Black pepper, Long pepper, *Embelia ribes*, *Woodfordia fruticosa*	Analgesic and anti-inflammatory	74
Rumalaya	*Mahagograj guggul*, *Shemkha bhasma*, Shilajiit, latakasturi, *Swarnamakshika bhasma*, Maharasnadi quath, Manjishtha, Shigres, Gokshura, Guduchi	Analgesic and anti-inflammatory	76
Rumalaya fort	Shallaki, Guggula, Rasna, Yashtimadhu, Gokshura, Guduchi, Nirgundi, Sunth	Analgesic and anti-inflammatory	76
Reosto	Guggula, godanti bhasma, rasna, arjuna, ashvagandha, bala, kukkutandatvak bhasma	Analgesic and anti-inflammatory	76
Poly-herbal ayurvedic formulation	*Sida retusa* (root), *Withania somnifera*, *Frillaria roylei*, *Paederia foetida* (prasarini)		75
Charak	Suvarna paan, muktashukti bhasma, kukkudtandwak, shallaki, guggul, nirgundi, shyonak, guduchi, bala mool, gokhsur, ashvagandha, shuddha, kupilu	Analgesic and anti-inflammatory	76

TABLE 9-3 *(Continued)*

Ayurvedic formulations	Composition	Action	Ref.
Arthrella	Suvarna paan, errand tel, shallaki guggul, nirgundi, shyonak, nagarmotha, shunthi, shuddha kupilu, khurasani ajwayan.	Analgesic and anti-inflammatory	76
Rymanyl	Abhrak bhasma, Suva rnamakshik bhasma, Vang bhasma, Nag bhasma, Ras sindur, Suvarna paan, Shyonaka, Nirgundi, Guggul shuddha,Errand mool, Nagarmotha, punarnava, guduchi, pippali mool, Ashwagandha, Mnishottar, Shunthi, Khurasani ajawayan, Kupilu shuddha, Bachanag Shuddha	Analgesic and anti-inflammatory	76
R-compound	Guggul, Vavdine, Haldi, Jatamanshi, Rasna, Nirgundi, Sunth, Bel Chal, Chitrak chal, Chop Chini, Devdasu, Gangrene, Ajwayan, Neem Chal, Sarson, White Naws adar, Swarn bhasma, Abrak bhasma, Bang bhasma, Yasada bhasma, Mandur bhasma, Loh bhasma, Pippli mool, Dared, Errand Mool, Vacha, Chavak, Amala, Vasaka, Aru Chal, Ashwagandha, Behra.	Analgesic and anti-inflammatory	76
Rumartho	Suvarna Makshik bhasma, Vyadhiharan, Kasis bhasma, Agmvatari ras, Ashwagandha churna, Chop chini, Sudha kuchla, Punarnava mool, Dasmula churna	Analgesic and anti-inflammatory	76
Jwarankush	Suddha parad, Suddha gandhak, Suddha vats Nabh, suddha Kanak seed, Suddha tankad, Suddha harital.	Analgesic and anti-inflammatory	76
Maharasnadhi quathar	Rasna (*Pluchea lanceolata*), Damasa (*Fagonia arabica*), Errand (*Ricinus communis*) Root, Devdaru (Deodar), Kachura (*Curcuma zeodoaria*), Mainphal (*Randia dumetorum*, Vansa (*Adhatoda vasika*), Ginger (*Zingiber officinalis*), Haritaki (*Terminalia chebula*), Chavya (*Piper chaba*), NagarMothan (*Cyperus rotundus*), Punarnava (*Boerhaavia diffusa*), Guduchi (*Tinospora cordifolia*), Vidari (*Ipomoea digitata*), Saunf (Fennel), Gokshuradi (*Tribulus terrestris*), Ashwagandha (*Withania somnifera*), Apamarga (*Achyranthes aspera*), Amaltas (*Cassia fistula*), Shatavari (*Aspargus racemosus*), Pippali (*Piper longum*), Piyabansa (*Barleria prionitis*), Coriander (*Coriandrum sativum*), Kantakari (*Solanum xanthocarpum*), Brahti (*Solanum indicum*), Dalchini (*Cinnamomum cassia*) (Cinnamon) Bark.	Analgesic and anti-inflammatory	77

TABLE 9-3 *(Continued)*

Ayurvedic formulations	Composition	Action	Ref.
Kaishore Guggulu	*Commiphora mukul, Terminalia cheb, Terminalia bellerica, Emblica officinalis, Tinospora cordifolia, Zingiber officinale, Piper nigrum, Embelia ribes, Operculina turpethu, Baliospermum montanum*	Analgesic and anti-inflammatory	78
Kutajarishta	*Holarrhena antidysenterica,* Dry grapes, *Madhuca indica, Gmelina arborea, Woodfordia fruticosa, Gmelina arborea, Madhuca indica*	Analgesic and anti-inflammatory	79
Punarnavasava	*Zingibar officinale,* Pepper *Piper longum, Capsicum annuum, Terminalia chebula, Terminalia belerica, Emblica officinalis, Berberis aristatam, Tribulus terrestris, Solanum indicum, Solanum xanthocarpum, Adhatoda vasica, Aurondo donax, Picrorrhiza kurroa, Piper chaba, Boerhavia diffusa, Azadirachta indica, Tinospora cordifolia, Trichosanthes dioica, Vitis vinifera, Woodfordia fruticosa*	Analgesic and anti-inflammatory	80
Rheumatil gel	*Cedrus deodara*	Analgesic and anti-inflammatory	81
Plugit capsule	*Maharasnadi kwath, Pathyadi kwath, Zingiber officinale, Ocimum sanctum, Vitex negundo, Commiphora mukul, Narsinh churna, Shulgajkesari gutti, Godanti bhasma, Shankh bhasma, Swarnamakshik bhasma*	Analgesic	82
Dashamoolarish	*Aegle marmelos, Oroxylum indicum, Stereospermum suaveolens, Premna integrifolia, Gmelina arborea, Solanum xanthocarpum, Solanum indicum, Esmodium gangeticum, Uraria picta, Tribulus terrestris*	Analgesic	83
Amrutanjan	*Cinnamomum camphora, C. zeylanicum, Cymbopogon citrates, Eucalyptus polybractea, Gaultheria* sp.	Cures pain	68
Divya arshkalpa vati	*Aloe vera, Azadirachta indica, Berberis aristata, C. camphora, Daemenorops draco, Sapindus* sp., *Solanum nigrum, T. chebula*	Cures colic pain	68
Divya ashmarihara rasa	*Hajarala yahuda, Hordeum vulgare, Raphanus sativus*	Relieves pains	68
Divya gaisahara choorna	*Citrus limon, Cuminum cymimum, Ferula foetida, Piper nigra, T. chebula, Trachyspermum ammi*	colic pain	68
Divya mukta vati	*Acorus calamus, Bacopa monnieri, C. paniculatus, C. pluricaulis, Inula racemosa, L. stoechas, N. jatamansi, Rauwolfia serpentina, T. arjuna, W. somnifera*	Chest pain	68

TABLE 9-3 *(Continued)*

Ayurvedic formulations	Composition	Action	Ref.
Divya pidantaka kvatha	*Cyperus rotundus, Nyctanthes arbortristis, Piper chaba, P. longum, Pluchea lanceolata, Ricinus communis, T. ammi, Vitex negundo, W. somnifera, Z. officinale*	Useful in joint pain, sciatica, osteo-arthritis, gout, rheumatoid arthritis, muscular and skeletal pains and oedema.	68
Divya udaramrita vati	*A. marmelos, A. vera, B. diffusa, E. officinalis, Mangifera indica, Operculina turpethum, Phyllanthus niruri, P. kurroa, Plumbago zeylanica, S. nigrum, T. belerica, T. ammi*	Cures jaundice, anaemia, chronic fever, diarrhoea and abdominal pain	68
Divya churna	*F. vulgare, Ipomoea nil, R. centifolia, T. chebula, Z. officinale*	Cures abdominal pain, flatulence, heaviness & nausea	68
Divya pidantaka rasa	*A. marmelos, Clerodendron phlomoides, Commiphora mukul, C. rotundus, Gmelina arborea, Moringa oleifera, Oroxylum indicum, P. lanceolata, Pseudarthria viscida, S. indicum, Stereospermum suaveolen, Strychnos nuxvomica, T. cordifolia, T. ammi, T. terrestris, Uraria lagopoides, V. negundo, W. somnifera*	Useful in joint pain, arthritis, lumbar pain, cervical spondylitis and sciatica	68
Divya pidantaka taila	*Aconitum ferox, A. calamus, A. marmelos, Allium sativum, Anethum sowa, A. racemosus, B. aristata, Butea mono-sperma, Calotropis procera, C. paniculatus, C. zeylanicum, C. phlomoides, C. longa, Datura metel, E. alba, F. vulgare, G. glabra, G. arborea, Hebenaria intermedia, I. racemosa, Lilium polyphyllum, Malaxis acuminate, M. ferrea, N. jatamansi, Oroxylum indicum, Paderia foetida, P. chaba, P. longum, P. lanceolata, P. zeylanica, Polygonatum verticillatum, Pseudarthria viscida, R. communis, Roscoea alpina, R. cordifolia, Sesamum indicum, S. indicum, Stereospermum suaveolen, Strychnos nuxvomica, T. ammi, T. terrestris, Uraria lagopoides, Valeriana wallichii, V. negundo, Z. officinale*	Relieves pain of lumbar region, knee-joints, cervical spondylitis, oedema & inflammation	68
Divya medohara vati	*B. diffusa, C. mukul, E. officinalis, E. ribes, Operculina turpethum, P. kurroa, T. belerica, T. chebula*	Thyroid disorders, rheumatic arthritis, joint pains, pain to lumbar region and knee joints.	68

TABLE 9-3 *(Continued)*

Ayurvedic formulations	Composition	Action	Ref.
Divya hriday-amrita vati	*B. diffusa, C. mukul, C. rotundus, P. lanceolatus, P. zeylanica T. arjuna, T. cordifolia, V. negundo*	Removes the arterial block, angina pain and palpitation	68
Divya vatari churna	*M. oleifera, P. kurroa, T. foenum-graecum, W. somnifera, Z. officinale*	Cures rheumatoid arthritis, sciatica, pain in back and lumbar region	68
Himalaya rumalaya forte	*Alpinia galanga, Boswellia serrata, C. wightii, G. glabra T. cordifolia, Tribulus terrestris*	Relieves pain from arthritis and traumatic inflammation	68
Rumalaya gel	*B. serrata, Cedrus deodara, Cinnamomum zeylanicum Gaultheria fragrantissima, M. arvensis, Pinus roxburghii V. negundo, Z. officinale*	Analgesic, relieves pain, joint mobility	68
Anqaruya-i-kabir	Main drug is *Semicarpus anacardium*	Anti-inflammatory	84
Bandiq-al-bazur	Main drugs are *Cucumis melo, Cucumis sativus*	Anti-inflammatory	84
Hab azraqui	*Strychnous nux vomica, Piper nigrum*	Joint pain and inflammation	84
Hab asgand	*Molasses, Asparagus racemosus, Asparagus adscendens, Zingeber officinale, Piper longum, Argyereia speciosa, Withania somnifera, Ptychotis ajowan*	Rheumatism and gout	84
Dawa-i-gulu	*Acacia catechu*, Glycerine, Iodine, Alcohol, Potassium iodide, *Mentha pipertia*	Tonsilitis	84
Roghan anaf	Menthol oil, Camphor oil, White oil, Eucalyptus oil	Nasal pain	84
Roghan aujakhas	*Calotropis gigantean* flower oil, *Celastrus paniculatus* oil	Muscular and neuralgic pains	84
Roghan babunah	*Matricria chamomilla* flowers, *Sesamum indicum* oil	Analgesic	84
Roghan badam talk	*Prunus amygdalus*	Analgesic	84
Roghan turb	*Raphanus sativus, Sesamum indicum* oil	Ear aches	84
Roghan henna	*Lawsonia inermis* leaves, *Sesamum indicum* oil	Gout	84
Roghan khaskhas	Poppy seeds	Headaches	84
Roghan darchini	*Cinnamomum officinalis*	Analgesic	84

TABLE 9-3 *(Continued)*

Ayurvedic formulations	Composition	Action	Ref.
Roghan dhatura	Dhatura metal, *Sesamum indicum* oil	Gout	84
Roghan kuchla	*Strychnous nux vomica, Sesamum indicum* oil, opium	Anti-rheumatic	84
Roghan kaddu	*Lagenaria siceraria*	Analgesic	84
Arq peppermint	Menthe piperita oil	Analgesic for stomachache	84
Arq dasmol	Ten different herbs	Analgesic (cold)	84
Roghan gul	*Rosa damacsena* petals (300 g), *Sesamum indicum* oil	Analgesic	84
Roghan gul akh	Dried *Zingiber officinale* (100 g), *Colchichum autumnale* (100 g), fresh *Caloptropis gigantean* flowers 200 g), *Sesamum indicum* oil	Analgesic for pain in leg joints	84
Roghan laung	Clove	Analgesic	84
Roghan malkangni	*Calastrus paniculatus* (6 g), *Prunus amygladus* (3 g)	Inflammation	84
Roghan mom	Bees wax acacia (1 kg), Arabica charcoal (50 g)	General analgesic	84
Itrifal saghir	*Emblica officinalis, Termenalis belerica, Potminalia chebula, Termenalia chebula*	Analgesic	84
Chandraprabha Vati	3gm (*Cinnamomum camphora, Acorus calamus, Cyperus rotundus, Andrographis paniculata, Tinospora cordifolia, Cedrus deodara, Curcuma longa, Aconitum heterophyllum, Berberis aristata, Piper longum, Plumbago zeylanica, Coriandrum sativum, Terminalia chebula, Terminalia bellirica, Emblica officinalis, Piper chaba, Embelia ribes, Zingiber officinalis, Piper nigrum,* Purified Copper, *Hordeum vulgare*, Rock salt, Sochal salt, Vida salt), 12 g (*Operculina turpethum, Baliospermum montanum, Cinnamomum tamala, Cinnamomum zeylanicum, Elettaria cardamomum, bambusa bambos*), 24 g (*Loha Bhasma*) + 96 gm (*Commiphora mukul*), 96 g (Shilajatu)	Analgesic and anti-inflammatory	84
Maha yogaraja guggulu (Baidyanath)	Sontha, Pipal, Chavya, Piplamul, Hing, Ajmod, Indrajau, Patha, Vidanga, Kutki, Atis, Vacha, Triphala, Guggulu, Vang bhasma, Lauh bhasma, Nag bhasma, Raupya bhasm, Abhrak bhasm, Mandoor bhasma, Ras sindoor.	Analgesic and anti-inflammatory	84

TABLE 9-3 *(Continued)*

Ayurvedic formulations	Composition	Action	Ref.
Dashanga ghana	Yashtimadhu, Tagara, Sukshmaila, Jatamamsi, Haridra, Daruharidra, Shirisha, Kushta, Rakta Chandana, Hribera	Analgesic and anti-inflammatory	84
Mahanarayan tail	*Withania somnifera, Solanum surattense, Sida cordifolia, Tribulus terrestris, Oroxylum indicum, Abutilon indicum, Sida veronicaepetia, Stereospermum suaveolens,* Til Oil, Cow's milk, *Asparagus racemosus, Cinnamomum camphora, Crocus sativus* etc.	Analgesic and anti-inflammatory	84
Mahavishgarbh tail	Made of 72 Ayurvedic herbs with sesame oil	Sciatica, Rheumatism	84

Current communication represents an updated review on plants with analgesic and AIA with special emphasis on those plants found in different parts of the India. For the first time, we have explored that all the reported mechanism adopted by phytoconstituents in relieving pain and inflammation. This article will be helpful to the common people for their primary health care and the researchers for further isolation and characterization of the active chemical constituents responsible for analgesic anti-inflammatory potential. The categorization of such plants according to their medicinal properties directs as well as decides its future plan related with their isolation, characterization, clinical evaluation and formulation, and development of a single or multiple components. Collection of several reports like this of a particular plant defines its prominent medicinal property, which could further help in conducting the specified research on that plant. On the basis of this survey, we have founded that there is a huge diversity of anti-inflammatory components. Compounds such as flavanoids, alkaloids, and terpenoids are the lead compounds against pain and inflammation. They adopt various mechanisms to reduce the pain as well as inflammation. To get the maximum yield it is very necessary to define their natural occurrence with their specified source which will help in further development of that plant in traditional as well as allopathic (derivatives) system. Ayurvedic formula for various medicinal plants reported for inflammation is mentioned in Figure 9-3.

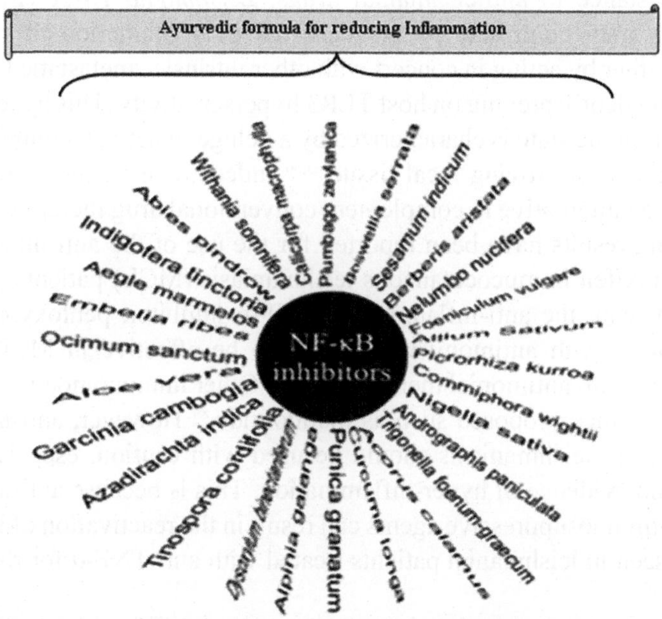

FIGURE 9-3 Anti-inflammatory plants that are responsible for NF-kappaB inhibition and can be used for the development and designing of Ayurvedic formulations.

9.6 ROLE OF ANTI-INFLAMMATORY PLANTS IN *LEISHMANIA*

Medicinal plants exerts great role in the discovery and development of new drugs. Inflammation is a frequent problem therefore majority of human population is currently affected worldwide. Synthetic drugs are not useful in all cases as they are having lot of side effects. Compounds such as flavanoids, alkaloids, and terpenoids are the potent source for anti-inflammatory drugs. Hence, there is an urgent need to explore such potent plants with their respective chemical diversity and their molecular mechanism involved in reducing inflammation and pain. Several reports confirm that *Leishmania* induces severe inflammatory reponses that may lead to the progression of disease, parasite persistence, and perhaps even resistance to antileishmanial drugs. This has been recently found in the case of *Leishmania guyanensis*. *L. guyanensis*, the nucleic acid of *Leishmania* RNA virus (LRV1) acts as a potent innate immunogen, eliciting a hyper-inflammatory immune response through toll-like receptor 3 (TLR3). The resultant inflammatory cascade has been shown to increase disease severity, parasite persistence, and perhaps even resistance to antileishmanial drugs. *Leishmania* RNA virus in this subgenus may contribute to the destructive inflammation of metastatic disease either by acting in concert with other intrinsic "metastatic factors" or by independently preying on host TLR3 hypersensitivity. This hyper-inflammatory immune state is characterized by a deluge of activated immune cells, swelling, and destroying local tissue.[85,86] Indeed, controlling inflammation could be an alternative to complement conventional drug therapies. Already, interesting results have been reported for the use of the anti-inflammatory drug tamoxifen in mucocutaneous leishmaniasis (MCL) patients.[87] Further, treatment with the anti-inflammatory TNF-α inhibitor, pentoxyphylline in combination with antimony was shown to be effective in MCL patients unresponsive to antimonial therapy alone.[88] Other immunomodulatory drugs have been since proposed such as thalidomide.[89] However, anti-inflammatory drugs in leishmaniasis should be used with caution, especially when there is no evidence of hyper-inflammation. This is because anti-inflammatory or immunosuppressive agents can result in the reactivation of leishmaniasis as seen in leishmanial patients treated with anti-TNF-α for rheumatoid arthritis.[90]

Recently found data have emphasized the role of an intrinsic parasite factor in the devolution of disease, that is, *Leishmania* dsRNA virus that, when present in *L. guyanensis*, acts as a potent innate immunogen, redirecting the immune response of the host by inducing a hyper-inflammatory reaction and possibly triggering dissemination.[91] Indeed, drugs countering the type of hyper-inflammation caused by LRV have been successful in the treatment of MCL. Tamoxifen[87] and a TNF–α inhibitor, pentoxyphylline[88] for example, were used in combination with antimony and were shown to aid in the resolution of disease. It would be interesting to determine whether these drugs have an independent or supporting role to antimony, perhaps only working to create an environment in which antimony is effective. Refractory and secondary MCL lesions often display antimony resistance and drugs reverting this process are obviously much desired.

Glycyrrhiza glabra, popularly known as liquorice, is one of the most ancient medicinal plants and has long been used in traditional Chinese, Tibetan, Indian, and Arabian medicine for the treatment of pulmonary diseases and inflammatory processes.[92,93] The strong antileishmanial protection was also imparted through the regulation of macrophage-released cyclooxygenase-2 (Cox-2)-dependent prostaglandin E2 (PGE2) levels. Effect of Gallic acid (GA) on pro-inflammatory and anti-inflammatory cytokine release in *L. donovani*-infected peritoneal macrophages was also observed.[94]

There are only very few reports available on the anti-inflammatory drugs that can administer to decrease the progressive inflammatory state during *Leishmania*. Our purpose is to introduce the natural anti-inflammatory class of medicinal plants that can used as potential drug to reduce inflammatory responses, progression of disease, parasite persistence, and may reduce the resistance to antileishmanial drugs. Various anti-inflammatory medicinal plants that are exploited from ancient times are discussed later.

KEYWORDS

- **Medicinal plants**
- **Ayurveda**
- **inflammation**
- **pain**
- **analgesics**
- **anti-inflammatory**

REFERENCES

1. Evans, W. C. *Trease and Evans Pharmacognosy*, 15th ed.; Elsevier Publisher: Haryana, India, 2002.
2. Aftab, K.; Sail, A. A. Phytomedicine: New and Old Approach. *Hamdard Medicus* **1999,** *42* (2), 11–15.
3. Shabbir, G. S.; Bahadur, Choudhry M. R. Botanical Description, Significance and Production Technology of Some Important Medicinal Herbs. *Hamdard Medicus* **2003,** *XLVI* (1), 23-26.
4. Sertie, J. A. A.; Bassile, A. C. Anti-inflammatory Activity and Subacute Toxicity of Artemetin. *Planta Med.* **1990,** *56* (1), 36–40.
5. Evans, W. C. *Trease and Evans Pharmacognosy*, 12th ed.; Elsevier Publisher: Haryana, India, 1983.
6. Prajapati, N. D.; Kumar, U. *Agro's Dictionary of Medicinal Plants*. Agrobiose: Jodhpur, 2003 pp 53–72.
7. Evans, W.C. *Trease and Evans Pharmacognosy*, 16th ed.; Elsevier Publisher: Haryana, India, 2009; pp 169–170.
8. Patel, N. J.; Gujarati, V. B.; Gouda, T. S.; Rao, N. V.; Nandakumar, K.; Shantakumar, S. M. Antidiarrhoeal Activity of Alcoholic and Aqueous Extracts of Roots of *Tylophora indica* (Wight & Arn.) in Rodents. *Pharmacology* **2006,** *1*, 19–29.

9. Nielsen, O. H.; Ainsworth, M.; Csillag, C.; Rask-Madsen, J. Systematic Review: Coxibs, Non-steroidal Anti-inflammatory Drugs or No Cyclooxygenase Inhibitors in Gastroenterological High-risk Patients. *Aliment. Pharmacol. Ther.* **2005,** *23,* 27–33.
10. Sharma, S. K.; Goyal, N.; Singh, S.; Vasudeva, N. Aanlgesic Activity of the Root of *Abutilon indicum* (Linn.). *Hamdard Medicus* **2006,** *XL* (4), 14–17.
11. Hindawi, A. I.; Al Deen, M. K.; Nabi, I. H.; Ismail, M. H. Anti-inflammatory Activity of Some Iraqi Plants Using Intact Rats. *J. Ethnopharmacol.* **1989,** *26* (2), 163–168.
12. Moura, A. C. A.; Silva, E. L. F.; Fraga, M. C. A, Wanderley, A. G., Afiatpour, P.; Maia, M. B. S. Antiinflammatory and Chronic Toxicity Study of the Leaves of *Ageratum conyzoides* L. in Rats. *Phytomedicine* **2005,** *12* (1-2), 138–142.
13. Kim, J. H.; Lee, K. W.; Lee, M. W.; Lee, H. J,; Kim, S. H.; Surh, Y. J. Hirsutenone Inhibits Phorbol Ester-induced Upregulation of COX-2and MMP-9 in Cultured Human Mammary Epithelial Cells: NF-κB as a Potential Molecular Target. *FEBS Lett.* **2006,** *580,* 385–392.
14. Ojewole, J. A. Potentiation of the Antiinflammatory Effect of *Anacardium occidentale* (Linn.) Stem-bark Aqueous Extract by Grapefruit Juice. *Methods Find. Exp. Clin. Pharmacol.* **2004,** *26* (3), 183–188.
15. Prieto, M.; Recio, M. C.; Giner, R. M.; Mánez, S.; Giner-Larza, E. M.; Ríos, J. L. Influence of traditional Chinese anti-inflammatory medicinal plants on leukocyte and platelet functions. *J. Pharm. Pharmacol.* **2003,** *55* (9), 1275–1282.
16. Dweck, A. C. Herbal Medicine for the Skin their Chemistry and Effects on Skin and Mucous Membranes. *Personal Care Magazine* **2002,** *3* (2), 19–21.
17. Ahamed, K. N.; Kumar, V.; Raja, S.; Mukherjee, K.; Mukherjee, P. K. Anti-Nociceptive and Anti-Inflammatory activity of *Araucaria bidwillii* Hook. *Iranian J. Pharmacol. Therapeutics* **2005,** 4 (2), 105–109.
18. Ahmad, F.; Khan, R. A.; Rasheed, S. Study of Analgesic and Anti-inflammatory Activity from Plant Extracts of *Lactuca scariola* and *Artemisia absinthium. J. Islamic Acad. Sci.* **1992,** *5* (2), 111–114.
19. Suba, V.; Murugesan, T.; Kumaravelrajan, R.; Mandal, S. C.; Saha, B. P. Antiinflammatory, Analgesic and Antiperoxidative Efficacy of *Barleria lupulina* Lindl. Extract. *Phytotherapy Res.* **2005,** *19* (8), 695–699.
20. Gupta, M.; Mazumder, U. K.; Gomathi, P.; Selvan V. T. Antiinflammatory Evaluation of Leaves of *Plumeria acuminate. BMC Complement. Altern. Med.* **2006,** *6,* 36.
21. Biren, S. N.; Nayak, B. S.; Seth, A. K.; Jalalpure, S. S.; Patel, K. N.; Patel, M. A.; Mishra, A. D. Search for Medicinal Plants as a Source of Anti-inflammatory and Anti-arthritic agents - A review. *Pharmacog. Mag.* **2006,** *2* (6), 77–86.
22. Mahmood, M. K. H.; Bachar, S. C.; Islam, M. S.; Ali, M. S. Analgesic and Diuretic Activity of *Curcuma xanthorrhiza. Dhaka University J. Pharm. Sci.* **2004,** *3,* 1–2.
23. Asongalem, E. A.; Foyet, H. S.; Ngogang, J.; Folefoc, G. N.; Dimo, T.; Kamtchouing, P. Analgesic and Antiinflammatory Activities of *Erigeron floribundus. J. Ethnopharmacol.* **2004,** *91* (3), 301–308.
24. Zhang, X. Traditional Medicine and WHO. *Hamdard Medicus* **1996,** *39* (3), 102.
25. Iskander, M. N.; Song, Y.; Coupar, I. M.; Jiratchariyakul, W. Antiinflammatory Screening of the Medicinal Plant *Gynura procumbens. Plant Foods Hum. Nutr.* **2002,** *57* (3-4), 233–244.
26. Srinivasa, U.; Neelakanta, S.A. R.; Rao, V. J. Analgesic Activity of *Clerodendrum phlomidis* Stem Bark. *Indain Drugs* **2010**, *47* (2), 57–59.

27. Shanmugasundaram, P.; Venkataraman, S. Anti-nociceptive Activity of *Hygrophila auriculata* (schum) Heine. *African J. Traditional CAM.* **2005,** *2* (1), 62–69.
28. Saha, A.; Masud, M. A.; Alimuzzamam, M.; Bachar, S. C.; Kundu, J. K.; Datta, B. K. Analgesic and Anti-inflammatory Activity of *Imperata cylindrical*. *Dhaka University J. Pharm. Sci.* **2005,** 4(1).
29. Belsare, D. P.; Pal, S. C.; Mandal, S. C. *Anti-inflammatory and Analgesic Activity of Stembark of Jacaranda mimosifolia Humb.*, ninth International Congress of the International Society of Ethnobiology, 2004; International Society of Ethnobiology: Canterbury, United Kingdom, 2004.
30. Ghule, B. V.; Ghante, M. H.; Upaganlawar, A. B.; Yeole, P. G. Analgesic and Anti-Inflammatory Activities of *Lagenaria siceraria* Stand. Fruit Juice Extract in Rats and Mice. *Pharmacognosy Magazine* **2006,** *2* (8), 232–235.
31. Owoyele, B. V.; Olaleye, B.; Oke, J. M.; Elegbe, R. A. Anti-inflammatory and Analgesic Activities of *nothospondias staudtii*. *Nigerian J. Physiol. Sci.* **2004,** *19* (1-2), 102–105.
32. Sener, B. Recent Results in the Search for Bioactive Compounds from Turkish Medicinal Plants. *Pure Appl. Chem.* **1994,** *66* (10/11), 2295–2298.
33. Abreu, P.; Matthew, S.; Gonza′lez, T.; Costa, D.; Segundo, M. A.; Fernandes, E. Anti-inflammatory and Antioxidant Activity of a Medicinal Tincture from *Pedilanthus tithymaloides*. *Life Sci.* **2006,** *78*, 1578–1585.
34. Otuki, M. F.; Lima, M. A.; Malheiros, A.; Yunes, R. A.; Calixto, J. A. Topical Anti-inflammatory Effects of the Ether Extract from *Protium kleinii* and α-Amyrin pentacyclic Triterpene. *Eur. J. Pharmacol.* **2005,** *507* (1-3), 253–259.
35. Ratheesh, M.; Helen, A. Anti-inflammatory Activity of *Ruta graveolens* Linn Oncarrageenan Induced Paw Edema in Wistar Male Rats. *African J. Biotechnol.* **2007,** *6* (10), 1209–1211.
36. Baricevic, D.; Sosa, D.; Loggia, R. D.; Tubaro, A.; Simonovska, B.; Krasna, A.; Zupancic, A. Topical Anti-inflammatory Activity of *Salvia officinalis* L. Leaves: The Relevance of Ursolic Acid. *J. Ethnopharmacol.* **2001,** *75* (2-3), 125–132.
37. Okoli, C. O.; Akah, P. A.; Ezugworie, U. Anti-inflammatory Activity of Extracts of Root Bark of *securidaca longipedunculata* Fres. *African J. Traditional CAM.* **2005,** *2* (3), 54–63.
38. Mesia-Vela, S.; Souccar, C.; Lima-Landman, M. T. R.; Lapa, A. J. Pharmacological Study of *Stachytarpheta cayennensis* Vahl in Rodents. *Phytomed.* **2004,** *11* (7-8), 616–624.
39. Sharma, S. K.; Perianayagam, J. B.; Pillai, K. K. Anti-inflammatory Activity of *Trichodesma indicum* Root Extract in Experimental Animals. *J. Ethnopharmacol.* **2006,** *104* (3), 410–414.
40. Galvez, J.; Gracioso, J. D. S.; Camuesco, D.; Galvez, J.; Vilegas, W.; Brito, A. R. M. S.; Zarzuelo, A. Intestinal Antiinflammatory Activity of a Lyophilized Infusion of *Turnera ulmifolia* in TNBS Rat Colitis. *Fitoterapia* **2006,** *77* (7–8), 515–520.
41. Cheeke, P. R.; Piacente, S.; Oleszek, W. Anti-inflammatory and Anti-arthriticE effects of *Yucca schidigera*: A Review. *J. Inflamm.* **2006,** *3*, 6.
42. Patil, S. S.; Bhide, A. A.; Gorle, A. M. Anti-ulcer and Antiinflammatory Studies on *Acacia catechu*. *Indian Drugs* **2010,** *47* (2), 50–53.
43. Rahman, M. A.; Bachar, S. C.; Rahmatullah, M. Analgesic and Anti-inflammatory Activity of Methanolic Extract of *Acalypha indica* Linn. *Pakistan J. Pharmaceutical Sci.* **2010,** *23* (3), 256–258.
44. Kokate, C. K.; Purohit, A. P.; Gokhale, S. B. *Pharmacognosy*, 41st ed.; Nirali Prakashan: Pune, India, 2008.

45. Ara, A.; Arifuzzaman, M.; Ghosh, C. K.; Hashem, M. A.; Ahmad, M. U.; Bachar, S. C.; Nahar, L.; Sarker, S. D. Anti-inflammatory Activity of *Adenanthera pavonina* L., Fabaceae, in Experimental Animals. *Brazilian J. Pharmacog.* **2010,** *20* (6), 929–932.
46. Saha, A.; Ahmed, M. The Analgesic and Anti-inflammatory Activities of the Extract of *Albizia lebbeck* in Animal Model. *Pakistan J. Pharmaceutical Sci.* **2009,** *22* (1), 74–77.
47. Das, A. K.; Shahid, I. Z.; Choudhuri, M. S. K.; Shilpi, J. A.; Ahmed, F. Anti-inflammatory, Antinociceptive and Diuretic Activities of *Amooracucullata* Roxb. *Orient. Pharm. Exp. Med.* **2005,** *5* (1), 37–42.
48. Ruppett, B. M.; Peveria, E. F. R.; Gonccalves, L. C.; Pereira, N. A. Pharmacological Screening of Plants Recommended by Folk Medicine as Anti-snake venom-1, Analgesic and Anti-inflammtory Activities. *Mem.Inst. Oswaldo Cruz.* **1991,** *86* (II), 203–205.
49. Uddin, M. N.; Begum, J.; Rahman, M. A.; Ahmed, N. U.; Akter, R.; Abdullah, A. M. Antinociceptive and Anti-inflammatory Properties of the Methanol Leaf Extract of *Argyreia argentea. J. Pharmaceutical Sci. Res.* **2010,** *2* (8), 465–471.
50. Mosaddek, A. S. M.; Rashid, M. M. U. A Comparative Study of the Anti-inflammatory Effect of Aqueous Extract of Neem Leaf and Dexamethasone. *Bangladesh J. Pharmacol.* **2008,** 3, 44–47.
51. Husni, T.; Hantash, A. E. J. Evaluation of Narcotic (Opioid Like). Analgesic Activities of Medicinal Plants. *Europ. J. Scientific Res.* **2009,** *33* (1), 179–182.
52. Alam, M. B.; Hossain, M. S.; Haque, M. E. Antioxidant and Anti-inflammatory Activities of the Leaf Extract of *Brassica nigra. Int. J. Pharmaceutical Sciences Res.* **2011,** *2* (2), 303–310.
53. Nagore, D. H.; Ghosh, V. K.; Patil, M. J.; Wahile, A. M. In *vitro* Antioxidant and *in vivo* Anti-inflammatory Activity of *Cassia sophera* Linn. *Int. J. Pharm. Pharm. Sci.* **2010,** *2* (1), 114–121.
54. Kadam, S. H., Dombe, S. A., Naikwadi, P. N., Patil, S. P., Lokhande, V. Y. Anti-inflammatory Activity of *Celosia Argentea* Leaves. *Intern. J. Drug Formulation Res.* **2011,** *2* (1), 105–108.
55. Harisha, C. R.; Ashok, B. K.; Acharya, R.; Sukla, V. J.; Ravishankar, B. Anti-inflammatory and Analgesic Activity of Roots and Stem of *Cissus repeda* vahl. *Pharmacog. J.* **2010**, *21* (18), 7–54.
56. Chakma, J. S.; Rahman, M. A.; Islam, S.; Rana, M. S.; Ahmed, N. U. Analgesic and Anti-inflammatory Effect of *Clausena suffruticosa* Root Extract in AnimalM model. *J. Sci. Res.* **2011,** *3* (3), 631–639.
57. Khatry, N.; Kundu, J.; Bachar, S. C.; Uddin, M. N.; Kundu, J. K. Studies on Antinociceptive, Antiinflammatory and Diuretic Activities of Methanol Extract of the Aerial Parts of *Clerodendron viscosum* Vent. Dhaka Univ. *J. Pharm. Sci.* **2005,** *5* (1–2), 63–66.
58. Howlader, M. A.; Alam, M.; Ahmed, K. T.; Khatun, F.; Apu, A. S. Antinociceptive and Anti-inflammatory Activity of the Ethanolic Extract of *Cymbidium aloifolium* (L.*). Pakistan J. Biol. Sci.* **2011,** *14* (19), 909–911.
59. Chowdhury, K. K.; Saha, A.; Bachar, S. C.; Kundu, J. K. Analgesic and Anti-inflammatory Activities of *Desmodium triflorum* DC. *J. Biol. Sci.* **2005,** *5* (5), 581–583.
60. Hoque, N.; Habib, M. R.; Imam, M. Z.; Ahmed, J.; Rana, M. S. Analgesic and Anti-inflammatory Potential of Methanolic Extract of *Glinus oppositifolius* L. *Aust. J. Basic Appl. Sci.* **2011,** *5* (8), 729–733.
61. Apu, A. S.; Bhuyan, S. H.; Prova, S. S.; Muhit, M. A. Anti-inflammatory Activity of Medicinal Plants Native to Bangladesh: A review. *J. App. Pharmaceutical Sci.* **2012,** *02* (02), 7–10.

62. Podder, M. K.; Das, B. N.; Saha, A.; Ahmed, M. Analgesic activity of bark of *Murraya paniculata*. *Int. J. Medicine Medical Sciences* **2011,** *3* (4), 105–108.
63. Sengupta, R.; Sheorey, S. D.; Hinge, M. A. Analgesic and Anti-inflammatory Plants: An Updated Review. *Int. J. Pharm. Sci. Rev. Res.* **2012,** *12* (2), 114–119.
64. Borikar, V. I.; Jangde, C. R.; Rekhe, D. S.; Philip, P. Study of Analgesic Activity of *Bauhinia racemosa lam* in Rats. *Vet. World* **2009,** *2* (4), 135–136.
65. Kim, H. P.; Son, K. H.; Chang, H. W.; Kang, S. S. Anti-inflammatory Plant Flavonoids and Cellular Action Mechanisms. *J. Pharmacol. Sci.* **2004,** *96*, 229–245.
66. Vane, J. R.; Botting, R. M. Mechanism of Action of Nonsteroidal Anti-inflammatory Drugs. *Am. J. Med.* **1998,** *104* (3), 2S–8S.
67. Shah, B. N.; Seth, A. K.; Maheshwari, K. M. A Review on Medicinal Plants as a Source of Anti-inflammatory Agents. *Res. J. Med. Plant* **2013,** *5*, 101–115.
68. Aggarwal, B. B.; Prasad, S.; Reuter, S.; Kannappan, R.; Yadev, V.R.; Park, B.; Park, B.; Kim, J. H.; Gupta, S. C.; Phromnoi, K.; Sundaram, C.; Prasad. S.; Chaturvedi, M. M, Sung, B. Identification of Novel Anti-inflammatory Agents from Ayurvedic Medicine for Prevention of Chronic Diseases. *Curr. Drug Targets* **2011,** *12* (11), 1595–1653.
69. Yadav, S. S.; Galib, R. B.; Prajapati, P. K.; Ashok, B. K.; Varun, B. Anti-inflammatory Activity of Shirishavaleha: An Ayurvedic Compound Formulation. *Int. J. Ayurveda Res.* **2010,** *1* (4), 205–207.
70. Ruknuddin, G.; Biswajyoti, P.; Kumar, P. P.; Krishnaiah, A. B.; Basavaiah, R. Anti-inflammatory and Analgesic Activities of *Dashanga Ghana*: An Ayurvedic Compound Formulation **2013,** *3* (3), 303–308.
71. Yamini, K.; Chalapathi, V. Pharmacological Screening of Anti-inflammatory Activity of Ayurvedic Formulation "nimbadi thailam." *Int.J. Pharm. Tech. Res.* **2010,** *2* (1), 485–448.
72. Koppikara, S. J.; Jagtapa, S. D.; Devarshia, P. P.; Jangleb, N. M.; Awada, V. B.; Welec, A. A.; Harsulkara, A. M. an Ayurvedic Formulation Improves the Antioxidant Status on TNBS Induced IBD in Rats. *Europ. J. Integrative Med.* **2014,** *6*, 12–15.
73. Singh, R. S.;Ahmad, M.; Wafai, Z. H.; Khan, Z. Y.; Sharma, M.; Seth, V. Analgesic Effect of Dashamula versus Diclofenac Sodium. *J. Clinical Diagnos. Res.* **2012,** *6* (3), 547–550.
74. Kabir, A. U.; Samad, M. B.; D Costa, N. M.; Hannan, J. M. Investigation of the Central and Peripheral Analgesic and Anti-inflammatory Activity of Draksharishta an Indian Ayurvedic Formulation. *J. Basic Clin. Pharm.* **2012,** *3* (4), 336–340.
75. Uddin, M. J.; Motaleb, M. A.; Mazumder, B. K.; Shohel, M.; Hossain, M. B.; Chowdhury, A. A.; Mazid, M. A. Evaluation of Analgesic and Anti-inflammatory Effects of a Poly-herbal Ayurvedic Formulation. *Bangladesh Pharm. J.* **2013,** *16* (1), 59–62.
76. Singh, M.K.; Nagori, K.; Tripathi, D. K. *Potential* Analgesic & Anti-Pyretic Herbal drugs: A Comparative Review of Marketed Products. *Int. J. Phytomed.* **2010,** *2*, 197–209.
77. Thabrewa, I.; Dharmasirib, M. G.; Senaratnec, L. Anti-inflammatory and Analgesic Activity in the Polyherbal Formulation Maharasnadhi Quathar M. *J. Ethnopharmacol.* **2003,** *85* (2–3), 261–267.
78. Lather, A.; Gupta, V.; Bansal, P.; Sahu, M.; Sachdeva, K.; Ghaiye, P. An Ayurvedic Polyherbal Formulation Kaishore Guggulu: A Review. *Int. J. Pharm. Biol. Arch.* **2011,** *2* (1), 497–503.

79. Ashraful, K. Investigation of the Central and Peripheral Analgesic and Anti-inflammatory Activity of Kutajarishta, an Indian Ayurvedic formulation. *Int. J. Phytopharmacy* **2012,** *2* (5), 129–134.
80. Samad, M. B.; D'Costa, N. M.; Kabir, A.; Hannan, J. M. A. Investigation on Central and Peripheral Analgesic and Anti-Inflammatory Activity of Punarnavasava, an Ayurvedic Preparation. *Eur. J. Med. Plants* **2013,** *3* (1), 146–162.
81. Dhaniwala, N.; Kohli, K. R.; Sharma, G. An Open, Prospective, Labeled Clinical Study to Evaluate and Compare the Efficacy of New Rhumatil Gel with Diclofenac Gel on Osteoarthritis & Other Musculo-skeletal Conditions. *Indian J. Trad. Knowledge* **2010,** *9* (4), 656–659.
82. Soni, H.; Shah, P.; Zaveri, M.; Patel, S.; Patel, G. Evaluation of Acute Toxicity and Analgesic Activity of Plugit Capsule: An Ayurvedic Formulation. *Int. J. Res. Ayurveda Pharm.* **2014,** *5* (3), 270–273.
83. Joshi, S. S.; Bhalerao, P. P.; Gajbhiye, S. V. Evaluation of Analgesic Activity of Dashamoolarishtha Formulation by Using Experimental Models of Nociception. *Int. J. Pharmacol. Therapeutics* **2013,** *3* (3), 1–9.
84. Panda, H. *Handbook onAayurvedic Medicines with Formulae, Processes and their Uses*; National Institute of Industrial Research: New Delhi, India, 2004.
85. Marsden, P. D. Mucosal Leishmaniasis ("espundia" Escomel, 1911). *Trans. R. Soc. Trop. Med. Hyg.* **1986,** *80*, 859–876.
86. Ronet, C.; Ives, A.; Bourreau, E.; Fasel, N.; Launois, P.; Masina, S. Immune responses to *Leishmaina guyanensis* infection in humans and animal models. In*Immune Response to Parasitic Infection*; Jirillo, E., Brandonisio. O., Eds.; Bentham Science Publishers: Bussum, 2010; Vol. 1, pp 165–175.
87. Miguel, D. C.; Zauli-Nascimento, R. C.; Yokoyama-Yasunaka, J. K.; Katz, S.; Barbieri, C. L.; Uliana, S. R. Tamoxifen as a Potential Antileishmanial Agent: Efficacy in the Treatment of *Leishmania braziliensis* and *Leishmania chagasi* Infections. *J. Antimicrob. Chemother.* **2009,** *63*, 365–368.
88. Lessa, H. A.; Machado, P.; Lima, F.; Cruz, A. A.; Bacellar, O.; Guerreiro, J.; Carvalho, E. M. Successful Treatment of Refractory Mucosal Leishmaniasis with Pentoxifylline Plus Antimony. *Am. J. Trop. Med. Hyg.* **2001,** *65*, 87–89.
89. Blackwell, J. M. Tumour Necrosis Factor Alpha and Mucocutaneous Leishmaniasis. *Parasitol. Today* **1999,** *15*, 73–75.
90. Franklin, G.; Greenspan, J.; Chen, S. Anti-tumor Necrosis Factor-alpha Therapy Provokes Latent Leishmaniasis in a Patient with Rheumatoid Arthritis. *Ann. Clin. Lab. Sci.* **2009,** *39*, 192–195.
91. Ives, A.; Ronet, C.; Prevel, F.; Ruzzante, G.; Fuertes-Marraco, S.; Schutz, F.; Zangger, H.; Revaz-Breton, M.; Lye, L. F.; Hickerson, S. M.; Beverley, S. M.; Acha-Orbea, H.; Launois, P.; Fasel, N.; Masina, S. *Leishmania* RNA Virus Controls the Severity of Mucocutaneous Leishmaniasis. *Science* **2011,** *331*, 775–778.
92. Davis, E. A.; Morris, D. J. Medicinal Uses of Licorice through the Millennia: The Good and Plenty of it. *Mol. Cell Endocrinol.* **1991,** *78,* 1–6.
93. Ody, P. *The Complete Medicinal Herbal;* Dorling Kindersley: New York, 1993.
94. Bhattacharjee, S.; Bhattacharjee, A.; Majumder, S.; Majumdar, S. B.; Majumdar, S. Glycyrrhizic Acid Suppresses Cox-2-mediated Anti-inflammatory Responses during *Leishmania donovani* Infection. *J. Antimicrob. Chemother.* **2012,** *67* (8), 1905–1914.

CHAPTER 10

MODERN TREATMENT FOR LEISHMANIASIS

CONTENTS

PART X MODERN TREATMENT FOR LEISHMANIASIS

ABSTRACT

Current part discusses the modern ways to treat leishmaniasis. In this study, we have reported for the first time the biochemical characterization of the drug-sensitive *Leishamnia* sp. and drug-resistant strains and natural drug-resistant strain. The role of sensitivity of electron transport inhibitors and ATPase inhibitors in drug resistance is also discussed. In addition, we have also explored succinate efflux transporter as a chemotherapeutic target.

10.1 INTRODUCTION

An infectious disease is a clinically evident disease resulting from the presence of pathogenic microbial agents, including pathogenic viruses, pathogenic bacteria, fungi, protozoa, multicellular parasites, and aberrant proteins known as prions. These pathogens are able to cause disease in animals and/or plants. Leishmaniasis, is a group of diseases caused by protozoan parasite belonging to family *Trypanosomatidae*. Clinical manifestations for leishmaniasis range from self-healing cutaneous and mucocutaneous skin ulcers. If not treated, this ulcerative condition may also progress in to a fatal visceral form, that is, visceral leishmaniasis (VL) or kala-azar (KA). Currently, leishmaniasis has affected the whole globe and become the significant cause of morbidity and mortality in several countries of the world. According to reports, its prevalence was found in 88 countries, with near around 400,000 new cases per year.[1] At present, this infectious tropical disease is influencing United States,[2] with approximately 500 parasitologically confirmed cases.[3] In contrast, VL has been reported in more than 60 countries.[4] Among these countries about 500,000 new cases annually of symptomatic VL were only found in the rural areas of only five countries: India, Nepal, Bangladesh, Brazil, and Sudan.[5] Among these five countries, 50% of all VL cases were found in Indian subcontinent. Association of leishmaniasis has also been reported with human immunodeficiency virus (HIV) among nearly 33 countries.[6] In addition, it has been also reported that acquired immunodeficiency syndrome (AIDS) patients are more vunerable against leishmaniasis.[7]

This endemic desease is caused by parasite *Leishmania,* which is transmitted by an invertebrate sandfly vector, *Phlebotomus*. This transmission of parasite leads a digenetic life cycle.[8] Treatment and control of leishmaniasis rely solely on chemotherapy since, vaccines against leishmaniasis are still under development.[9] It has been reported that first-line drug for all forms of leishmaniasis, which is being utilized for more than 60 years is organic salt of pentavalent antimony Sb(V).[10] Nevertheless, recently a large-scale increase in clinical resistance to pentavalent antimonials has been reported.[11,12] This type of resistence is chiefly found in India where 65% of previously untreated patients fail to respond promptly or relapse after therapy with antimony drugs.[13]

Potential chemotherapeutic agents that are potentially utilized as second-line drugs include pentamidine and amphotericin B. However, their serious side effects and high cost limit their use.[14] Neoplastic agent called as miltefosine (hexadecylphosphocholine) has now been approved as the first oral drug for leishmaniasis, which can be used for both antimony-responding and nonresponding patients.[15] However, cost and long life in the body limits its usage. In addition, it has been also reported that a single point mutation may also lead to develop miltefosine resistance in the parasite.[16] Aminosidine (parenteral formulation of aminosidine in phase IV trials) has recently been approved for leishmaniasis treatment in India.[17–19] Paromomycin, an aminoglycoside antibiotic, has been used for the treatment of both VL, in a parenteral formulation, and cutaneous leishmaniasis (CL) in both topical and parenteral formulations.[20,21] Both cytoplasmic and mitochondrial protein synthesis were inhibited following paromomycin exposure. But a cell line selected for resistance to the drug showed reduced paromomycin accumulation associated with a significant reduction in the initial binding to the cell surface. The drug induced reduction in membrane potential and inhibition of protein synthesis are less pronounced in the resistant strain in comparison to the wild type.[22]

Studies of the pharmacology of antileishmanial agents have been hampered by the insensitivity in promastigote of *Leishmania* to commonly used drugs. In this chapter, I will demonstrate that the parasites are sensitive to antileishmanial drugs in drug-sensitive strain, but not sensitive to drug-resistant strain.

In search of new antileishmanial agents, in this chapter, I have also explored the electron transport system of plasma membrane and mitochondrion in the *Leishmania* parasite[23–25] The physiological consequences of targeting the *Leishmania* parasite electron transport chain are not well understood. Part of this problem is that the function of *Leishmania* parasite mitochondria is regarded as somewhat enigmatic.[25]

This chapter also explores a new method for in vitro differenciation of *Leishmania donovani*, which is a modification of the method by Debrabant et al.[26] These axenic amastigotes resembles animal-derived amastigotes, they express the amastigote specific A2 gene; they down regulate lipophosphoglycan, mitochondrial- and plasma membrane-related electron transport system, as well as downregulation of adenosinetriphosphatase (ATPase). In this chapter, I have explored the ability of axenically grown amastigote to be used in a relevant drug-screening procedure. The chemosensitivities of extracellular amastigote form to different drugs, including those currently used for leishmaniasis, were evaluated and compared with those of promastigote form. At last, I have tried to evaluate their mode of action in amastigote form.

These findings on the respiratory changes and the patterns of growth inhibition of wild *L. donovani* and its drug-resistant strains are particularly important in order to evaluate the resistance mechanisms. Knowledge regarding the comparative sensitivities of drugs and other effectors involved in energy metabolism of both drug-sensitive and drug-resistant parasite forms could lead to the identification of new sensitive lead compounds for further targets as chemotherapeutic agents.

10.2 CURRENT SCENARIO ON LEISHMANIASIS

10.2.1 PROTOZOAL PARASITIC DISEASE: CURRENT SITUATION AND NEW PERSPECTIVE

Parasitic diseases continue to be major causes of human misery and death in the world. By a conservative estimate, there are more than 65,000 described species of protozoa distributed among seven named phyla.[27] Of those, only a few species cause disease in humans, but these few inflict much misery and death on millions of people. Enteric fever, malaria, trypanosomiasis, leptospirosis, HIV, and leishmaniasis are exponentially increasing and life-threatening. Among these, malaria, trypanosomiasis, and leishmaniasis are caused by parasitic protozoa. These diseases occur in area far from the main stream of medical research of the industrial world, and the only substantial contact of the later with these diseases has been during military operation.[28] In addition, there was little wealth in these areas to attract commercial interest in their problems. All of the above may seem quiet disheartening; but now the scene is changing. First, moral obligations of the developed nation to assist the less fortunate have been recognized; second, an economic strength of many nations of the tropics has meant that their voices can not be ignored; and third, their standard of living are raising. On the other hand, the World Health Organization (WHO) has established a special research programme into the most important parasitic diseases such as malaria, schistosomiasis, trypanosomiasis, and leishmaniasis. Some of the main objectives of the scientific working group on leishmaniasis are epidemiology, vaccine studies, and development of novel compounds in addition to the existing drugs.[29,30] Due to the widespread resurgence of the above-mentioned diseases, the fresh interests have regained during the last decade, and have placed the subject of parasitology in a new phase.

10.2.2 THE LEISHMANIASIS: A GLOBAL PROBLEM

Leishmaniasis is a major health problem in many tropical and desert climates. It is the cause of considerable morbidity and mortality in terms of World Health. It is one of the major parasitic diseases in the developing world. Leishmaniasis usually strikes the poorest of the poor. As a disease, it more often debilitates than kills and makes people dependent on others. People who work in various farming practices, forestry, mining, and fishing have a great risk of being bitten by sandflies. Members of the genus *Leishmania* of the parasitic protozoans are the etiological agents responsible for a group of human diseases. *Leishmania* may infect many vertebrates, but in human hosts the infection most frequently stems from the bites of sandfly vectors. There may be a tremendous loss of man-working hours in the endemic regions, which may hold up developmental programs in many countries. It may be relatively effective when the disease is of a domestic nature and apparently an anthroponosis (e.g., Indian KA). But the vast majority of the leishmaniasis is zoonosis, with reservoir in wild animals. This complicates their control in many parts of the world. There is no recognized, reliable mean of chemoprophylaxis or vaccination against infections with different forms of leishmaniasis. Chemotherapy is still, in many respects, unsatisfactory.[31]

10.2.2.1 LEISHMANIASIS*: AN OVERVIEW AND GEOGRAPHICAL DISTRIBUTION*

The origins of *Leishmania* are unclear.[32,33] One possible theory proposes an African origin, with migration to the Americas. Another migration from the Americas to the Old World about 15 million years ago, across the Bering Strait land bridge. Another proposes a Palearctic origin.[34] Such migrations would entail migration of vector and reservoir or successive adaptations along the way. A more recent migration is that of *Leishmania infantum* from Mediterranean countries to Latin America (there named *Leishmania chagasi*), since European colonization of the New World, where the parasites picked up its current New World vectors in their respective ecologies. This is the cause of the epidemics now evident. One recent New World epidemic concerns foxhounds in the United States.

Leishmaniasis can be transmitted in many tropical and sub-tropical countries, and is found in parts of about 88 countries of which 67 are in the Old World and 21 in the New World.[35] Approximately 350 million people live in these areas. The settings in which leishmaniasis is found range from rain forests in Central and South America to deserts in West Asia. More than 90% of the world's cases of VL are in India, Bangladesh, Nepal, Sudan, and Brazil.

Leishmaniasis is found through much of the Americas from northern Argentina to southern Texas, though not in Uruguay or Chile, and has recently been shown to be spreading to North Texas.[36] During 2004, it is calculated that some 3,400 troops from the Colombian Army, operating in the jungles near the south of the country (in particular around the Meta and Guaviare departments), were infected with leishmaniasis. Apparently, a contributing factor was that many of the affected soldiers did not use the officially provided insect repellent, because of its allegedly disturbing odor. It is estimated that nearly 13,000 cases of the disease were recorded in all of Colombia throughout 2004, and about 360 new incidents of the disease among soldiers had been reported in February 2005.

The disease in found across much of Asia, though not Southeast Asia, and the Middle East. Within Afghanistan, in particular Kabul is a town where leishmaniasis occurs commonly—because of the bad sanitation and waste left uncollected in streets, allowing parasite-spreading sandflies an environment that they find favorable.[37,38] In Kabul, the number of people infected was estimated at least 200,000, and in three other towns (Herat, Kandahar, and Mazar-i-Sharif) there may be about 70,000 more, accordinxg to WHO figures from 2002 (Figure 10-1).[38]

Africa, in particular, the East and North, is the home for cases of leishamaniasis. The disease is spreading to Southern Europe but is not found in Australia or Oceania.

Leishmaniasis is mostly a disease of the developing world, and is rarely known in the developed world outside a small number of cases, mostly in instances where troops are stationed away from their home countries. Leishmaniasis has been reported by U.S. troops stationed in Saudi Arabia and Iraq since the Gulf War of 1990, including VL.[39] In September 2005, the disease was contacted by at least four Dutch marines who were stationed in Mazari Sharif, Afghanistan, and subsequently repatriated for treatment.

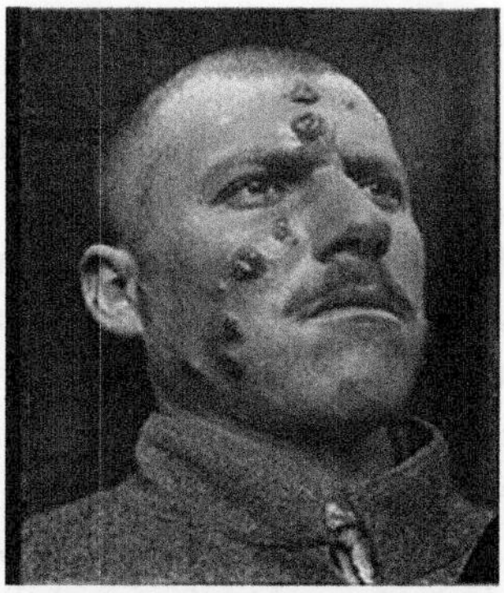

FIGURE 10-1 A case of cutaneous Leishmaniasis in the Middle East (1917), known then locally as "Jericho Buttons" for the frequency of cases near the ancient city of Jericho.

Leishmaniasis affects at least 12 million individuals each year, with about 300 million people at risk, both in the developed and developing world. In the last decade, VL has surged in epidemic proportions in new areas in Sudan, Pakistan, and China. It has also become a major problem in AIDS patients in Europe and South America (Figure 10-2).

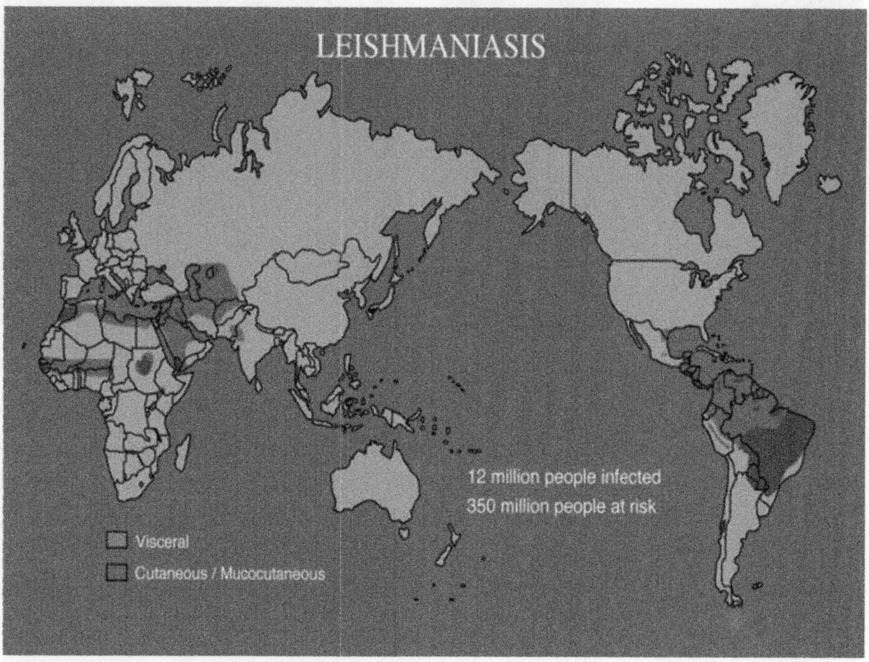

FIGURE 10-2 Distribution of leishmaniasis.

The disease, leishmaniasis, was named in 1901 for the Scottish pathologist William Boog Leishman. This disease is also known as Leichmaniosis, Leishmaniose, and formerly, Orient Boils, Baghdad Boil, KA, black fever, sandfly disease, Dumdum fever or espundia.

Most forms of the disease are transmissible only from animals (zoonosis), but some can be spread between humans. Human infection is caused by about 21 of 30 species that infect mammals. These include the *L. donovani* complex with three species (*L. donovani, L. infantum*, and *L. chagasi*); the *Leishmania mexicana* complex with three main species (*L. mexicana, L. amazonensis*, and *Leishmania venezuelensis*); *Leishmania tropica; Leishmania major; Leishmania aethiopica*; and the subgenus *Viannia* with four main species (*Leishmania (V.) braziliensis, Leishmania (V.) guyanensis, Leishmania (V.) panamensis*, and *Leishmania (V.) peruviana*). The different species are morphologically indistinguishable, but they can be differentiated by isoenzyme analysis, DNA sequence analysis, or monoclonal antibodies.Three important diseases are caused by three different species of *Leishmania*. Infections are regarded as CL, mucocutaneous leishmaniasis and VL (Figure 10-3).

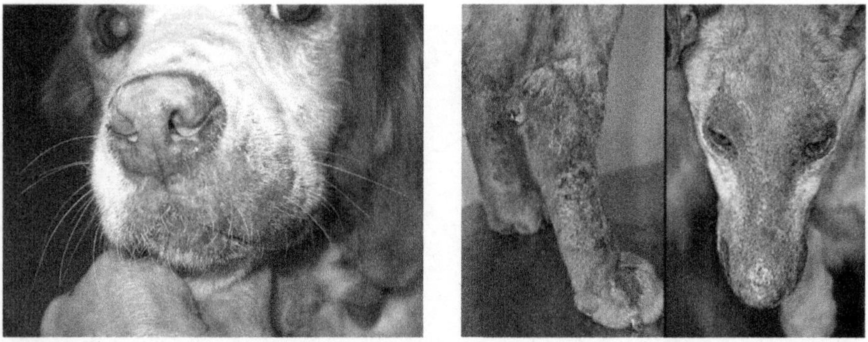

FIGURE 10-3 Canine leishmaniasis.

Cutaneous (localized and diffuse) infections appear as obvious skin reactions (Figure 10.4). The most common is the oriental sore (caused by Old World species *L. major*, *L. tropica*, and *L. aethiopica*). In the New World, the most common culprits are *L. mexicana* and *L. (Viannia) braziliensis*. Cutaneous infections are most common in Afghanistan, Brazil, Iran, Peru, Saudi Arabia, and Syria.

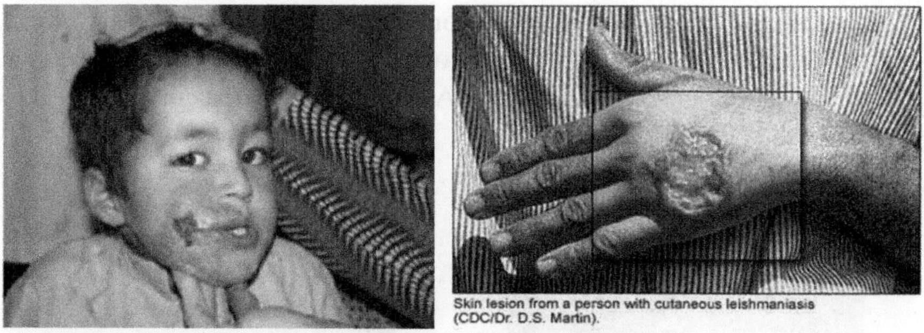

FIGURE 10-4 Infection with cutaneous leishmaniasis.

Mucocutaneous (espundia) infections start as a reaction at the site of bite, and can enter via metastasis into the mucous membrane and become fatal.

Mucocutaneous infections are most common in Bolivia, Brazil, and Peru. Mucocutaneous infections are also found in Karamay, China Xinjiang Uygur Autonomous Region (Figure 10.5).

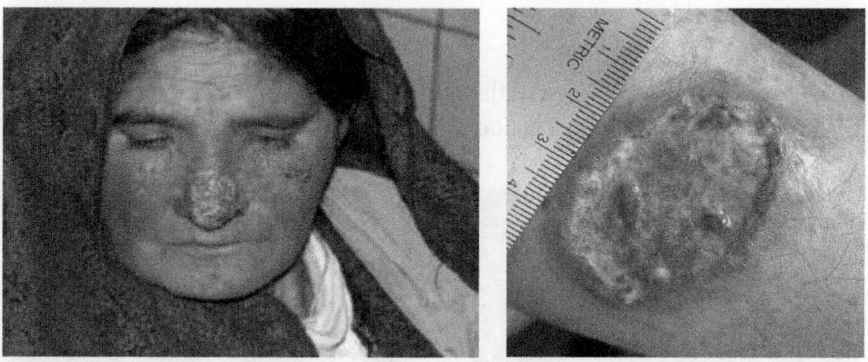

FIGURE 10-5 Infection with mucocutaneos lLeishmaniasis.

Visceral infections are often recognized by fever, swelling of the liver and spleen, and anemia. They are known by many local names, of which the most common is probably KA,[40] and are caused exclusively by species of the *L. donovani* complex (*L. donovani*, *L. infantum* syn., and *L. chagasi*)[41] found in tropical and subtropical areas of all continents except Australia.

Visceral infections are most common in Bangladesh, Brazil, India, Nepal, and Sudan.[41] It is also found in part of China, such as Sichuan Province, Gansu Province, and Xinjiang Uygur Autonomous Region (Figure 2.6).

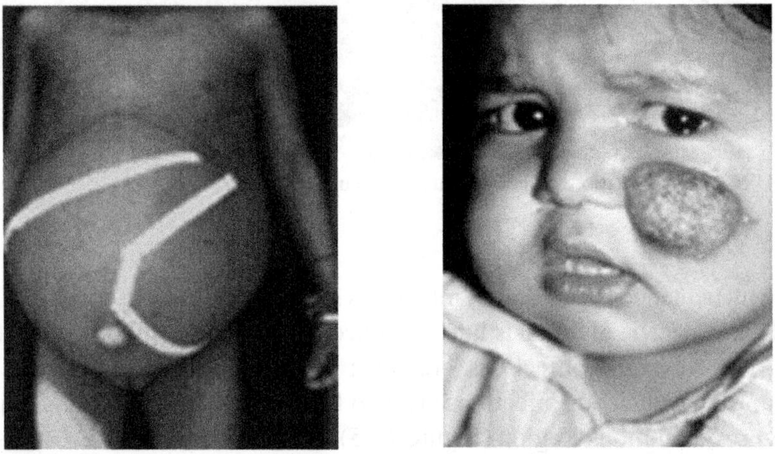

FIGURE 10-6 Infection with visceral leishmaniasis.

Another form is diffuse CL that produces widespread skin lesions, which resemble leprosy and is particularly difficult to treat (Figure 10.7).

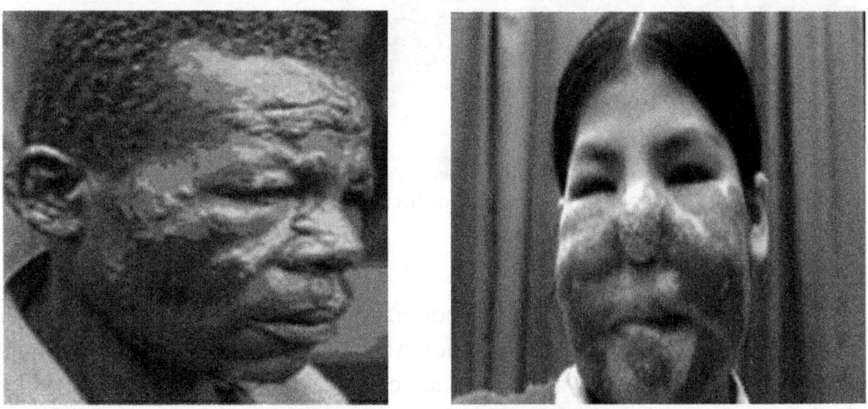

FIGURE 10-7 Infection with diffuse cutaneous leishmaniasis.

VL, also known as KA and black fever, is the most severe form of leishmaniasis. Several species of *Leishmania* are known to give rise to the visceral form of the disease. The "Old World" (Africa, Asia, and Europe) species are *L. donovani* and *L. infantum* and the "New World" (South America) species is *L. chagasi*.

The parasite, *Leishmania*, is the second-largest parasitic killer in the world (after malaria), responsible for an estimated 60,000 deaths among the half-million infections that occur each year worldwide.[42] The parasite migrates to the internal organs such as liver, spleen (hence "visceral") and bone marrow and if left untreated will almost always result in the death of the host. Signs and symptoms include fever, weight loss, anemia, and substantial swelling of the liver and spleen. According to the WHO, HIV/VL coinfection is the emerging problem.[42]

VL is endemic in many areas, with mortality reaching 98% in untreated cases. In India, VL or KA has its home in plains of the Ganges and Brahmaputra. It has been known to occur epidemically and endemically in well-defined areas in the eastern sector of India, namely, Assam, Bihar, West Bengal, eastern districts of Uttar Pradesh, foothills of Sikkim, and to a lesser extent in Tamilnadu and Orissa.[43] One of the largest epidemics occurred in 1978 in north Bihar where over half a million people fell victim to KA. In 1982, 7500 cases were reported in India and in 1 year alone between 1987 and 1988, 22,000 cases of KA were recognized. In Pakistan, 239 cases of VL due to *L. infantum* were reported between 1985 and 1995.[44] More than 90% of visceral cases appear in India, Nepal, Bangladesh, Sudan, and Brazil.[35,45,46] In Bangladesh, cases of VL greatly declined within 1953 to 1970, probably as a result of mass chemotherapy with pentavalent antimonial and widespread spraying with dichlorodiphenyltrichloroethane to control malaria. Following the end of the malaria control program in 1970, sandfly vector population increased and so did the cases of VL, and currently appears at a rate in excess of 15,000 per year. Recent cases of canine VL of man have been registered in the southern states of United States, Oklahoma and Kansas (Figure 10.3). In sporadic and epidemic cases of VL, people of all ages are susceptible with males at least twice more likely to contact the disease than females, except those who have conferred immunity due to past infection. Figure 10-8 represents the widespread geographical distribution of VL.

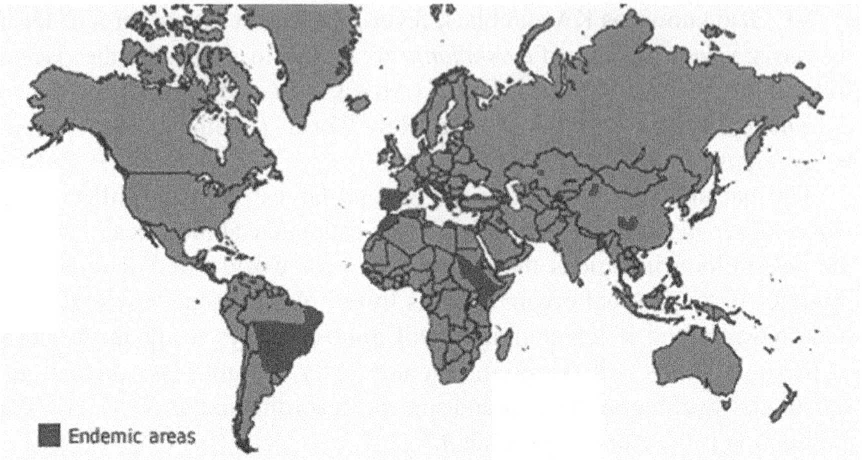

FIGURE 10-8 Geographic distribution of visceral leishmaniasis.

Post-kala-azar dermal leishmaniasis (PKDL) occurs in India and mainly in Sudan and Kenya. Reports of PKDL in China and Iraq have also been documented. In the New World, PKDL is extremely rare. About 1 to 1.5 million new cases are reported annually worldwide.[35] The large number of endemic countries illustrates the global importance of the problem. The overall prevalence is 13 million cases and the estimated population at risk is about 350 million. The number of cases of leishmaniasis is increasing, mainly because of man-made environmental changes that increase human exposure to the sandfly vector. Removal of forest, mining, building dams, widening areas under cultivation, creation of new irrigation scheme, expanding road construction in primary forest such as the Amazon, continuing widespread migration from the rural to urban areas, and continuing fast urbanization are among the primary causes for increased exposure to the sandfly. Another risk factor is the movement of susceptible population into endemic areas, including large-scale migration of population for economic reason. Renewed interest on the subject over the past 40 years, however, has lead to a recognization that the diversity and complexity of leishmaniasis and their positive parasites, is far beyond what we had previously imagined.

The traditional treatment is with pentavalent antimonials such as sodium stibogluconate and meglumine antimoniate. Resistance is now common in India,[13,47] and the treatment of choice for VL acquired in India is now Amphotericin B[48] in its various preparations (Ambisome,[49] Abelcet, Amphocil[50]). Ambisome dose: total dose 21 mg/kg (Mediterranean/Brazilian VL), total dose 7.5 mg/kg over 6 days (Indian VL); Amphocil dose: total dose

7.5 mg/kg over 6 days (Indian VL). A low dose (0.5mg–1 mg/kg) is given on the first day, increasing to 1 mg–2mg/kg on the second day, followed by 1.5 mg–3 mg/kg on the third and subsequent days.

Miltefosine (Impavido) is the first oral treatment for this disease. The cure rate of miltefosine in phase III clinical trials is 95%; studies in Ethiopia showed that it is also effective in Africa. In HIV immunosuppressed people who are coinfected with leishmaniasis it has shown that even in resistant cases, two-third of the people responded to this new treatment. Miltefosine has received approval by the Indian regulatory authorities in 2002 and in Germany in 2004. It is now registered in many countries. The drug is generally better tolerated than other drugs. Main side effects are gastrointetinal disturbance in the first or second day of treatment (a course of treatment is 28 days), which does not affect the efficiency. Because it is available as an oral formulation, the expense and inconvenience of hospitalization is avoided, which makes it a drug of choice.

Paromomycin, an aminoglycoside antibiotic, has been used for the treatment of both VL, in a parenteral formulation, and CL in both topical and parenteral formulations.[20,21] The drug had originally been identified in the 1960s, but had been abandoned because it would not be profitable, as the disease mostly affects poor people.[42] The Indian government approved paromomycin for sale in August 2006.[51]

10.2.2.2 COINFECTION OF LEISHMANIASIS WITH AIDS

Leishmaniasis is spreading in several areas of the world as a result of rapidly spreading of endemic AIDS. The deficiency of immunity leads to increased susceptibility to infections, including leishmaniasis.[52,53] Coinfection with HIV has lead to the spread of leishmaniasis, typically a rural disease, into urban areas. Coinfections have been reported in 33 countries worldwide (Figure 10-9). In Asia, coinfections are increasingly being reported from India, Bangladesh, and Nepal that are facing antimonial resistance.[54] In southern Europe 25–70% of adult VL cases are related to HIV and 1.5–9% of AIDS cases suffer from newly acquired or reactivated VL, of the first 1,700 cases of coinfection that have been reported by WHO in 1998, 1,440 cases belong to southwestern Europe.[55] The *Leishmania* accelerate the onset of AIDS by cumulative immunosuppression and by stimulating the replication at several areas of the world as a result of rapidly spreading epidemic AIDS. According to the data of WHO[56] the areas where HIV/*Leishmania* coinfection is distributed are extensive. Most of the coinfections in the America are reported in Brazil, where the incidence of AIDS has risen from 0.8 cases per 1,00,000 inhabitants in 1986 to 10.5 cases per 1,00,000 inhabitants in 1997.

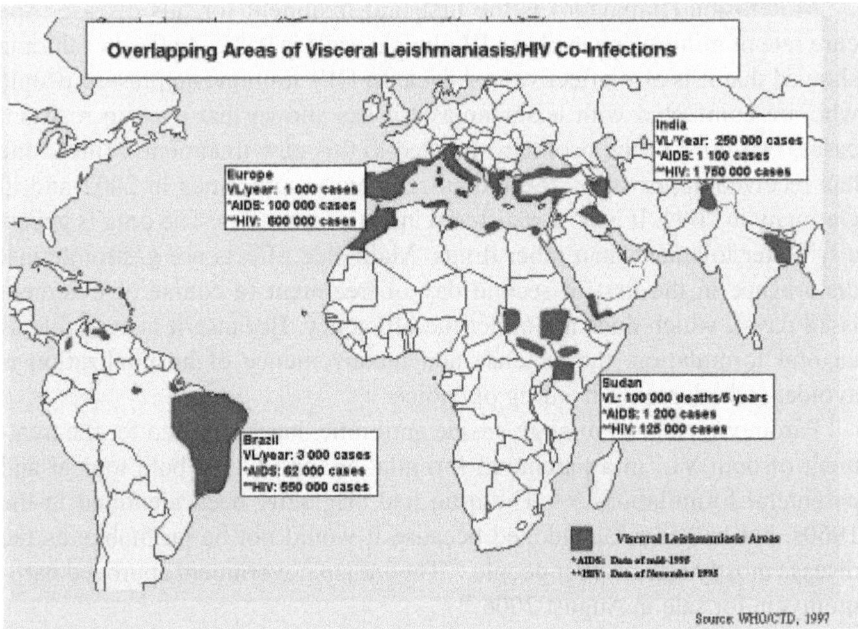

FIGURE 10-9 Overlapping areas of visceral leishmaniasis/HIV coinfections.

India launched the KA elimination program in 2001. WHO in partnership with South Asian Association for Regional Cooperation (SAARC) and the Environmental Health Project (EHP), has initiated a Joint Plan on cross-border control of KA, HIV/AIDS, tuberculosis, and malaria.

10.2.2.3 KALA-AZAR: HISTORY AND CLINICAL PERSPECTIVE

Descriptions of conspicuous lesions similar to CL has been discovered on tablets from King Ashurbanipal from the seventh century B.C., some of which may have been derived from even earlier texts from 1500 to 2500 B.C. Moslem physicians including Avicenna in the 10th century gave detailed descriptions of what was called Balkh sore.[57] In 1756, Alexander Russell, after examining a Turkish patient, gave one of the most detailed clinical descriptions of the disease. Physicians in the Indian subcontinent would describe it as KA (pronounced *kālā āzār*, the Urdu, Hindi, and Hindustani phrase for *black fever*, *kālā* meaning black and *āzār* meaning fever or disease). As for the New World, evidence of the cutaneous form of the disease was found in Ecuador and Peru in pre-Inca potteries depicting skin lesions and deformed faces dating back to the first century CE. The 15th- and 16th-century texts from the Inca period and from Spanish colonials mention "*valley sickness*," "*Andean sickness*," or "*white leprosy*" which are likely to be CL.[58]

Who first discovered the organism is somewhat disputed. It is possible that Surgeon major Cunningham of the British Indian Army saw it first in 1885 without being able to relate it to the disease.[59,60] In 1901, Leishman identified certain organisms in smears taken from the spleen of a patient who had died from "Dumdum fever" (Dum Dum is an area close to Kolkata) and in 1903, Captain Charles Donovan (1863–1951) described them as being new organisms.[58] Eventually Ronald Ross established the link with the disease and named the organism *L. donovani*. By linking this protozoan with KA, Leishman and Donovan discovered the genus, *Leishmania*.

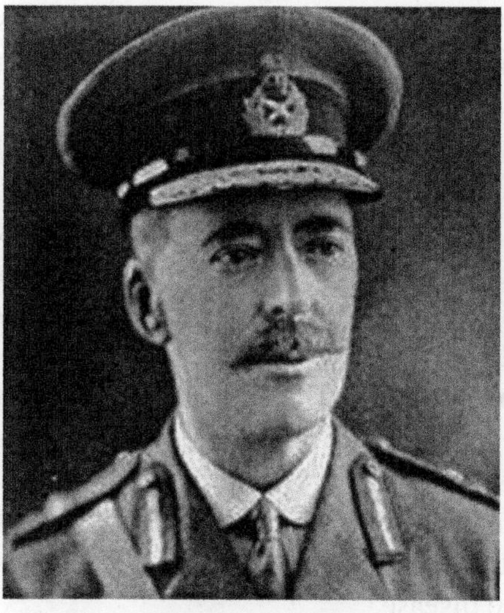

William Leishman

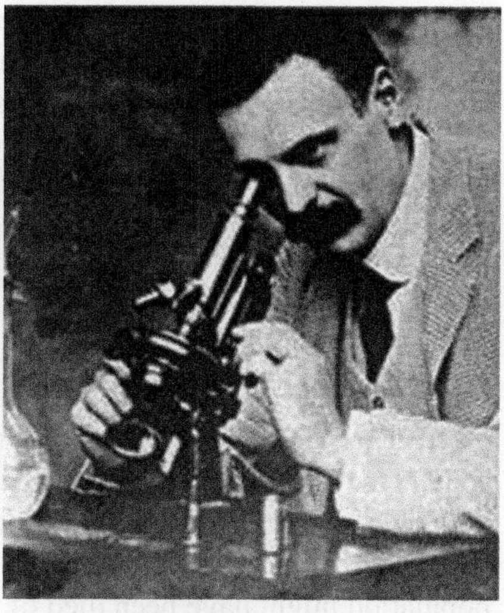

Charles Donovan

The genus *Leishmania* most probably arose from a monoxenous flagellate of the ancestors of phlebotomine sandflies.[61] The first species of *phlebotominae* were found in Lower Cretaceous in the Lebanon, south of the Tethys Sea. A *phlebotomus* was found in amber in the Baltic area in the Upper Eocene belonging to about 30 million years ago. From then on, various phlebotomine sandflies have been found in East Africa.

According to Baker,[62] a vector-borne infectious disease of humans is frequently one which commences as an infection of blood-sucking invertebrates and progresses to an infection of a vertebrate animal. From this state it may infect humans via the invertebrate, eventually dispensing with the animal reservoir and becoming a human disease transmitted human to human (anthroponotic) by the blood-sucking invertebrate. As the disease builds up in humans, it finds a more direct form of transmission between humans, such as a droplet infection or via an ectoparasite of humans. This stage will normally be the most virulent form of the disease in humans. It may then fall away and become only a mild disease of humans.

Acceptance of the Baker's concept[62] which means that zoonoses will tend to be older than anthroponoses, leads to the concept that infection in humans with *L. infantum* is older than infection with *L. donovani*.

Kala-azar endemic areas in India is illustrated in Figure 10.10. The first description of KA that is acceptable is that of Twining.[63] He found cancrumoris, anaemia and the characteristic skin pallor. In the 1860s, it began to become obvious that a considerable infectious fever was rife in Garo hills of Assam, and then progressed steadily up the Brahmaputra valley over a 10-year period. More local synonyms include kala-jwar, kala-dukh, Burdwan fever, Sahib's disease and Shirkari disease in India, Ponos in Greece, and Semieh in Sudan. The origin and spread of the disease was traced by Dr. J. Eliot, the Civil Surgeon of Burdwan. He was able to trace the disease back to 1824–1825 to a village called Mahomedpore east of Jessore, infamous as the starting point of the first great pandemic of Cholera in 1817. He mentions the inefficacy of quinone and the splenomegaly. It was a disease of fearsome mortality and seems to have been a disease of swifter mortality than at present, but then the apparent celerity would depend on how soon patients sought the infective help. The disease travelled slowly westward, totally depopulating some villages, and reached Burdwan in 1860. The government of Bengal wrung its hands and reported that as many as 30% of the areas population might have been died of the disease.

At the end of the 19th century, KA was reported in Assam. At this time, many still thought of KA as a form of malaria and the severity of the Assamese outbreak persuaded the government of India to set up a team to enquire into episode. The first investigation led to a conclusion that the disease was beriberi and caused by *Ankylostoma*, but this view was soon discarded. A second investigation by Surgeon-Captain (later "Sir") Leonard Rogers made the link between the Assamese disease and Burdwan fever. Rogers concluded that the disease was a highly virulent form of malaria.

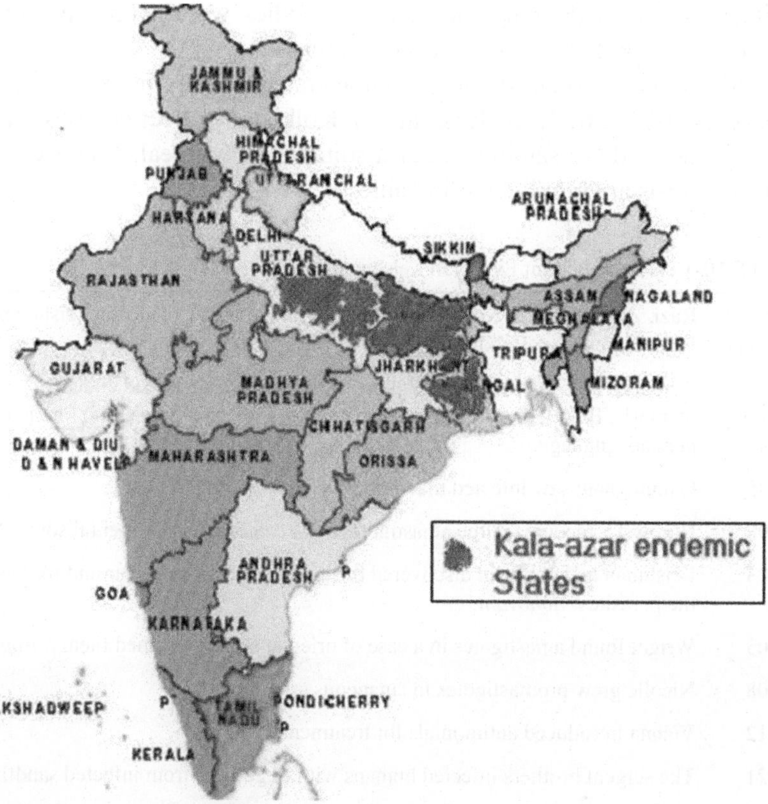

FIGURE 10-10 Kala-azar endemic areas in India.

In 1903, Leishman[64] noted that soldiers invalided home to Britain from the cantonment of Dumdum (the place of the present Kolkata airport) had a characteristic illness, "an extreme degree of cachexia," irregularly intermittant fever, anaemia, muscular atrophy, and great enlargement of the spleen. He referred to these patients to as cases of Dumdum fever. He had no immediate explanation for these bodies of spleen, but 3 years later he found similar bodies in the internal organs of a rat that had died from experimental trypanosomiasis, he proposed that Dumdum fever might be a form of Indian trypanosomiasis. This possibility was published in the British Medical Journal of May 30, 1903. In the same year, Professor Donovan from Madras Medical College, on reading Leishman's article, immediately realized the significance of the bodies, which he had found similar bodies in a postmortem spleen smears. He first thought that they might be a resting form of a malaria parasite, but had then decided they were probably postmortem artifacts. He later demonstrated that the bodies were neither postmortem artifact nor an Indian form of trypanosomiasis.[65]

Phlebotomus argentips was demonstrated to be the vector for the organism in 1924 by Knowles et al.[66] in Kolkata by direct demonstration of the parasite in these sandflies after a suitable blood meal. Major events of Leishmaniasis are highlighted in Table 10.1.

TABLE 10-1 The Important Events in Leishmaniasis[67]

9th century	Razi, Zakarya (Also Known As Al–Rhazi) Described Cutaneous Leishmaniasis; Later Known As 'Balkh Sore'.
10th Century	Avicenna and independently abu mansour bokharai described cutaneous leishmaniasis. Bokharai called it "pasheh gazidegi" meaning mosquito bite in the persian language.
1885	Cunningham saw infected macrophages from an oriental sore.
1898	Borowsky recognized the amastigotes of *Leishmania* in an oriental sore.
1903	Leishman and donovan discovered the amastigotes in kala-azar and ross named the parasite *l. donovani.*
1903	Wright found amastigotes in a case of oriental sore and named them *l. tropica.*
1908	Nicolle grew promastigotes in cutaneous culture.
1912	Vianna introduced antimonials for treatment.
1921	The sergent brothers infected humans with flagellates from infected sandflies.
1923	Shortt and sen introduced brahmachari's antimonial for the cure of kala-azar.

10.2.2.4 DIFFERENT GEOGRAPHICAL FORMS OF KALA-AZAR

The different types of KA exist, which vary considerably in clinical symptoms, severity, and response to antimony treatment.[68] It can be suggested that these variations have come about as the disease has developed from its primitive state as a zoonosis (Table 10-2). They are as follows:

- Indian KA
- Acute toxic KA
- Infanite or Mediterranean KA
- Chinese KA
- Russian KA
- Sudanese KA
- East African KA

TABLE 10-2 The Main Difference between Important Forms of Kala-Azar

	Symtoms	Indian KA	Sudanese KA	E. African KA
1.	Skin lesions with visceral diseases	Do not occur	Fairly common on legs and head	Sometimes seen on legs
2.	Frequency of *Leishmania* in blood	Often seen	Rarely seen	Rarely seen
3.	Response to penta–valent antimony	Good	Little or none	Little or none
4.	Incidence of relapse	Not common	Common	Common
5.	Post–kala-azar dermal leishmani-asis (PKDL)	Latent period 1–2 years. Duration long. Found in 5%–10% of cases.	Little or no latent period. Duration long. Found in 30% of cases.	Latent period 5–9 months. Duration not known. Found in small proportion of cases

10.2.3 PROTOZOOLOGY OF THE GENUS LEISHMANIA

In the animal kingdom, protozoa may be regarded either as a phylum or as a group of microorganisms within the protista having the basic characteristics of animal cells.[69] Still there is controversy over which of each pair of definitions is more correct. Eukaryotic cells are the basic cellular organization of protozoa. The cell contents are delineated into large number of membrane-bound organelle such as nuclei, mitochondria, glycosomes (microbodies), Golgi apparatus, lysosomes, and food vacuoles. This organism is quite distinct from that of prokaryotic microorganisms, which lack membrane-bound organelles, but is similar to other lower eukaryotes such as algae and fungi.[70] Absence of mechanically rigid cell wall, external to the plasma membrane distinguishes protozoan cells from that of algae, fungi, and higher plants and underlies their similarity to those of multicellular animals.

10.2.3.1 CLASSIFICATION OF THE GENUS LEISHMANIA

The animal kingdom has been divided into two groups; one is metazoa and another is protozoa. The metazoas are multicellular; different groups of cells perform different biochemical reactions to fulfil the diverse physiological requirements of life process. The protozoas are unicellular performing all functions of life within the cell. Some important characteristics of protozoa are the following.

- Protozoa are generally larger than bacteria and yeast.
- Protozoa has well defined nucleus with nuclear membrane.
- Protozoa are generally motile throughout the life cycle or at least during certain period of life cycle.

The phylum protozoa was classified by Doflin[71] into two subphyla–plasmodroma and ciliophora. The classification can be enumerated as below.

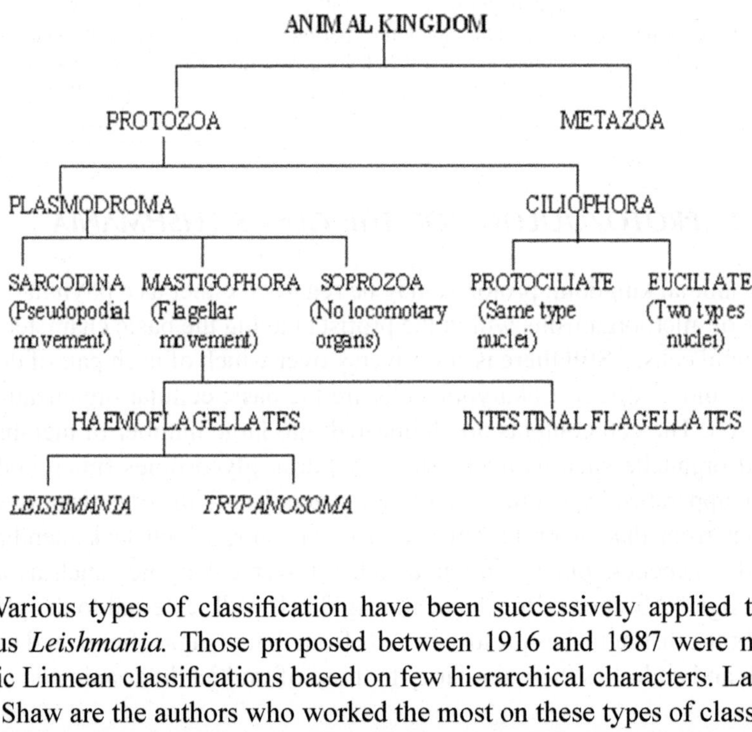

Various types of classification have been successively applied to the genus *Leishmania.* Those proposed between 1916 and 1987 were monothetic Linnean classifications based on few hierarchical characters. Lainson and Shaw are the authors who worked the most on these types of classification and who made them evaluative. Their last classification (1987) divided the genus *Leishmania* into two sub-genera: *Leishmania* sensu stricto (Table 10-3.A) present in both Old and New World, and Viannia (Table 10-3.B), restricted to New World. Within these two sub-genera various species complexes were individualized.

TABLE 10-3A Sub-genus *Leishmania Ross,* 1903[72]

L. donovani complex	*L. donovani* (Laveran & Mesnil, 1903) *L. archibaldi* Castellani & Chalmers, 1919
L. infantum complex	*L. infantum* Nicolle, 1908 (syn. *L. chagasi* Cunha & Chagas, 1937)
L. tropica complex	*L. tropica* (Wright, 1903)
L. killicki complex	*L. killicki* Rioux, Lanotte & Pratlong, 1986
L. aethiopica complex	*L. aethiopica* Bray, Ashford & Bray, 1973
L. major complex	*L. major* Yakimoff & Schokhor, 1914
L. turanica complex	*L. turanica* Strelkova, Peters & Evans, 1990
L. gerbilli complex	*L. gerbilli* Wang, Qu & Guan, 1964
L. arabica complex	*L. arabica* Peters, Elbihari & Evans, 1986
L. mexicana complex	*L. mexicana* Biagi, 1953 (syn. *L. pifanoi* Medina & Romero, 1959)
L. amazonensis complex	*L. amazonensis* Lainson & Shaw, 1972 (syn. *L. garnhami* Scorza et al., 1979) *L. aristidesi* Lainson & Shaw, 1979
L. enriettii complex	*L. enriettii* Muniz & Medina, 1948
L. hertigi complex	*L. hertigi* Herrer, 1971 *L. deanei* Lainson & Shaw, 1977

TABLE 10-3B Sub-genus *Viannia* Lainson and Shaw, 1987[73]

L. braziliensis complex	*L. braziliensis* Vianna, 1911. *L. peruviana* Velez, 1913
L. guyanensis complex	*L. guyanensis* Floch, 1954 *L. panamensis* Lainson & Shaw, 1972 *L. shawi* Lainson et al., 1989
L. naiffi complex	*L. naiffi* Lainson & Shaw, 1989
L. lainsoni complex	*L. lainsoni* Silveira et al., 1987

Haemoflagellates infect the vascular system and various tissues of the body. This group is well marked for its parasitic nature. Most of the protozoan diseases in man are caused by this group of organisms. Thus haemoflagellates are responsible for the diseases such as KA, sleeping sickness, oriental sore, espundia, and so forth.

10.2.3.2 MORPHOLOGY AND ULTRASTRUCTURE OF LEISHMANIA

The outcomes of electronic microscopic studies on *Leishmania* have revealed many differences between amastigote form and promastigote form (Figure 10.11 & 10.12). It has been observed that during the transformation of amastigote to promastigote, there was the lengthening and elaboration of the mitochondrion,[74] except for some exceptions where a long and tortuous mitochondrion have been observed in amastigotes.[75,76] Many scientists have confirmed that the mitochondrion was extended during amastigote to promastigote transformation.[77,78]

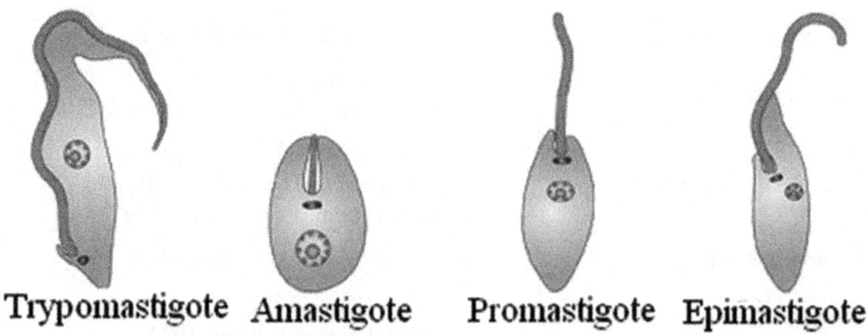

FIGURE 10-11 The main cellular forms of trypanosomatids as defined by cell shape, flagellum presence and attachment, and position of the basal body, kinetoplast and nucleus. In general, the epimastigote and promastigote forms of digenetic trypanosomatids are found in the vector, the trypomastigote form is found in the mammalian host and the amastigote form is intracellular.

The number of subpellicular microtubules in amastigotes is not same in all the species in *Leishmania*. In case of *L. donovani*, 80–120 subpellicular microtubules have been found,[79] whereas in case of *L. mexicana* their number is 180–200.[80] The microtubules of the promastigotes radiate in all directions from a point near the flagellar base, unlike in other trypanosomatids in which they are spiralled.[81]

The distance between the microtubules differs between mammalian and reptilian species.[82] The subpellicular microtubules have been used as a potential means of separating *Leishmania* species.

Lysosomes were absent in promastigotes, but present in amastigotes.[83] All species of *Leishmania,* except *L. tropica*, contain rough endoplasmic reticulum.[75] Four isolated tubules were observed in the reservoir region that may serve to anchor the subpellicular tubules to the flagellar apparatus.[75] The amastigote–promastigote transformation in *Leishmania* is associated with an increase in the number of mitochondrial profiles per section, the relative mitochondrial volume was decreased, and the concentration of the DNA fibrils to the centre of the kinetoplast with a wider disposition of the cytoplasmic RNA granules has been observed.[84]

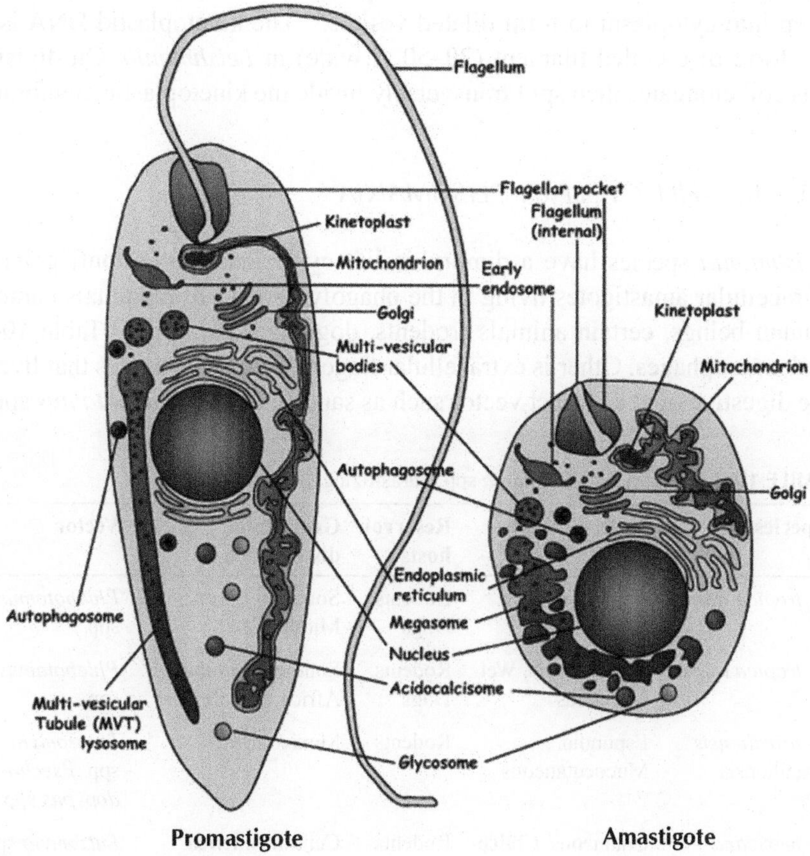

FIGURE 10-12 Changes in cell shape during the *Leishmania* life cycle.

(a) Scanning electron microscope images of the main *Leishmania major* life-cycle stages, the procyclic and metacyclic promastigotes were grown in culture, the amastigote was isolated from an infected macrophage isolated from a mouse.

(b) Schematic representation of the main intracellular organelles from *Leishmania* promastigote (left) or amastigote (right) forms. The flagellar pocket marks the anterior end of the cell.

Kinetoplast has been found to be connected to the basal body by a band of amorphous material.[85] Promastigotes may sometimes contain pigment granules and lipid bodies.[86] Both amastigotes and promastigotes contain peroxisomes, which contain all the glycolytic enzymes in their vesicle.[87]

The nucleus of *Leishmania* is covered with two nuclear membranes of 7 nm thickness, and having a prominent nucleolus (endosomes), situated centrally with 0.6–1 μm in diameter. The nuclear membrane remains intact during division. Nuclear membrane may contain extensions that penetrate deep into cytoplasm to form dilated vesicle.[77] The kinetoplastid DNA is in the form of a coiled filament (20–50 Å wide) in *Leishmania.* On division this coil elongates then split transversely inside the kinetoplastic membrane.

10.2.3.3 LIFE CYCLE OF LEISHMANIA

Leishmania species have a dimorphic life cycle, one is the nonflagellated intracellular amastigotes living in the phagolysosomes of mammals namely, human beings, certain animals (rodents, dogs, jackals, foxes) (Table 10-4) and macrophages. Other is extracellular flagellated promastigotes that live in the digestive tract of insect vector such as sandfly that is, *Phlebotomus* spp.

TABLE 10-4 Important *Leishmania* spp. Parasitizing Humans

Species	Type of disease	Reservoir hosts	Geographic distribution	Vector
L. tropica minor	Dry cutaneous	Rodents, Dogs	Southern Europe, Middle East	*Phlebotomus* spp.
L. tropica major	Oriental sore, Wet cutaneous	Rodents, Dogs	Southern Europe, Africa, Middle East	*Phlebotamus* spp.
L. braziliensis braziliensis	Espundia, Mucocutaneous	Rodents	Mexico, Brazil	*Lutozomyia* spp. *Psychodopypus* spp.
L. mexicana mexicana	Cutaneous, Chilcero ulcer	Rodents	Central America	*Lutzomyia* spp.
L. mexicana amazonensis	Diffuse cutaneous	Rodents	Amazonas region	*Lutozomyia* spp.
L. peruviana	Uta, Cutaneous	Dogs	Peru	*Lutzomyia* spp.
L. donovani	Kala-–azar, Dum-dum fever, Visceral	Dogs, Foxes	Africa, Asia, Middle East, Southern Russia, South America	*Phlebotomus* spp.

TABLE 10-4 *(Continued)*

Species	Type of disease	Reservoir hosts	Geographic distribution	Vector
L. donovani chargasi	Visceral	Foxes, Cats, Dogs	South America	*Lutzomyia* spp.
L. donovani infantum	Visceral infantile	Dogs	Miditerranean countries	*Phlebotomus* spp.

Sandflies are the principal agent of transmission in nature. The female sandfly feed on blood and transmit the infection. The male sandfly does not suck blood but feed on plant juices and takes no part in transmission. Different stages are demonstrated in Figure 10.13–10.18.

The nonflagellated intracellular amastigotes proliferates in the acid pH of lysosomes of human macrophages.[88,89] The infective promastigotes enter into the subcutaneous tissue in the human host during the bite of an infected sandfly vector. They are phagositosed by mononuclear phagocyte after which they convert into intracellular nonflagellated amastigote form.

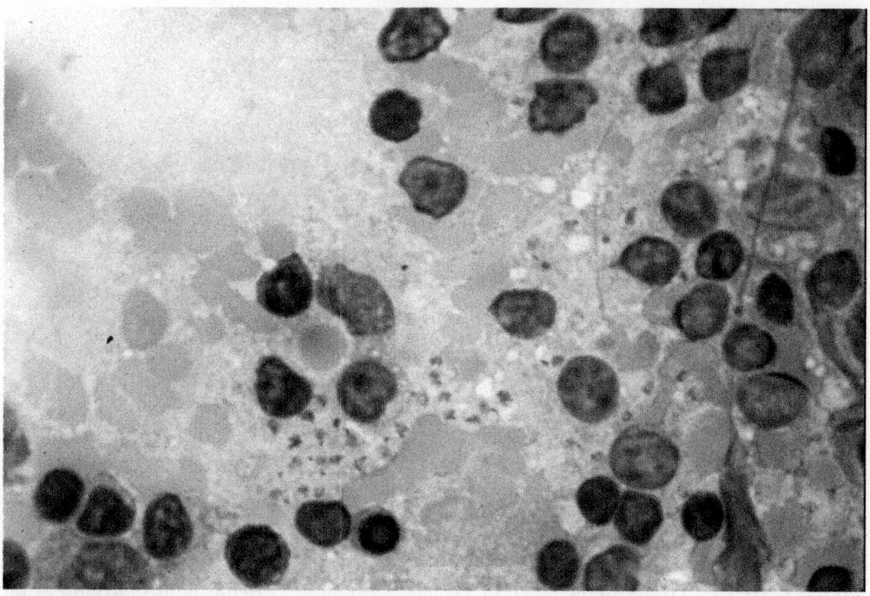

FIGURE 10-13 *Leishmania* amastigotes. The parasite has this morphology when residing in the phagolysosomes of mammals and macrophages.

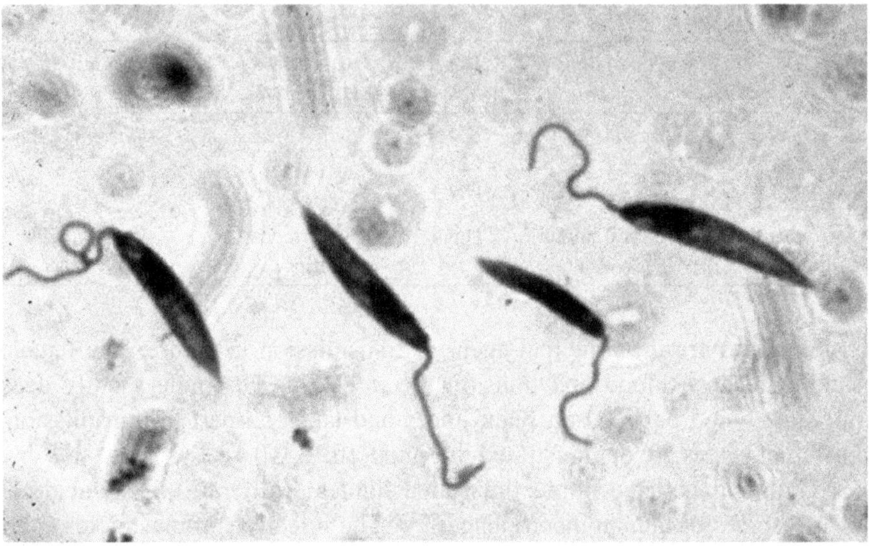

FIGURE 10-14 *Leishmania* promastigotes. The parasite has this morphology when residing in the sandfly vector.

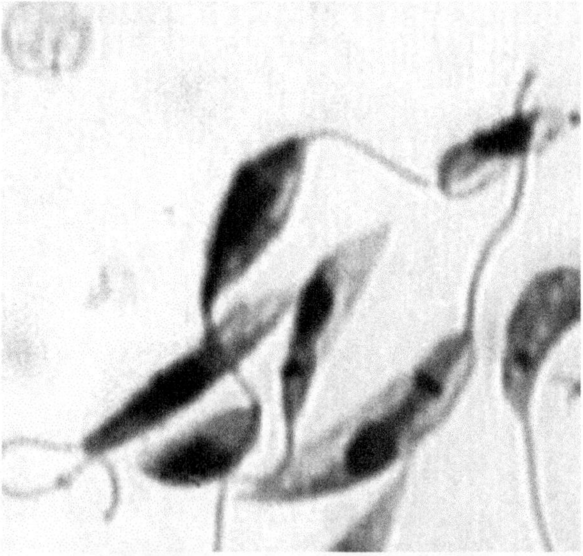

FIGURE 10-15 Promastigote stage of *Leishmania* culture: Promastigotes develop in the insect midgut and move to the salivary glands and proboscis of the sandfly where they become metacyclic insect stages capable of infecting the mammalian host.

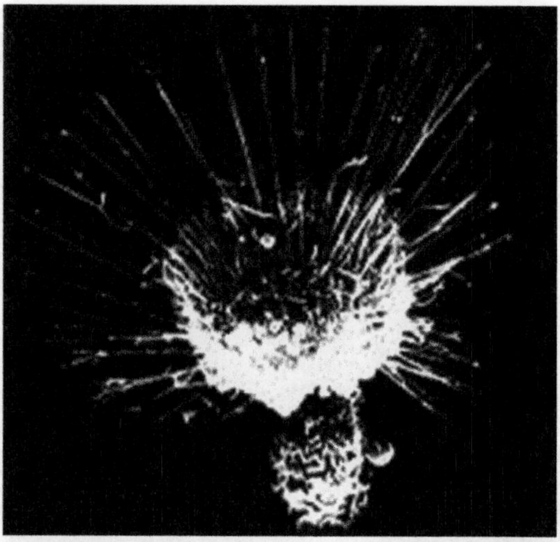

FIGURE 10-16 Macophages actively taking up promastigotes: The parasites enter the macrophages by a mechanism of phagocytosis and end up in vacuoles called phagosomes. These phagosomes then fuse with the lysosomes to form phagolysosomes and it is here that the promastigotes transform to amastigotes which survive and multiply inside these organelles.

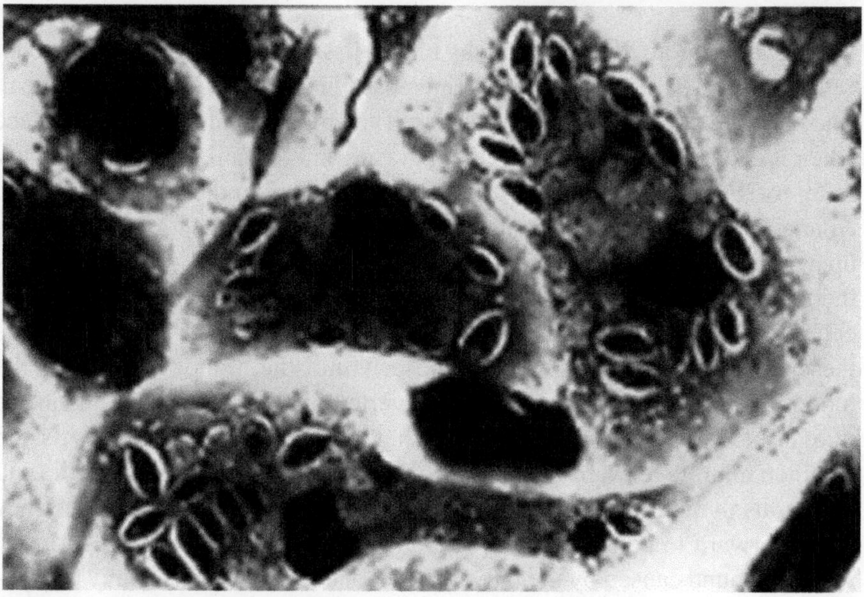

FIGURE 10-17 Infected macrophages, in culture amastigotes are visible inside phagolysosomes.

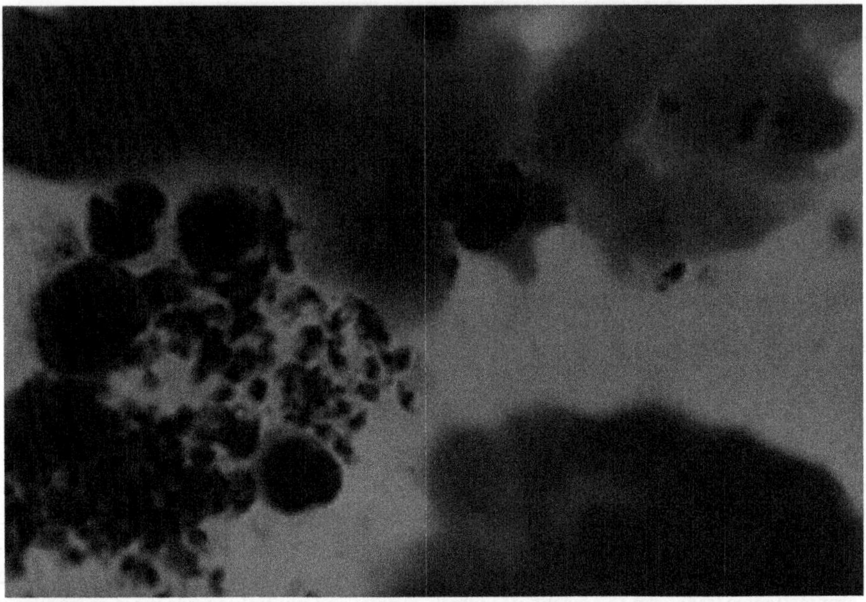

FIGURE 10-18 Impression smear of infected liver stained with giemsa. Amastigotes in the infected macophages (kupfer cells) are visible as small binary dots representing nucleus and kinetoplast.

The amastigote form multiply by binary fission inside reticuloendothelial cells (Figure 10-19). The parasites increases in size and becomes spherical. The cells are packed with the parasites. The enlargement of cell takes place when it is unable to hold any further parasite and the cell ruptures. As many as 50 to 200 or even more may be found embedded in the cytoplasm of the enlarged host cells. The parasites enter into circulation and are again taken up by or invade fresh cells and the cycle repeats. In this way, the whole endothelian system becomes progressively infected. Some of the free *Leishmania* cells are phagocytosed by macrophages in the blood stream. The insect sucks these free amastigotes as well as those within the monocytes during the blood meal. These amastigotes are converted into the promastigotes in the midgut of certain species of sandfly. They again multiply by binary fission and then migrate forward to the anterior part of thoracic midgut or cardia and enormous number of flagellates appears (Figure 10-19). From midgut, they move forward to contaminate the mouth parts of the sandfly to regurgitate into the wound caused by the bite of the second blood meal. A heavy pharyngeal infection of the sandfly is observed between the sixth and ninth day of its infective blood meal.

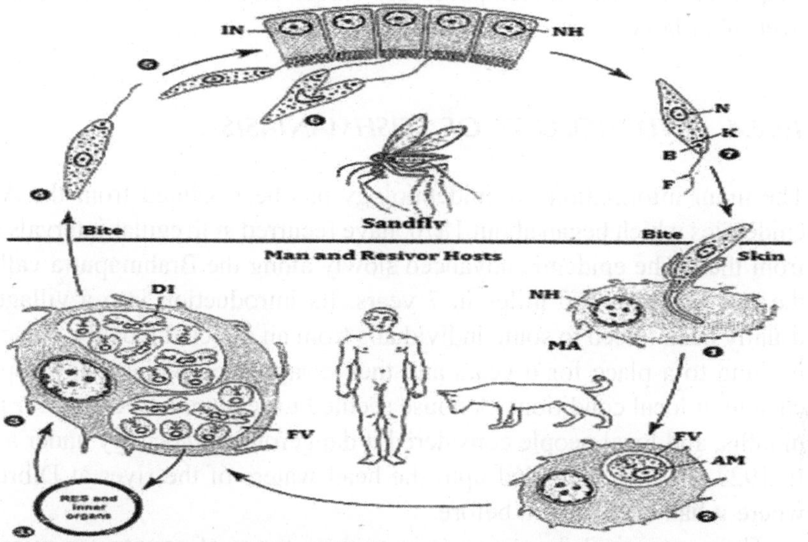

FIGURE 10-19 Life cycle of *Leishmania* spp.

(1) After bite of the sandfly vector the injected promastigote state is engulfed by macrophages in the skin of the vertebrate host. (2) Transformation of promastigotes into amastigote states (2–4 μm in diameter) requires 1–4 hours; reproduction proceeds as binary fission inside a parasitophorous vacuole, which later breaks down. (3) When macrophages are almost filled with amastigotes (after 48 hours), they finally burst and set free the parasites, which may enter other macrophages in the skin, leading to a CL. (3.1) Amastigotes of the *L. donovani* group are carried to inner organs and may enter various host cells, where they are reproduced by repeated binary fissions and lead to a VL within 4–6 months. (4) When a sandfly (*Phlebotomus*) ingests amastigotes along with its blood meal, (5) the latter are transformed into slender promastigotes (910–920 μm in length) in the midgut, where they multiply by repeated binary fission. (6) Quickly they block up the gut of the vector and move to the pharynx and buccal cavity, where they are injected to a new host with the fly's next bite. (7) All stages have a slight surface coat. AM-amastigote stage; B-basal body of flagellum; DI-dividing stage; F-free flagellum; FV-food vacuole; INB-intestinal cell; K-kinetoplast; MA-macrophages; N-nucleus; NH-nucleus of host cells.

The ingestion of promastigotes into mononuclear phagocyte mediated by receptor is accompanied by an oxidative burst of the phagocyte, during which oxidants such as superoxide and hydrogen peroxide are formed.[90–92] Hydrogenperoxide can be converted into hydroxyl radical ($\dot{O}H$) through the Fenton reaction in the presence of a source of iron: $H_2O_2 + Fe^{2+} \rightarrow \dot{O}H + OH^- + Fe^{3+}$.

Mitotic cycle of *L. donovani* has been found to have a sequence of 15.2 hours resting phase, 1.1 hours prophase, 3.9 hours metaphase, 0.9 hour anaphase, and 1.8 hours telophase and binucleate phase to make a total turnover of 24 hours.

10.2.4 EPIDEMOLOGY OF LEISHMANIASIS

The main information on epidemiology has been gained from the Assam epidemics which began about 1870, have recurred at irregular intervals since from then. The epidemic advanced slowly along the Brahmaputra valley at the rate of some 100 miles in 7 years. Its introduction into a village has usually been traced to some individuals from an infected locality. Generally, it clung to a place for 6 years and then disappeared without any apparent change in local conditions. A house seemed to retain the infection for many months, and local people considered it dangerous to reoccupy under a year. In 1922–1923, it extended upto the head waters of the river at Dibrugarh where it had been known before.

The neotropical form occurs in various types of country–in miserable hovels, in dense forests, in desert country, and on river banks.

The outstanding epidemiological features of the disease in India and China are that it is confined to rural district, especially alluvial plains and does not usually occur above 2,000 feet. The temperature conditions are a monthly mean maximum below 100°F, and a monthly mean minimum above 45°F. In India, a high degree of humidity is a common factor; not so in China. In the Mediterranean, the greatest number of cases occurs from March to May; in Assam in the cooler months, from November to February; in the Sudan, after the rains between August and December; in China no seasonal incidence has been observed. The patchy distribution in Sudan resembles the epidemiological features of the South American disease.[93] Both sexes are equally affected, although in certain areas higher incidence may be noticed among the males. Age of the victims is a factor in the course of the disease, and fatal outcome is most frequent in infants and small children. Poor nutrition, concomitant infection with other pathogens, and other stress factors predispose the patient to lethal consequences.

The epidemiology of vector-borne disease is evolving toward quantitative epidemiology. The vast development of quantitative epidemiology requires the knowledge of all the parameters of the transmission cycle of the parasite, which may be incorporated into complex mathematical models. Study of the mathematical model in parallel with field observations is one of the important ways of testing the adequacy of current epidemiological concepts and control strategies.

The quantitative epidemiology of leishmaniasis is still descriptive compared to malaria, which reached a fairly advanced level. The main reasons are a great heterogeneity of epidemiological or epizoological pattern and poor knowledge of many factors of the natural history of the parasites, vectors, and vertebrate hosts. From the point of view of quantitative epidemiology, clinico-epidemiological parameters may be compared to differentiate between the different *Leishmanias*.

10.2.4.1 ZOONOTIC FORM VERSUS ANTHROPONOTIC FORM

In case of zoonotic form, the role of humans is usually negligible, and the force of infection does not depend on nonimmunes in the community. Whereas, in case of anthroponotic, the proportion of nonimmunes is very important. Hence, the description of the accumulation of the infection in human beings may be simplified in zoonotic models, the movement of the pathogen from the reservoir to human beings independent from the amount of the leishmaniasis in population.

10.2.4.2 VISCERAL FORM VERSUS CUTANEOUS FORM

The main difference between two forms are in the fatality rate (severity) of the disease, susceptibility and diagnosis. In visceral form, the severity or fatal rate is high and differential mortality is taken into picture in the model. Since cutaneous form does not cause mortality, the model will be simpler.

The susceptibility of human varies greatly in VL. Not all the individuals exposed to Mediterranean form are susceptible.[94,95] In case of CL, all the individuals are susceptible. Each act of transmission result in overt disease and because each infective bite occurring over the weeks between the first bite and the development of a protective immunity produces a separate leishmanioma multiple acts of transmission in the same person may sometimes be recognized.

The diagnosis of VL is comparatively expensive than CL, in which it is easy, safe, and more definite.

10.2.4.3 ACUTE FORM VERSUS CHRONIC FORM

The infection is self-limiting and of short duration in many forms of leishmanaisis; but in others, it is chronic and may go on for years. In zoonotic CL of central Asia, the lesions heal in 3–4 months, but in few cases they persist upto 1 year. The same *Leishmania* may behave differently in different hosts. For example, zoonotic CL is self-limiting in human beings, but chronic and lifelong in gerbils.

10.2.5 TRANSMISSION AND VECTORS

The probable evolutionary history of *Leishmania*, from a parasite of insects and eventually to one of mammals, implies that infected sandflies are primary hosts, which are known as vectors. Other much rarer modes of transmissions are congenital, blood transfusion, or by direct (sometimes sexual) contact or inoculation.

10.2.5.1 SANDFLY TRANSMISSION

Many vectors transmit leishmaniasis to people who make contact with them through agriculture, road-building, military monoeuvers, herding, charcoal burning, and other activities.[96–98] The activity of sandflies which may enhance their role as vectors, is increased flight range under certain conditions.[81] Killick–Kendrick et al.[99] showed that *Phlebotomus ariasi* is sufficiently mobile to spread the infection (leishmaniasis) to neighbouring areas within a radius of 1–2 km. The peridomestic or domestic habits of species such as *Phlebotomus papatasi*, *Phlebotomus sergenti,* and *Phlebotomus argentipes* and *Lutzomyia longipalpis* ensure close association with human being.

Following the observation that there was a correlation between the distribution of *P. argentipes* in India and KA, it was found that there was a rapid development of promastigote forms in *P. argentipes,* and in 1942 KA was successfully transmitted to human volunteers by the bite of *P. argentipes.*[100]

Sandflies are the principal agents of transmission in nature. Sandflies are small hairy flies with long hairy legs (Figure10-20). The female sandfly feeds blood and transmits the infection (Figure 10-21). One or more blood meals are necessary to complete the maturation of each batch of eggs. The male sandfly does not suck blood but feeds on plant juices and does not take part in transmission. Sandflies are inactive in day light, seeking shelter in dark moist places and coming out at night time. Usually, the normal fly covers less than a meter, but sandflies can cover more than a kilometer overnight.

Female sandflies feed on a variety of both cold- and warm-blooded animals and do not specially feed on man, but a few species such as *P. argentipes* in India have become domestic and dependent on man.

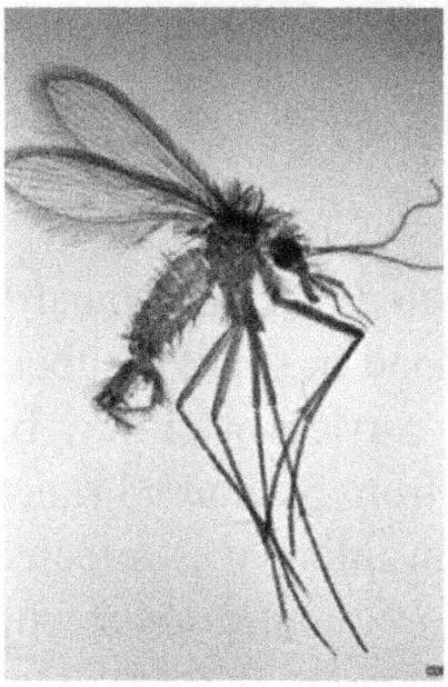

FIGURE 10-20 Sandfly.

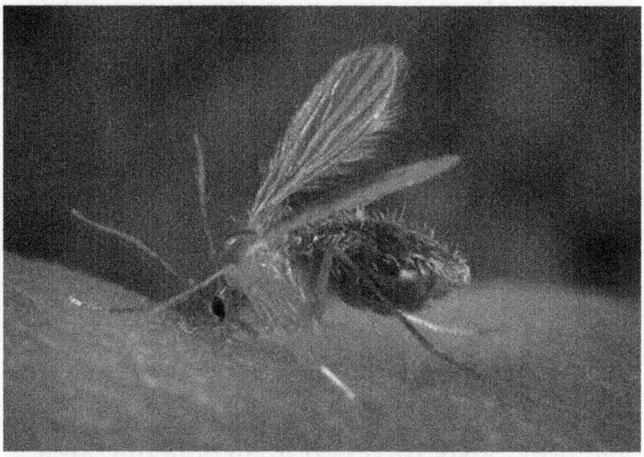

FIGURE 10-21 Sandfly biting a victim.

Breeding sites are dark damp places rich in organic matter and female flies are ready to lay eggs within 3–10 days after a blood meal. The eggs are laid and larvae hatch that require high humidity to compete their development in less than 3 weeks; but species that live in colder climate may take up to 3 months. Flies emerge during the hours of darkness and mate, the female storing sufficient sperm to lay eggs at intervals throughout life, which in nature is rarely more than a few weeks. The life cycle from egg to adult varies from 1 to 3 months.

A sandfly is infective to a new host from 5 to 10 days after the infective blood meal and remains infected for the rest of its life. Infection of a new host occurs with the second blood meal after egg laying has taken place.

In other epidemic centers, different species of sandfly are involved: *Phlebotomus major* in Eastern Mediterranean; *Phlebotomus orientalis* and *Phlebotomus clydei* in the Sudan; *Phlebotomus perniciosus* in Western Mediterranean and North Africa; *Phlebotomus arpaklensis* in Tajikistan and Transcaucasia; *Phlebotomus chinese* and *P. sergenti* var. mongolicus in China; *Phlebotomus longeroni* in Sudan; *Phlebotomus garnhami* in Eastern Africa; and *Phlebotomus longipalpis* and *Phlebotomus intermedius* in South America.

10.2.5.2 CONGENITAL TRANSMISSION

That KA may occasionally be a congenital infection has been proved by Low et al. in 1925, who diagnosed this disease in a 7-month-old child, born in England of a mother who suffered severely fromKA during pregnancy.[101–104]

10.2.5.3 BLOOD TRANSFUSION

KA is one of the protozoal diseases that can be transmitted by blood transfusion.[105–108] Amastigotes may occur in the peripheral blood in small numbers in the early stages of infection and in asymptomatic carriers who may be infective for a short period. Cases have been recorded from Southern France during incubation period and in Scandivania where an infant was infected from blood given in exchange transfusion from an asymptomatic donor who had previously travelled in an endemic area.

10.2.5.4 DIRECT CONTACT

Since amastigotes can be demonstrated in stools containing blood and mucus in a patient with dysentry; and in nasal mucosa and nasal discharges, direct transmission via these routes is possible.[109,110] Direct transmission by the sexual route has also been described.[111]

A case of accidental infection with *L. donovani* in a laboratory worker, whose fingers had been bitten on several occasions by experimentally infected animals, had been recorded by Terry et al.[112]

10.2.6. BIOCHEMISTRY OF *LEISHMANIA*

10.2.6.1 MORPHOLOGICAL TRANSFORMATION OF *LEISHMANIA*

Some work has been done on transformation biology of amastigote form to the motile promastigote form and vice versa. The transformation of promastigote to amastigote forms has been claimed to be triggered off by withdrawing riboflavin from a medium without any change in cell growth at 25°C.[113] The intracellular amastigotes of mammalian *Leishmania* have been produced in vitro by adopting the organism to grow at 34°C.[114] But *L. torentolae* does not respond to elevated temperature in this way; growth of this organism in a defined medium is inhibited at 33°C. Addition of red blood cell extract allows growth at this temperature, but the formation of amastigotes has not been observed.[115]

The promastigote form can readily be grown on a variety of complex media at a temperature ranging from 16° to 32°C. Morphologically intermediate forms can be produced by the inoculation of *L. donovani* bodies in a media having red blood cell extract and human or hamster serum at 37°C.[116,117]

Cultures of spleen from hamsters infected with *L. donovani* contained initially the amastigotes at 37°C.[118] In older cultures the parasites, after having escaped from the destroyed cells, multiply as promastigote forms. In the system of Lomy et al., the intracellular stages of *L. donovani* in the presence of carcinosarcoma cells could be maintained several months by serial transfers.[119]

Formation of promastigotes from amastigotes in the body is accompanied by the highly developed chondriome structures.[120] The effect of temperature upon the conversion of culture to blood stream forms have been observed by many scientists and seem to play an important role in reciprocal transformation.[121–125] An additional nutritional requirement due to elevated temperature has been due to the inactivation of certain enzymes.[126] The flagellates of crithidia develop lipid requirements when maintained at increased temperatures 32.5°C–33.5°C to maintain normal growth.[127] The sensitivity of *L. donovani* culture form to high temperature has been shown to be mainly due to increased template RNA degradation.[128]

The tubulin biosynthesis was severely restricted during the transformation to the amastigote form.[129] Tubulin was shown previously to be a component of functional microtubules that are present in axonemal, subpellicular, and nuclear structure of trypanosomatid protozoa.[130] *L. donovani* surface membrane was specifically shown to have tubulin by Dwyer et al. in 1980.[131]

Amino acids and glucose have been found to be necessary for the transformation of amastigote form to promastigote form.[132] This transformation is accompanied by an increase in polyamine levels and mitochondrial volume[84,133] with substantial proliferation (Figure 10-22), respiratory rates,[134] and cyclic adenosine 5′-monophosphate, adenosine 5′-phosphate (cAMP) levels.[135] Cyclohexamide, actinomycin D, puramomycin,[136] antileishmanial drugs,[137] and lymphocyte factors[138,139] have been reported to inhibit this transformation. Amastigotes and promastigotes differ in their surface coat,[140] antigenic properties[141] and in the levels of cAMP catabolizing enzymes.[135] The effect on tubulin biosynthesis during this transformation is controlled at the post-transcriptional level.[142]

10.2.6.2 CULTURAL REQUIREMENT

A systemic evaluation of growth of the haemoflagellates is very difficult problem as they require complex media. Only a few leishmanial species can be cultivated in a well-defined media outside the host.[143–145] (Figure 10-22). The requirement of blood in haemoflagellate culture was first initiated by Novy and McNeal.[146] Nicolle grew *L. tropica* and *L. donovani* in the blood agar media.[147] Later many scientists confirmed that no *Trypanosoma* or *Leishmania* can grow in a completely haemoglobin-free medium.[148,149] It was observed that the requirement of hemin in the haemoflagellates was due to their inability to synthesize it.[150,151] (Figure 10-22). Subsequent research proved that along with hemin, other components of blood were also required for haemoflagellate growth.[152] Some of the vitamins were found to to be involved in promoting the growth of haemoflagellates. Ascorbic acid is required as a growth promoting agent in some strains of *Leishmania* and *Trypanosoma*.[152–154]

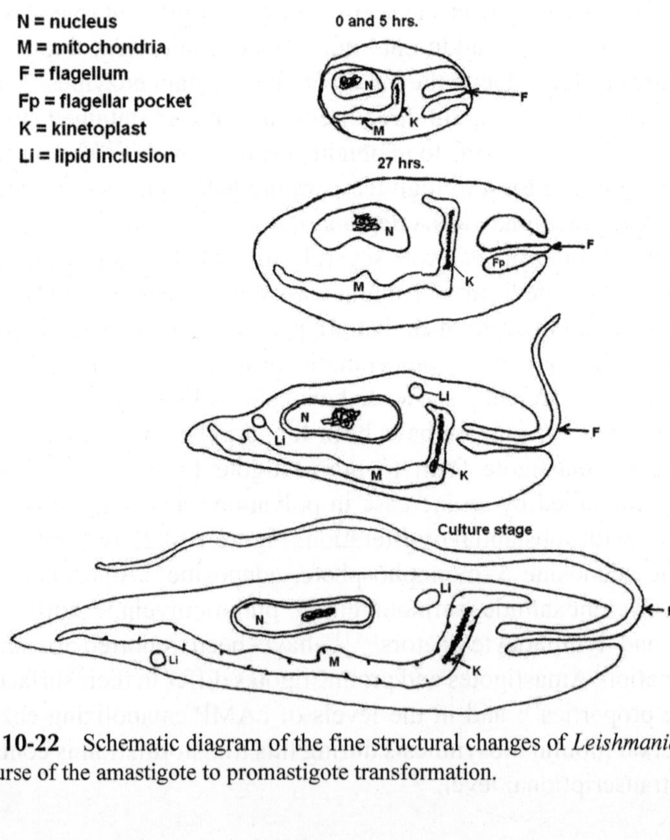

FIGURE 10-22 Schematic diagram of the fine structural changes of *Leishmania donovani* in the course of the amastigote to promastigote transformation.

Some of the amino acids are very essential for flagellates.[155] At least 10 amino acids are essential for the growth of *L. torentolae*. However, amino acid requirement varies in different protozoal classes and species. Glucose could be completely replaced by high amount of L-proline in promastigotes of *L. donovani.*[145] L-proline may be the major energy substrate of *L. donovani*. The earlier biochemical and nutritional work done by Krassner and Flory[156] showed rapid catabolism of L-proline for the promastigotes. The promastigotes of *L. donovani* does not require any lipid material at lower growth temperatures and the organism may have de novo synthetic and desaturase pathway.[143–145] This conclusion was consistent with work done by Beach et al. in lipid metabolism of promastigotes of *L. donovani*, earlier.[157]

At least one purine derivative is required for most of the organisms.[158] Some of the trypanosomatids inter-convert purines and its derivatives.[159–161] Uracil can be used as supplement in the place of other pyrimidine requirements in some ciliates and flagellates.[162–166]

The need of additional nutrient at increased temperature has been observed. There was a good growth at 33°C and stimulation at 28°C for *L. torentolae* grown on the medium fortified with red blood cell extract.[115] It was also observed that chick embryo extract in the medium is required for the good growth of *L. donovani* and *Trypanosoma cruzi*, at environmental temperatures.[117,167]

10.2.6.3 UTILIZATION OF SUBSTRATES

Von Brand[168,169] and Chang[170] studied on the utilization of substrates for *L. donovani*. Chang working with four haemoflagellates of *L. donovani, L. braziliensis, L. tropica,* and *L. cruzi* showed that, they could oxidize glucose and fructose; but not maltose and lactose. But Mukherjee showed that *L. donovani* promastigotes could effectively use mono and disaccharides.[171] They are glucose, fructose, mannose, maltose, glycerol, sucrose, ribose, erythritol, arabinose, galactose, and erythrose.[172] Glucose only being metabolized when the culture reaches the stationary phase[156] and both proline and glutamate support the growth of promastigotes of *L. donovani*, but in some species the proline is more preferred substrate.

The breaking down of complex protinaceous substances such as peptone and gelatin by *L. tropica*, is less pronounced when glucose is present. This suggests that the glucose is the preferred substrate.[148]

10.2.6.4 ENERGY METABOLISM

The glycolysis is fully established in the promastigotes of *L. donovani.*[173] Chattarjee and Datta studied the formation of succinate from glucose via pathways that involve pyruvate.[174] Hexokinase, phosphofructokinase have been shown to be present in *L. donovani* and *L. brazilliensis.*[175] Furthermore, the enzymes of glycolysis have also been studied as potential pathway regulatory sites in *L. tropica, L. mexicana, L. donovani,* and *L. tarentolae*. Glycolytic chain is sensitive to iodoacetate, arsenite, malonate, and fluoroacetate.

Promastigotes of *L. donovani* have many large mitochondria with plate-like cristae, a functional tricarboxylic acid (TCA) cycle and glyoxylate cycle.[176,177] The terminal respiratory chain is localized in the kinetoplast–mitochondrion complex of *L. tropica*. Mukkada showed that electron transport chain enzymes such as reduced nicotinamide adenine dinucleotide (NADH) dehydrogenase, succinate dehydrogenase, cytochrome *b*, cytochrome c_1, cytochrome *c*, cytochrome *a*, cytochrome a_3, and cytochrome *o*, are present in the promastigotes of *L. donovani.*[178] Oxygen utilization is sensitive to cyanide, azide, and antimycin A.

Not much work was done on the pentose phosphate pathway in *L. donovani*. Cell-free extract is not able to oxidize glucose-6-phosphate.[179] Ghosh has reported that ketopentoses and sedoheptuloses are formed during the metabolism of *L. donovani.*[180] Beren et al. has observed the pentose phosphate shunt activity in *L. donovani* and *L. braziliensis.*[175] The presence of large amounts of glucose-6-phosphate dehydrogenase has been shown by Mukherjee.[171,181]

The enzymes of the glycolytic pathway are located in microbody called glycosome in *Trypanosoma brucei.*[182] Further kinetic work with U^{14}–C–D–glucose has revealed evidence for the existence of two pools of glycolytic metabolites or intermediates.[183] Application of modern biochemical techniques like carbon-13 nuclear magnetic resonance.[184] and advanced enzymology[185] are revealing may complexities in the catabolism of glucose that were not expected earlier.

10.2.7 DRUGS AVAILABLE FOR TREATMENT OF LEISHMAIASIS

The most widely used first-line drugs available for all forms of leishmaniasis are pentavalent antimony preparations such as Pentostam (sodium stibogluconate; Wellcome, Beckenham, United Kingdom) and Glucantime

(N-methylglucamine antimonate). These drugs are administered parenterally for 10 to 30 days. Both formulations are equally effective but also equally toxic when efficacy is expressed in relation to the amount of antimony administered. Pentostam contains the preservative 4-chloro-3-methylphenol (chlorocresol). No information on the effects of chlorocresol on Old World *L. donovani* is available. The only available data shows that promastigotes of *Leishmania panamensis* are susceptible to chlorocresol and are apparently resistant to sodium stibogluconate.[186] Chlorocresol antiamastigote activity could not be assessed due to the cytotoxic effect of this compound on macrophage cell lines. The pentavalent antimony needs to be reduced to the trivalent state by either host or parasite metabolism in order to exert its activity.[187] In bacteria and yeast, metal reduction can be mediated by enzymes,[188] and this may be the case in *Leishmania* too. Shaked-Mishan et al.[189] have reported that the reduction of Sb(V) to Sb(III) occurs in both stages of the parasite, but that the activity is much higher in the amastigote stage, which explains the severalfold higher sensitivity of the amastigote to Sb(V) and the role of reduction in sensitization of the parasite. Further, the ability to reduce Sb(V) to Sb(III) is lost in Pentostam-resistant mutants, supporting the role of reducing activity in antimony resistance. Recently, a parasite-specific enzyme, namely thiol-dependent reductase (TDR1) has been shown to catalyse the enzymic reduction of pentavalent antimonials to trivalent.[190] The enzyme is a tetramer protein, containing domains of the omega class of the glutathione S-transferases (GSTs), and uses reduced glutathione (GSH) as the reductant. Although TDR1 has been found to be highly abundant in the amastigote stage of the parasite, a direct relationship between the enzyme activity and antimony sensitivity in *Leishmania* amastigotes cannot be established. Although antimony-based drugs have been used since 1947, their mode of action is still far from understood; they may disrupt the parasite's energy production or interfere with trypanothione metabolism. Unfortunately, in many parts of the world, the parasite has become resistant to antimony and failures and relapses occur in all forms of leishmaniasis and constitute approximately 10–25% of cases. The route of entry of antimonials Sb(V) into *Leishmania* (or into macrophages) is not well understood, although pentavalent arsenate As(V), a metal related to Sb(V), is known to enter via a phosphate transporter.[188] The transport of antimony was first studied by using ^{125}Sb Pentostam Sb(V) in both stages of the *Leishmania mexicana* and *L. donovani* parasites,[191,192] but more recently Mass spectroscopy (MS) approaches have been used to demonstrate the accumulation of two forms of antimony,that is, Sb(V) and Sb(III), in both stages of the parasite. In a number of species, the accumulation of Sb(V) is higher in axenic amastigotes than in promastigotes.[192,193] It has been speculated that Sb(V) enters via a protein that recognizes a sugar moiety-like structure shared with gluconate, as gluconate has been shown to inhibit competitively the uptake of Sb(V) in axenic amastigotes.[193] Further, neither As(V) nor phosphate can compete with the uptake of Pentostam, ruling out the possibility of the use of an As(V) transporter by Sb(V). Although Sb(V) is accumulated by both stages of the parasite, at pharmacological concentrations, it has no antileishmanial activity.[186,194–196] However, in some studies, axenic amastigotes have been found to be as sensitive to Sb(V) as intracellular parasites.[189,197,198] This discrepancy needs to be resolved. Indeed, several factors, such as species, axenization status, pH, and thiol concentration, are likely to affect the drug assay and/or the rate of Sb(V) reduction.[199,200] The high antileishmanial activity of Sb(III) against both stages of *Leishmania* and the selective activity of Sb(V) against the intracellular parasite further support the hypothesis that the reduction of Sb(V) to Sb(III) is necessary for activity.

If antimony-based drugs are not effective, the second-line drugs include pentamidine (Lomidine) and amphotericine B (Fungizone), which have been introduced in 1940 and 1959, respectively. The mode of action of pentamidine is not clear although there are some indications that it may act on the parasite's mitochondrion.[201,202] Amphotericin B is a polyene antimycotic drug, which is believed to interact with membrane sterols, such as ergosterol present in *Leishmania*'s plasma membrane, to produce an aggregate that forms a transmembrane channel resulting in the loss of intracellular solutes and ions. But severe side effects and high cost limit their use.[14] Ambisome (introduced in 1994) is a formulation of amphotericine B in liposomes. Owing to the high capacity of cells of the reticuloendothelial system for phagocytosis, the drug is specifically targeted and taken up by the host cells of the *Leishmania* parasite. This will increase the efficacy and reduce toxicity of the drug. An important drawback of this formulation is its high cost. A new first-line oral drug for the treatment of VL was introduced in 2002. It is the ether-lipid analogue miltefosine (hexadecylphosphocholine, Impavido). This lysophospholipid, originally used for the treatment of certain types of cancer, has been shown to interfere with the synthesis of phospholipids and sterols in *Leishmania*.[203,204] The advantage of this drug is that it is given orally and is very effective. Miltefosine was originally tested for VL in India. The cure rate by miltefosine is 95%. Studies in Ethiopia showed that it is also effective in Africa and clinical trials in Colombia demonstrated a high efficacy for CL as well. It is now registered in many countries and is the first orally administered breakthrough therapy for both visceral and CL. A side effect is gastrointestinal disturbance. However, miltefosine resistance in laboratory strains of *Leishmania* has already been reported. Although it shows good efficacy, it is very expensive and has a long life in the body. Preliminary data from phase IV clinical trials in India involving domiciliary treatment with miltefosine along with weekly supervision suggests a doubling of the relapse rate.[205] This provides a warning that resistance could develop quickly in the future, and therefore plans are required to prevent it. A parenteral formulation of aminosidine (paromomycin) has recently been approved for leishmaniasis treatment in India,[17–19] where it is in phase IV trials. It is an aminoglycoside antibiotic that has been used for various clinical infections. The drug is used against Gram-positive and Gram-negative bacteria[206] and parasitic infections, including giardiasis, amoebiasis,[207] and cryptosporidiosis.[208] It has been used for the treatment of both VL, in a parenteral formulation, and CL in both topical and parenteral formulations.[20,21] The mechanism of antibacterial effect of paromomycin has been well documented, with the drug acting to inhibit protein synthesis through its interaction with ribosomal RNA subunits.[206] Moreover, at least three mechanisms of aminoglycoside resistance are recognized in prokaryotes: reduced uptake or decreased cell permeability, alterations at the ribosomal binding sites, or production of aminoglycoside modifying enzymes.[209] Previous studies have suggested the involvement of mitochondrial membrane potential, ribosomes, and respiratory dysfunction in the mode of action of paromomycin in *Leishmania* species.[210–212] Several other drugs, in particular the antifungal azoles itraconazole, ketoconazole, and fluconazole, have been on limited clinical trials. These drugs are supposed to act via inhibition of cytochrome P450, essential in the synthesis of ergosterol. So far, the results were equivocal. Allopurinol, a drug in use for the treatment of gout, probably functions as an alternative substrate for *Leishmania*'s hypoxanthine-guanine phosphoribosyl transferase, an enzyme located inside glycosomes. The allopurinol riboside produced is then incorporated into RNA causing inhibition of protein synthesis in the parasite. It has been used experimentally for human leishmaniasis, with variable degrees of success, and is also on trial for the treatment of Chagas' disease. This drug is now widely used for the treatment of leishmaniasis in dogs. Despite the fact that several drugs are available for the treatment of leishmaniasis, new and better drugs are urgently required. Most available drugs are costly, require long treatment regimes and are becoming more and more ineffective.

10.2.8 OUTLINE OF PROMASTIGOTE AND AMASTIGOTE METABOLISM

Biochemical analysis on *Leishmania* promastigotes has shown that these stages can use both glucose and amino acids, such as proline, as energy sources.[213] The catabolism of these substrates appears to involve both glycolysis, compartmentalized in peroxisome-like organelles called glycosomes, and mitochondrial metabolism with an active TCA cycle and linked electron transport chain. There is evidence that sugars other than glucose could also be used. This would especially be important in the case of midgut stages where plant sugars should be abundant. The presence of a glyoxylate cycle once reported, seems to be absent which would mean that fatty acids may not serve as the sole substrates for gluconeogenesis. In addition to carbon dioxide, other end products of promastigote metabolism include succinate and smaller amounts of acetate, pyruvate, D-lactate, alanine, ammonia, or urea. Considerably more fragmentary is our knowledge of the energy metabolism of amastigotes. The main reason for this is that these intracellular stages have been less available for study. The limited number of studies carried out show that *L. mexicana* amastigotes isolated from in vivo lesions have an increased beta-oxidation of fatty acids and a reduced need for proline and glucose consumption.[214] The full complement of TCA-cycle enzymes and respiratory chain are present. Glycosomes are less abundant in amastigotes than in promastigotes,[215,216] but have a bigger arsenal of enzymes such as malate dehydrogenase and phosphoenolpyruvate carboxykinase.[217,218] Results of recent studies carried out on in vitro-cultured amastigotes largely agree with the findings with lesion-derived amastigotes, thus opening the opportunity for more extensive analysis of the energy metabolism of the infectious stages of these parasites.

From previous studies, it is well known that the *Leishmania* promastigote relies mainly on glycolysis and amino acid metabolism for energy generation. Glucose and other hexose sugars, such as fructose and mannose, are converted to carbon dioxide, alanine, succinate, and acetate which are excreted as the major end products.[219] While promastigotes feed mainly on sugars, the amastigote stage in the phagosome feeds probably mainly on fatty acids and amino acids and may have limited access to glucose and other sugars generated from glycosylated proteins and glycolipids being degraded in the phagosomal compartment. Sugar residues required by *Leishmania* for protein glycosylation, glycophospholipid-anchor formation, and polysaccharide biosynthesis thus have to be formed de novo from oxaloacetate via the gluconeogenic pathway (Figure 10-23).

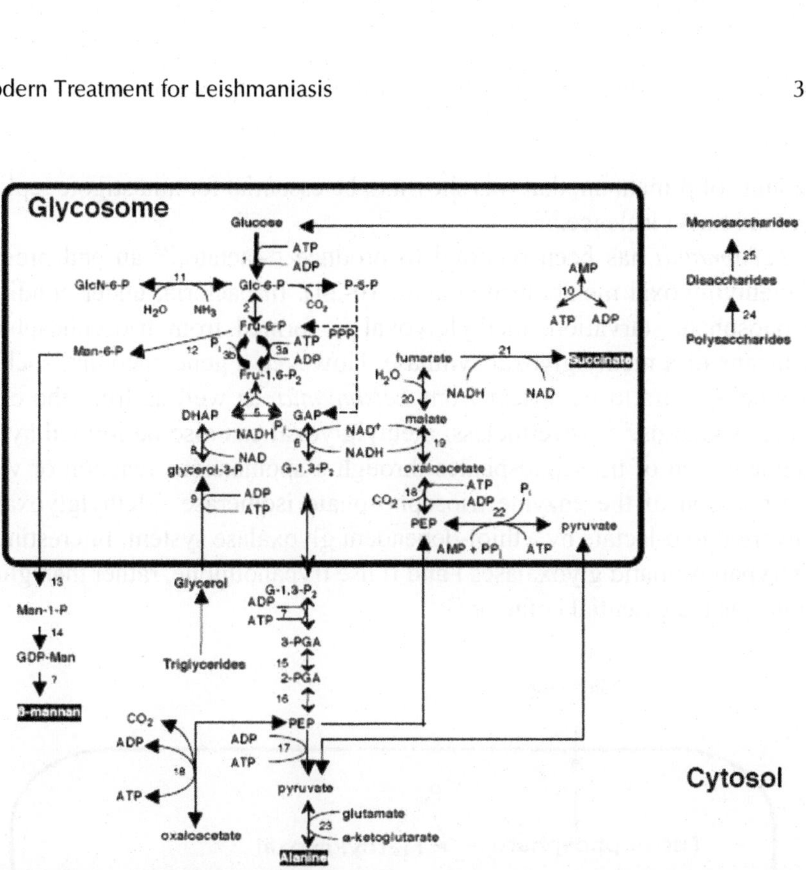

FIGURE 10-23 Gluconeogenic pathway.

The capacity of glucose uptake of amastigotes is considerably less than that of promastigotes.[220] Uptake is mediated via three glucose transporters encoded by homologous genes (LmGT1-3). Each glucose transporter isoform has a distinct biological function in the parasite.[221] These transporters are capable of importing a variety of hexoses (glucose, mannose, fructose, and galactose) into the cells.[222] Thus also the amastigote is capable of catabolizing hexose sugars via the glycolytic and pentose-phosphate pathways although at a reduced rate. Because of the apparent low pyruvate kinase activity in the intracellular stage, glucose degradation does not necessarily result in the production of pyruvate, but rather succinate via the phosphoenolpyruvate carboxykinase/malate dehydrogenase branch in the glycosome, which also comprises fumarate hydratase and NADH-dependent fumarate reductase. This enzyme that is involved in an essential pathway of glycosomal NADH reoxidation, is not found in higher eukaryotes and thus could be an interesting drug target. Indeed a number of inhibitors of fumarate reductase have been shown to exert potent antileishmanial activity.[223] Both infectious metacyclic promastigotes and amastigotes synthesize large amounts of β-mannan, that was shown to be essential for amastigote replication and thus virulence.[224]

Leishmania has been reported to produce D-lactate,[225] an end product of methylglyoxal metabolism (Figure 10-24). In bacteria, under condition of phosphate starvation, methylglyoxal is formed from triosephosphates by means of a methylglyoxal synthase. However, a gene encoding such an enzyme appears to be absent from *Leishmania*, as well as from the other trypanosomatids.[214] Nevertheless, methylglyoxal can also be formed by the fragmentation of triosephosphates through a spontaneous reaction or via a side reaction of the enzyme triosephosphate isomerase. Methylglyoxal is converted to D-lactate by a thiol-dependent glyoxalase system. Interestingly, the trypanosomatid glyoxalases I and II use trypanothione, rather than glutathione, as the essential cofactor.[226]

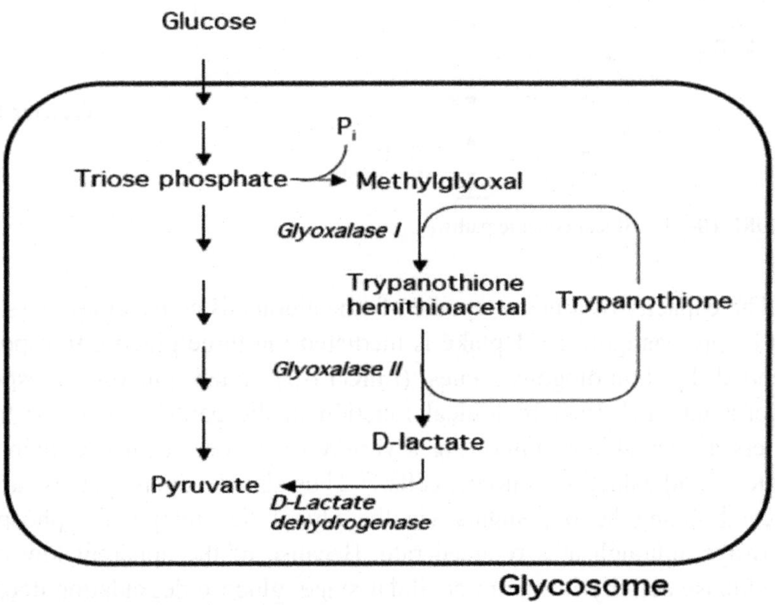

FIGURE 10-24 Methylglyoxal bypass.

The glycolytic end product pyruvate is further metabolized in the mitochondrion to acetyl-Co-A. A large part of the acetyl-CoA is converted to acetate by the TCA-cycle enzyme succinyl-CoA ligase and a unique acetate:succinate-Co-A transferase.[227,228] Together, the latter two enzymes catalyse a cycle leading to the net production of one mole of adenosine 5′-triphosphate (ATP) per mole of acetate produced.[227,229]

10.2.9 AN OVERVIEW OF *LEISHMANIA DONOVANI* AMASTIGOTE

The parasitic protozoa, *L. donovani,* cycle between phagolysosomes of mammalian macrophages and alimentary tract of sandflies.[230,231] In the vector, they grow as extracellular flagellated promastigotes, in the host they proliferate as intracellular aflagellated amastigotes. Normally, in the insect midgut, the actively dividing, immature, procyclic promastigotes differentiate into nondividing metacyclic forms, which migrate to the thoracic midgut and proboscis. These latter forms have been shown to be the infective stage of the parasite.[232] They are introduced into the host during a vector's blood meal and are subsequently phagocytosed by macrophages, where they differentiate into amastigotes.[231] Both the forms are adapted to live in hostile hydrolytic environments, and it is believed that specific molecules expressed on the parasite cell surface membrane play a key protective role.[233]

During transition through these different extra and intracellular environments, *Leishmania* are exposed to many changes in their living conditions. These changes include the elevated temperature of the mammalian host, toxic oxidants produced during phagocytosis by macrophages, acidic pH and proteases encountered in the macrophage phagolysosome, variations in the availability and type of nutrients, as well as the availability of oxygen. The mechanism that allows parasites to withstand these noxious stimuli is probably critical for their survival.[234]

The treatment of choice of human VL is the administration of a pentavalent antimony (SbV)-containing drug, amphotericin B and chalcone derivatives. Evidences showed that intracellular amastigote form of *Leishmania* was more susceptible than promastigote to pentavalent antimony containing drugs,[235] amphotericin B,[236] and chalcone derivative.[237] Differential sensitivity of these drugs with respect to amastigotes and host cells clearly indicates the presence of a distinguishable cell biological and biochemical processes in amastigote. There have been extensive studies on the biochemistry, cell biology, and immunology of promastigote forms of *Leishmania.*[238] In contrast to promastigotes, our knowledge of amastigote forms are poorly known, mainly because of difficulty in isolating large amount of viable pure intracellular forms of the parasite free of host tissue contamination.[187] Further amastigotes isolated from infected tissues represent heterogenous populations at any given time during infection, which differ presumably with regard to their age and stage of development in their cell cycle.[239] In fact, few laboratories attempted to grow axenic amastigotes with biochemical and molecular characteristics similar to those of macrophage-derived amastigotes.[26,240] Characterization of stage-specific metabolic steps, is an important step in the development of new therapeutic agents against the intracellular stage, which is responsible for the maintenance of leishmaniasis in mammals.

Studies during the past decade indicated that shifting promastigotes to an intralysosomal-like environment (e.g. 37°C and pH 5.5 at 5% CO_2 environment for visceral species) induced differentiation into amstigotes in host-free culture.[26,241,242] However, neither of these environmental conditions alone induced complete differentiation of promastigotes to amstigotes. Heat-induced growth arrest in promastigotes and acidic pH help the heat adapted promastigotes to differentiate into amastigotes.[243] Such an experimental system has already been used by several laboratories to investigate various stage-regulated functions in *L. donovani.*[235,244,245] Characterization of axenic amastigotes of the *Leishmania* species has demonstrated that they resemble the animal-derived amastigotes.[26,246] Regardless of the method used for differentiation, all axenic amastigotes express the known stage-specific proteins including A2, amastin, specific proteases, nucleotidases, phosphatases; downregulate the expression of surface coat lipophosphoglycan, and upregulate the expression of heat shock protein 70 (HSP 70)[247] peroxiredoxin[248] and malate dehydrogenase along with phosphoenolpyruvate carboxykinase.[249] Axenic amastigotes are virulent as they infect hamsters and macrophage cell lines. Moreover, differentiation in host-free culture resumes virulence of long-term attenuated promastigotes.[26]

The leishmaniae and other trypanosomatids are unique in that they contain a single mitochondrion per cell, which convolutes and ramifies in situ and occupies around 12% of the cell volume, and is associated with the kinetoplast to form a kinetoplast–mitochondrial complex.[78,250] The kinetoplast itself is a unique structure that contains nearly 10–20% of the total cell DNA. Quantitative morphometry of electron micrographs of *Leishmania* spp. demonstrated that after 3 hour of heat treatment there was no change in mitochondrial morphology, but after 6 hour of heat treatment the mitochondria lost their cristae and no longer possessed a clearly defined mitochondrial double membrane.[251,252] The ultrastructural complexity of these organelle and some basic features of its bioenergetics processes are not well understood. Studies on these aspects have been greatly hampered by difficulties in isolation of intact mitochondria from trypanosomatids.[253,254] Isolation of this organelle requires breakage of cells under harsh conditions, which are known to have adverse effects on mitochondrial membranes. In fact, damage is difficult to avoid because of the large size and ramifications of the single mitochondrion and the presence of microtubule arrays adhering to the inner side of the cell membranes of the trypanosomatids.[255] As a consequence, greater force is required to break the cells than that necessary to disrupt mitochondrial membrane.[255,256] To overcome these difficulties, digitonized cells have been useful as an experimental model.[254] Alternatively, several gentle cell rupture procedures and isolation method have yielded well-sealed phosphorylating vesicles resulting from rearrangement of mitochondrial fragments.[257] In spite of these efforts, information on the respiratory chain in *Leishmania* is incomplete and somewhat controversial. Martin and Mukkada[256] reported the evidence for the presence of complexes I, II, III, and IV in the respiratory chain of *L. tropica* promastigote. In contrast, Santhamma and Bhaduri claimed[258] that complex I is absent from the respiratory chain of *L. donovani* promastigote. No data is available on electron transport chain, energy coupling, and oxidative phosphorylation in amastigote form of *Leishmania.*

Recent reports have indicated that the plasma membrane of *L. donovani* promastigote can carry out plasma membrane electron transport.[23,24] In contrast to the mitochondrial electron transport in *Leishmania,*[256,259] studies in this laboratory have indicated that redox enzymes of the plasma membrane electron transport system orderly transfer electron from one redox carrier to the next with the molecular oxygen as the final electron acceptor. The redox carriers mediate the transfer of electrons from metabolically generated reductant to nonpermeable electron acceptors and oxygen. The redox chain appears to be branched at several points and it was suggested that this redox chain incorporate iron–sulphur centre, *b*-cytochromes, cyanide insensitive redox site, Na^+ and K^+ channel, capsaicin inhibited energy coupling site, and trifluoperazine inhibited energy-linked P-type ATPase. The results also indicated that chlorbiumquinone and ubiquinone[9] mediated the plasma membrane electron transport between cytosolic reductant and oxygen as well as nonpermeable electron acceptors. The finding that heat transformed, acidic pH stabilized *L. donovani* cell downregulate plasma membrane and mitochondrial electron transport as well as oxygen uptake prompted us to investigate the nature of energy metabolism in *L. donovani* amastigote. Although, environmental factors that trigger *Leishmania* differentiation in vitro were recognized many years ago, relatively little is known about the molecular processes that mediated the culture remodelling. It is likely that a series of changes in gene expression are instrumental in the morphological and metabolic changes associated with differentiation to the individual developmental forms.

Fumarate reductase and succinate dehydrogenase occupy central positions in cellular energy metabolism; fumarate reductase serves as the terminal acceptor for a major anaerobic respiratory pathway, while succinate dehydrogenase participates in both the Krebs cycle and as complex II of the aerobic respiratory chain. Although fumarate reductase and succinate dehydrogenase catalyze the same reaction (but in different physiological directions) and are not predicted to have similar structures, organisms with both types of respiratory chains use distinct proteins for each purpose for reasons not understood. In terms of the overall process of respiration, exciting progress has been made in structurally characterizing membrane-associated members of respiratory pathway. Fumarate reductase now joins structures available for cytochrome bc_1 complex III, cytochrome *c* oxidase complex IV, and the F_1 component of the ATP synthase complex V.[260] Given the lack of information on mitochondrial metabolism in *L. donovani* amastigotes and the apparent relevance of mitochondrial and plasma membrane biochemistry for its differentiation and for the chemotherapy of leishmaniasis, it is extremely important to develop strategies to study the bioenergetics of this cell.

10.3 REVIEW ON TRANSPLASMA MEMBRANE ELECTRON TRANSPORT SYSTEM

10.3.1 INTRODUCTION

Transmembrane electron transport is clearly recognized as the components and functional element in bacteria. Other prokaryotes (e.g., blue green algae) have plasma membrane electron transport, although not as well defined. For bacteria the importance is clear, because the plasma membrane has the entire energy coupling machinery for oxidative ATP synthesis. The situation is not clear in prokaryotic algae, since they have thylakoid membranes, which have ATP-synthesizing machinery,[261] In most eukaryotic cells, the mitochondria handles the major high efficiency ATP synthesis, so there is a need for an ATP-synthesizing system associated with plasma membrane electron transport. If ATP can supply energy for all plasma membrane transport function and if transport is the only energy requiring function of plasma membranes, then energy-coupled redox system will be redundant in the outer membrane. There have been proposals for direct coupling of electron transport to ion or nutrient transport activity, but these have not developed clearly.[262] The question is : Do eukaryotic plasma membranes have electron transport systems coupled to proton transport or ion movement, and if not, is the electron transport related to the energy coupling process or does it serve another function? Clearly, the presence of masses of thiol groups on receptors requires electron transfer across the membrane to maintain the thiol state.[263]

Other types of redox function are found in plasma membranes for special roles. The peroxide generating reduced nicotinamide adenine dinucleotide phosphate (NADPH) oxidase in neutrophils used for killing bacteria,[264] the xanthine oxidase that may have similar functions in addition to purine residue,[265] and the cytochrome b_5-dependent fatty acyl Co-A desaturase[266] are the examples. Proton transfer across the plasma membrane by the activation of a channel has been associated with the neutrophil transmembrane NADPH oxidase.[267] This enzyme may serve as a model for other eukaryotic plasma membrane redox systems associated with proton release. The NADH–cytochrome b_5 reductase, fatty acid desaturase, or methemoglobin reductase are exclusively on the cytoplasmic side of the plasma membrane, so these enzymes have not been associated with any proton transport.[268]

10.3.2 THE EVIDENCE FOR TRANSPLASMA MEMBRANE ELECTRON TRANSPORT

Evidence for transplasma membrane electron transport is found in all animal cells examined, ranging from protozoa to man.[269–272] It is detected by the reduction of impermeable dyes or complex ions by intact cells and by histochemistry.[273,274] Electron transport reactions based on oxidation of NADPH by oxygen or the same impermeable compounds can be detected in isolated plasma membranes in nonvesicular form.[275] If the isolated membranes form sealed vesicles, then either the impermeable reductant or impermeable oxidant will not be available at its reaction site or the oxidoreductions observed will represent internal and external dehydrogenases, which may or may not be connected to the transmembrane enzyme. Insertion of substrate into vesicles followed by resealing has been successful with electroporation of NADH into right side out plant plasma membrane vesicles.[276] The NADH in these vesicles can then be oxidized by external ferricyanide. Ascorbate has been inserted successfully by other methods.[277,278]

Oxygen is permeable to membranes, so a transmembrane NADH oxidase can be measured if the plasma membrane vesicles are inside out with the NADH dehydrogenase on the exposed face. On the other hand, impermeable hormones or other ligands for external surface site will not be able to influence the oxidase reaction in the inside-out sealed vesicles. Fortunately, isolated liver plasma membranes do not vesiculate easily because of desmosomes.[279]

If liver plasma membranes are not homogenized too vigorously, they show NADH dehydrogenase activity which is consistent with the transmembrane electron transport.[275] Erythrocyte membranes must be prepared in the open ghost form to show transmembrane electron transport.[280]

Plasma membranes also have sites for NADH oxidation on their external surface.[281] NADH oxidase or ferrocyanide reductase observed with right side out vesicles will measure this outer surface activity, so it cannot represent the transmembrane activity which is seen with whole cells. It could, however, represent an external feed to a part of the transmembrane electron transport chain analogous to the external NADH site on mitochondrial cristae in plants.[282]

Since, substrate-loaded vesicles of proper orientation have not been obtained with animal plasma membranes, studies on proton transport accompanying the transmembrane electron transport have been restricted to intact cells.

With intact cells, the shift in the redox state of NADH/NAD$^+$ when an external oxidant is reduced is consistent with the idea of a transmembrane electron transport.[283] It does not necessarily mean that NADH is the primary substrate since the NADH may reduce the primary substrate. For example, NADH may reduce semidehydroascorbate to ascorbate, and ascorbate may be the primary electron donor to the transmembrane electron transport.[284]

10.3.3 THE PROPERTIES OF ANIMAL CELL TRANSMEMBRANE ELECTRON TRANSPORT

With intact cells or perfused tissue, the rate of transplasma membrane electron transport measured by ferricyanide reduction can be quite rapid.[285,286] For example, rat liver cells have ferricyanide reduction rate as high as 260 nmol per min per g fresh weight of cells. If 4% of the liver cell protein is in the plasma membrane, then the rate of electron transport through the membrane would approach 100 nmol per min per mg membrane proteins. Rates of NADH–ferricyanide reductase up to 1,000 nmol per minute for mg protein have been reported for erythrocyte membranes, and 780 nmol per min per mg for rat liver plasma membranes, but part of this activity will come from internal or external enzymes. Ofcourse, ferricyanide is not a natural electron acceptor, so these rates only give maximum electron transport capacities of the transplasma membrane enzyme.

Isolated rat liver plasma membranes have a unique NADH oxidase which is not sensitive to cyanide and is stimulated by azide, transferrin, and hormones.[287–290] In isolated membranes the activity is up to 20 nmol per min per mg protein, unless it is stimulated by diferric transferrin or hormones. The measurement of the plasma membrane oxidase in cells is difficult because of the multifarious nature of cellular oxygen uptake. Since it is a cyanide-insensitive enzyme that may transfer electrons to impermeable external electron acceptors, transmembrane oxidase can be identified by measuring the effect of ferricyanide on cyanide-resistant oxygen uptake. The inhibition is postulated on the basis of ferricyanide-accepting electrons before the site where oxygen accepts electrons. In an experiment with well–oxygenated liver cells, it was found that 20% of respiration was insensitive to 1 mM KCN and one-half of that oxygen uptake was inhibited by 0.2 mM ferricyanide. In the absence of cyanide, 0.1 mM ferricyanide inhibits 10% of oxygen uptake by rat liver cells. The overall indication is that with well-aerated liver cells the transplasma membrane oxidase activity can be 10% of the total respiration.[291] Studies on the effect of diferric transferrin and growth factors on cyanide-resistant, ferricyanide-inhibited respiration of cells have not been done.

There are many reports in the literature about the complete inhibition of oxygen uptake by cyanide which actually should be unexpected, since internal endosomal cyanide-resistant oxidase (P_{450}) are known in addition to the plasma membrane enzyme. If the plasma membrane enzyme is involved in specialized functions or growth control, then it may be undetectable, unless diferric transferrin and growth factors are present. Transmembrane NADH–ferricyanide reductase activity is not necessarily connected to the oxidase activity, since open erythrocyte ghosts have no NADH oxidase activity, despite the high level of NADH–ferricyanide reductase.[288,289] Mammalian erythrocytes also have no transferrin receptors and diferric transferrin does not activate NADH oxidase in these membranes.[292] However, if transferrin receptors are inserted into the erythrocyte membranes by *Falciparum* infection, then cells show a transmembrane diferric transferrin reductase activity.[293] Whether this is coordinated to introduction of transmembrane oxidase and proton release remains to be seen.

The stimulation of the transmembrane oxidase by diferric transferrin brings up the question of the transferrin's acts. Does it act as a terminal oxidase by catalyzing the reoxidation of ferrous iron with oxygen as soon as the iron is reduced by the transmembrane electron transport[294] or does the binding of the diferric transferrin to the transferrin receptor activate the oxidase in the membrane by a conformational changes in the redox system? In support of the terminal oxidase hypothesis, we have demonstrated that the transmembrane electron transport system can act as ferric transferrin reductase.[295,296] Reduction of iron in diferric transferrin by cells can be demonstrated by direct spectrophotometric measurement of decrease in the absorbance of diferric transferrin at 465 nm under aerobic conditions (unpublished), or by formation of ferrous bathophenanthroline disulfonate (BPS) is the media, when cells are incubated with diferric transferrin. BPS is an impermeable ferrous chelator. Reduction of the transferrin iron at the membrane can also be measured with formation of ferrous dipyridyl trapped in the membrane.[297] The requirement for the transferrin receptor in these reactions with HeLa cells is indicated by inhibition with B3/25 and GB16 monoclonal antibodies to the transferrin receptor.[296]

NADH diferric transferrin reductase activity can also be demonstrated using isolated liver membrane.[275] Three types of assay can be used to measure the activity. (1) Direct measurement of a decrease of the diferric transferrin at 465 nm absorbance in the presence of NADH and membranes under anaerobic conditions. The absence of oxygen is essential in this assay because the ferrous iron formed is immediately reoxidized by oxygen to reform diferric transferrin. (2) Oxidation of NADH by membranes is greatly increased when diferric transferrin is added.[275,290] This reaction can be interpreted as a stimulation of an NADH–oxygen: oxidoreductase by diferric transferrin binding to the membrane. If the assay is for an NADH transferrin reductase, then it should work under anaerobic conditions, which has not been tested. The requirement for the transferrin receptor in this reaction is likely, since the reaction does not occur in erythrocyte membrane.[293] (3) Ferrous BPS is formed when diferric transferrin is added to liver plasma membranes with NADH. This type of assay has been criticized by Thorstensen and Aisen[290] on the basis that the BPS effectively raises the redox potential of the ferric transferrin to the point that it can be reduced by the transplasma membrane electron transport. Since diferric transferrin in simple solution at pH 7.0 has a redox potential at –500 mV and NADH has a potential at –320 mV, it is quite clear that they are correct that NADH cannot reduce diferric transferrin in simple solution. However, the presence of plasma membrane transferrin receptor and a complex transmembrane electron transport system introduces factors which do not allow a simple theoretical analysis of the possibility for reduction of external differic transferrin by cytosolic NADH. Both the surface of cells and isolated membranes has negative ζ potential, which can modify surface pH. Transferrin iron is released at pH below 7.0 and reduced by ascorbate (+56 mV). The redox potential of diferric transferrin bound to the transferrin receptor is unknown and it may be much higher than the free transferrin if the conformation of the transferrin is changed by binding. If a transferrin site is not important, then reduction of ferric desferrioximine would also be expected (–430 mV) in the presence of BPS. This reduction is not seen with HeLA cells.[291] Finally, the reduction of NAD^+ by succinate in mitochondria would be impossible, except for the fact that the cristae membrane can carryout reversed electron transport energized by the proton gradient created by the electron transport system. The plasma membrane may have an energy-linked reverse electron transport.

Actually, on thermodynamic grounds diferric transferrin reduction at the plasma membrane is even less likely than Thorstensen and Aisen[290] proposed because the redox potential of the electron carrier on the outer surface of the plasma membrane has been titrated at –160 mV,[298] which means that reduction of diferric transferrin at that site is less energetically favored than with NADH directly. The study of reduction of diferric transferrin by cells or membranes in the presence of BPS obviously will not answer the question whether diferric transferrin can be a natural acceptor for the plasma membrane electron transport. The fact that ferrons BPS formation occurs even in Thorstensen and Aisen experiments, is evidence for a transmembrane electron transport system, at least to high redox potential acceptors.

Differic transferrin in the presence of BPS can act as a high redox potential acceptor for the transmembrane electron transport. It should be noted that Thorstensen and Aisen[290] do confirm diferric transferrin stimulation of the plasma membrane NADH oxidase. In their studies, they do not consider the direct measurement of diferric transferrin reduction by decline in absorbance at 465 nm under anaerobic condition.[275] The erythrocyte sedimentation rate evidence that they present as direct assay for reduction is by no means conclusive, since it is done in the presence of 1 mM BPS, which at this concentration acts as an inhibitor of the transmembrane.[289] A more decisive answer could have been obtained if the experiment has been done under anaerobic conditions in the absence of BPS so that the loss of the transferrin iron signal could have been observed directly.

If not a redox carrier, then the diferric transferrin can act by binding to the transferrin receptor to activate the oxidase. The binding site at which diferric transferrin stimulates the NADH oxidase in the isolated plasma membrane appears to have much lower affinity for diferric transferrin than does the high-affinity binding site involved in iron uptake by endocytosis. Iron uptake is saturated at 1 μM diferric transferrin, whereas the stimulation of NADH oxidase by diferric transferrin is saturated at 40 μM.[299] This low-affinity site is also involved in diferric transferrin reduction by cells and is probably the site involved in the "nonsaturable" iron uptake by liver.[300] In other words, NADH oxidase stimulation and diferric transferrin reduction require 40 μM diferric transferrin to each saturation, which suggests that each of these activities occur at the same site on the membrane. The inhibition of diferric transferrin reduction by intact HeLA cells with B3/25 and GB16 monoclonal antibodies but not by GB18 or 42/6 further indicates binding and reduction at a site different from the high-affinity binding site. GB18 and 42/6 bind an epitope at the high-affinity site on the transferrin receptor but B3/25 and GB16 bind elsewhere on the receptor. Cooperative effects of B3/25 and 42/6 on cell proliferation have been described.[301]

In conclusion, the relationship between the plasma membrane NADH oxidase and diferric transferrin appears to involve a direct stimulation of the NADH oxidase when transferrin binds to a low-affinity site on the transferrin receptor, as well as slow reduction of iron in the diferric transferrin. The slow reduction at the low-affinity site may add to the total oxidase activity by recycling the ferric-ferrous iron by oxidation on the transferrin after the ferric iron is reduced by transmembrane electron transport.

10.3.4 COMPONENTS OF THE TRANSPLASMA MEMBRANE ELECTRON TRANSPORT SYSTEM

Plasma membranes have been reported to contain flavin, cytochromes of the *b* type, nonheme iron, coenzyme Q, α–tocopherol, thiol groups, and possibly copper.[277,289,302–304] Coenzyme Q is the only component for which there is good evidence for participation in the transmembrane electron transport.

10.3.5 EVIDENCE FOR COENZYME Q FUNCTION

Reductions of ferricyanide and diferric transferrin are inhibited by analogs of coenzyme Q and the inhibition is reversed by addition of coenzyne Q.[305,306] Piericidin A is the most effective inhibitor among the coenzyme Q analogs. 2, 3-dimethoxy-5-chloro-6-naphthyl-mercaptobenzoquinone and 2-methoxy-3-ethoxy-5-methyl-6-hexadecyl mercaptobenzoquinone are also good inhibitors of diferric transferrin reduction by cells.[305] The NADH–ferricyanide reductase and NADH oxidase activity of rat liver plasma membranes are inhibited by the same concentrations of the above inhibitors and addition of coenzyme Q_{10} partially restores the activity.

Extraction of coenzyme Q from lyophilized plasma membranes with heptane partially inhibits NADH-ferricyanide reductase activity. Activity is restored by addition of coenzyme Q in heptane membranes, followed by evaporation of the heptane by the Norling et al. procedure.[307] Loss of activity is proportional to the amount of coenzyme Q removed.[308]

A precedent for coenzyme Q function is transmembrane electron transport is seen in mitochondria.[309,310] A similar function as electron and proton carrier in the lipid phase may be possible in plasma membranes. It should be emphasised that the coenzyme Q appears to function before the site of external ferricyanide reduction by plasma membrane, whereas in mitochondria it functions after the site of ferricyanide reduction by NADH dehydrogenase For example, piericidin A inhibits ferricyanide reduction in the plasma membrane, whereas it does not inhibit ferricyanide reduction by mitochondrial cristae.[311] Antimycin A and rotenone do not inhibit electron transport in plasma membranes.[312,313] Since they act as coenzyme Q binding site in mitochondria, the coenzyme Q binding site in the plasma membrane must differ from those in mitochondria.[314]

10.3.6 INHIBITORS OF TRANSPLASMA MEMBRANE ELECTRON TRANSPORT

Inhibitors at specific sites in electron transport systems are useful in defining the sequence of the system or to see if the system contributes to a cellular function. The transmembrane electron transport from cells or the NADH dyhydrogenase activity of plasma membranes has been found to respond to some unique inhibitors.

For ferricyanide or diferric transferrin reduction by cells atebrin and chloroquinine are effective at high concentrations,[238,312,315,316] whereas adriamycin, cis-dichlorodiamine platinum II, actinomycin D, and bleomycin inhibit at low concentrations.[317] These same compounds are good inhibitors of NADH-ferricyanide reductase or NADH diferric transferrin with isolated plasma membranes. Atebrin and chloroquinine are effective against malaria and the other compounds are used as antitumor agents, so the inhibitions may point to a vital role of the redox system in cancer and infections by protozoa.

The important antitumor drugs that are strongly inhibitors of transplasma membrane electron transport include adriamycin and related anthracyclines-bleomycin, cis-diaminodichloro platinum II (cisplatin), actinomycin D, anthramycin, and retinoic acid.[306,317] Electron transport by transformed cells or tumor cells is more sensitive to these compounds than with normal cells and inhibition occurs at a concentration that inhibits cell growth.[318] Except for retinoic acid,[319] proton release associated with the redox activity is also inhibited at the same concentration starting at 10^{-7} M.[317] Adriamycin coupled to transferrin with glutaraldehyde is more effective than adriamycin alone in inhibition of transmembrane electron transport and redox-induced proton release. Good inhibition is seen with HeLa cells at 10^{-8} M adriamycin equivalent. Since the effect is seen in 3 minutes, the effectiveness of the conjugate suggests that the adriamycin acts at the plasma membrane and redox enzyme is close to the transferrin receptor.[320–322] The time is too short for the conjugate to release adriamycin to the nucleus.

10.3.7 PROTON RELEASE ASSOCIATED WITH TRANSPLASMA MEMBRANE ELECTRON TRANSPORT ANIMAL CELLS

Transplasma membrane electron transport is associated with proton release from cells, as measured by a change in the external pH.[298,323,324] Reduction of both ferricyanide and diferric transferrin is accompanied by proton release. The ratio of proton release to electron transfer is much lower for ferricyanide than for diferric transferring.[291] Because, ferricyanide and apotransferrin do not stimulate proton release, an electron acceptor is necessary. Inhibitors of transplasma membrane electron transport, such as adriamycin,[292] bleomycin,[325] cis-platin and piericidin A, as well as monoclonal antibodies to the transferrrin receptor,[326] inhibit the proton release at the same concentrations that inhibit electron transport; the redox system appears responsible for activation or driving the proton movement.

There are several known mechanisms by which proton transfer across the membrane could be coupled to the transplasma membrane electron transport. It could be based on (1) anisotropic arrangement protonated and protonated electron carriers as proposed by Mitchell[264] for mitochondria or (2) the electron transport protein could act as a redox-controlled proton channel as proposed by Wikstrom,[327] Wikstrom and Krab,[328] and Wikstrom et al.[329, 292] for cytochrome oxidase, or (3) the Q cycles with oxidation and reduction of coenzyme Q on opposite sides of the membrane might apply to plasma membrane, since coenzyme Q is present in the membrane.[304]

As an alternative, the redox-generated proton release could be based on activation of a channel or pump, such as the Na^+/H^+ antiport or proton-pumping ATPase.

The analysis of how redox-induced proton release occurs in the plasma membrane is far from complete. In early studies with ferricyanide as an electron acceptor, the stoichiometry of protons released during ferricyanide reduction was around two or three, which could be consistent with proton transfer through redox carriers during their oxidation–reduction cycle.[324] Later studies found 5 to 15 protons released per ferricyanide reduced, which would be more appropriate for activation of a channel.[291] Evidence that the Na^+/H^+ antiport could be the channel activated by ferricyanide was developed by Garcia-Canero et al.[330] when they showed that ferricyanide reduction stimulated Na^+ uptake by liver cells. They also showed Na^+ dependence and amiloride inhibition of the ferricyanide reduction. With HeLa cells the ferricyanide-induced electron transport was inhibited by amiloride and increased in Na^+ containing media.[331] Fuhrmann et al.[332] have also reported Na^+ influx into erythrocytes in presence of 5 mM ferricyanide.

The lack of inhibition of proton release by 4,4'-diisothiocyanatostilbene-2,2'-disulfonic acid (DIDS) and 4-acetamido-4'-isothiocyanato-2-2'stilbenedisulfonic acid disodium salt hydrate (SETS) treatment of cells indicates that the HC O_3^- / Cl^- anion exchanger is not the basis for ferricyanide-induced proton transfer.[326]

Diferric transferrin reduction is accompanied by a much greater proton release than with ferricyanide.[291] These are transformed which will tend to have high levels of transferrin receptor and may optimize the transferrin-related redox function. The stoichiometry of proton release to ferrous BPS formation as a measure of diferric transferrin reduction is often over 100. The H^+/e^- ratio is consistent with the activation of a H^+ channel rather than a carrier-dependent H^+ transfer.

These observations are subject to two major caveats. (1) The transferrin-stimulated NADH oxidase has not been measured as part of the diferric transferrin-stimulated electron transport, so the ferrous BPS formation may represent only a part of the electron transfer, which is inducing H^+ release. (2) Some preparations of diferric transferrin have adventitious loosely bound iron, which greatly stimulates the rate of ferrous BPS formation by cells. An indication of the effect of extra iron is seen where ferrous BPS formation is 140 nmol^{-1} gww^{-1} for HeLa cells with 10 μM diferric transferrin. The addition of 10 μM apotransferrin to convert all iron to the tightly bound form decreases the reduction rate to 80 nmol min^{-1} gww^{-1}. A further decrease may be achieved by incubating with ferric transferrin with apotransferrin before starting the reaction.[299,333]

An extensive series of studies on redox-induced proton release by rat pineal cells in the transformed and untransformed phenotype based on temperature-sensitive SV40[334] is consistent with dependence of a major part of the proton release on the Na^+/H^+ antiport activation with a small part possibly dependent on some other pathway.[326]

10.3.8 INHIBITION OF PROTON RELEASE

Good evidence for the requirement for electron transport to activate the antiport is seen in the specific inhibition of oxidant-induced proton release by agents that inhibit the transplasma membrane electron transport. These agents include adriamycin, cisplatin, bleomycin, and actinomycin[307,317] as well as inhibitory coenzyme Q analogs, piericidin A, and 2-methoxy-3-ethoxy-6-hexadecyl mercapto-1,4-benzoquinone. The effects of the coenzyme Q analogs are reversed by added coenzyme Q 300.

Retinoic acid is a special case. It inhibits transmembrane electron transport without the inhibition of proton release.[335] Retinoic acid also stimulates proton release in the absence of oxidants or other agonists to activate the antiport by direct acidification of the allosteric site.[336] The continued proton release with retinoic acid, even with the inhibition of transmembrane electron transport, is in contrast to the inhibition of both functions by adriamycin and other antitumor drugs. This difference may relate to the ability of retinoic acid to induce differentiation of transformed cells.[337]

The lack of retinoic acid inhibition of electron transport in SV40 transformed cells is further evidence that the portion of large T-antigen inserted into the plasma membrane modifies the electron transport system.[319]

10.3.9 MECHANISM OF ELECTRON TRANSPORT-DRIVEN ANTIPORT

The mechanism for the activation of Na^+/H^+ antiport by the transmembrane electron transport is not known. There are logical consequences of electron transport or some experimental observations that suggest mechanisms for the transfer of a stimulus from the redox system to the antiport based on the current ideas concerning the site of activation on the antiport itself. These mechanisms could be (1) activation of a protein kinase to phosphorylate the antiport, (2) localized protein increases as a result of oxidation of a protonated electron transport carrier (e.g., coenzyme Q) with subsequent direction of the proton to the allosteric activation site on the antiport through a closed channel, (3) changes in pH set point of the antiport by conformational changes in a closely associated redox protein during oxidation–reduction,[338] or (4) reduction of disulfide bonds that controls antiport activity.[332,339]

The evidence that the antiport is regulated by phosphorylation on a serine[340] opens up a new approach to control the antiport through the plasma membrane redox system. Tyrosine kinase can activate serine/threonine kinase [protein kinase C (PKC) or mitogen-activated protein]. Isolated tyrosine kinase is activated by low levels of H_2O_2.[341] Low et al.[248] have shown that band 3 in erythrocytes (note that the erythrocyte antiport at 110 KDa should be included in band 3 protein) is phosphorylated when H_2O_2 is added to the cells and that external ferricyanide can also cause phosphrylation of band 3. H_2O_2 has long been known to increase phosphorylation of other membrane proteins, for example, the insulin receptor to mimic the action of insulin.[342] Quinones, such as coenzyme Q, can generate H_2O_2 in membranes by autooxidation of semiquinones formed during the electron transport.[305,308] Since there is now evidence that coenzyme Q functions in the plasma membrane electron transport,[305,308] and H_2O_2 generation occurs during NADH oxidation with isolated liver plasma membrane,[343] one must consider if generation of a low level of H_2O_2 is the basis for antiport activation by the plasma membrane redox system.[285]

The redox state of quinone in a membrane has been shown to control protein kinase activity. The redox state of plastoquinone in chloroplasts controls phosphorylation of the high-harvesting complex protein.[344, 345]

Addition to permeant acids to cells also activates the antiport.[338] The protons are considered to act at an allosteric activator site on the cytosolic domain of the antiport, which may be associated with phosphorylated site. Oxidation of NADH on the cytosolic side produces protons, which is close to the allosteric activator site. Oxidation of cellular NADH by external ferricyanide and diferric transferrin has been shown.[283] If the protons from the redox activity are released into a closed channel, which communicates with the activator site, then activation by redox action can occur without decreasing the bulk cytosolic pH. A channel of this type, controlled by calcium has been described in chloroplasts.[308]

The possible relation between the transmembrane electron transport system, the transferrin receptor, and the Na^+/H^+ antiport is illustrated in Figure 10-25. Redox activation of a proton channel has also been described during the respiratory burst of erythrocytes, where rapid H_2O_2 formation occurs.[267] A role of PKC in this process has also been indicated.[346]

Figure 10-25 shows the proposed relation between the transplasma membrane electron transport system, the transferrin receptor, and the Na^+/H^+ antiport for mammalian cells. Electron transport across the membrane is stimulated by ferric transferrin associated with the transferrin receptor. As a consequence of the electron transport activity, the antiport associated either by proton release from protonated electron carriers or by generation of peroxide from superoxide to activate protein kinase to phosphorylate the antiport. Oxidation of a coenzyme Q semiquinone is the most likely source of superoxide. External NADH may also be oxidized by the redox enzyme. "X" may be flavoprotein.

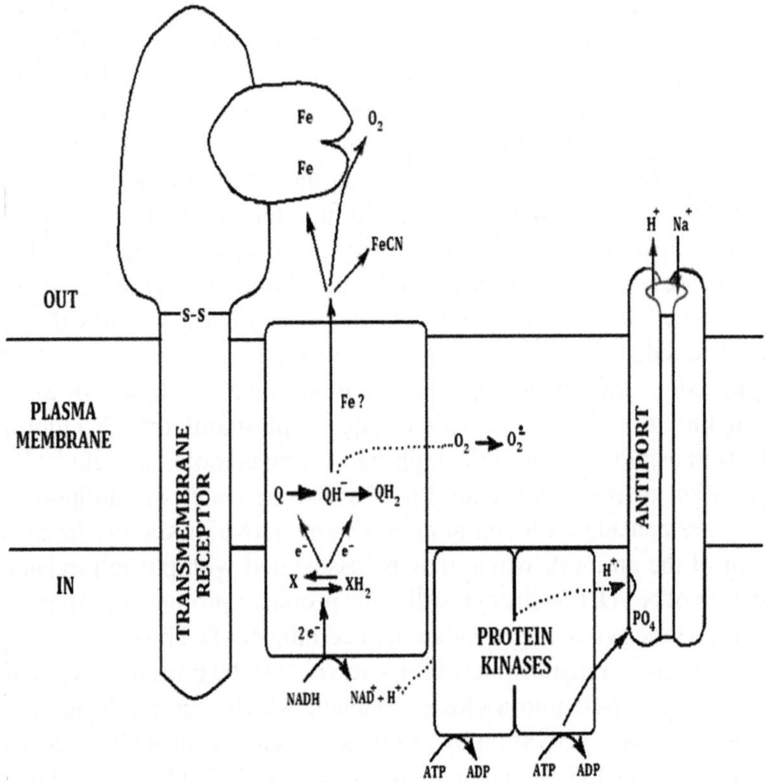

FIGURE 10-25 Transplasma membrane electron transport systems.

10.4 ELECTRON TRANSPORT CHAIN

An electron transport chain couples a chemical reaction between an electron donor (such as NADH) and an electron acceptor (such as O_2) to the transfer of H^+ ions across a membrane, through a set of mediating biochemical reactions. These H^+ ions are used to produce ATP, the main energy intermediate in living organisms, as they move back across the membrane. Electron transport chains are used for extracting energy from sunlight (photosynthesis) and from redox reactions such as the burning of sugars (respiration).

10.4.1 INTRODUCTION

The cells of almost all eukaryotes (animals, plants, fungi, algae, protozoa—in other words, the living things except bacteria, archaea, and a few protists) contain intracellular organelles called mitochondria, which produce ATP. Energy sources such as glucose are initially metabolized in the cytoplasm. The products are imported into mitochondria. Mitochondria continues the process of catabolism using metabolic pathways including the Krebs cycle, fatty acid oxidation, and amino acid oxidation. The end result of these pathways is the production of two kinds of energy-rich electron donors, NADH and succinate. Electrons from these donors are passed through an electron transport chain to oxygen, which is reduced to water. This is a multi-step redox process that occurs on the mitochondrial inner membrane. The enzymes that catalyze these reactions have the remarkable ability to simultaneously create a proton gradient across the membrane, producing a thermodynamically unlikely high-energy state with the potential to do work (Figure 10-26).

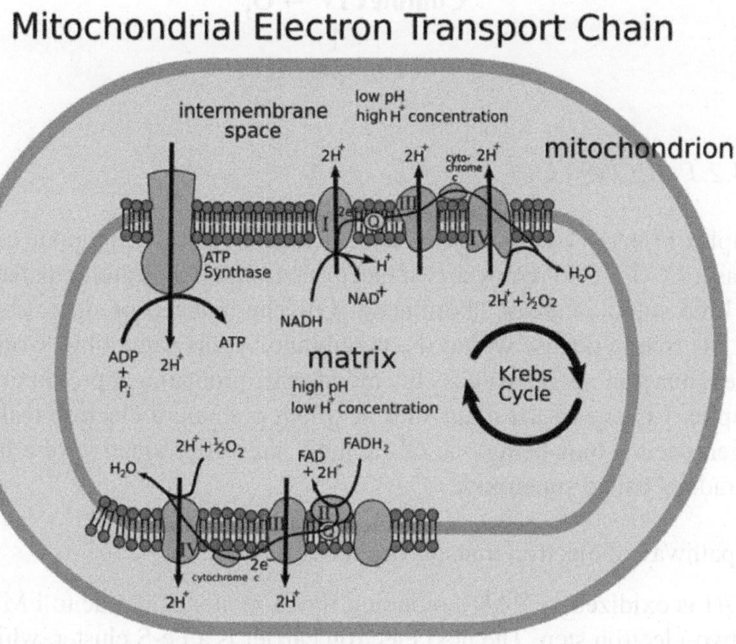

FIGURE 10-26 The electron transport chain in the mitochondrion is the site of oxidative phosphorylation in eukaryotes. the NADH and succinate generated in the citric acid cycle are oxidized, providing energy to power ATP synthase.

Although electron transport occurs with great efficiency, a small percentage of electrons are prematurely leaked to oxygen, resulting in the formation of the toxic free–radical superoxide. The similarity between intracellular mitochondria and free-living bacteria is striking. The known structural, functional, and DNA similarities between mitochondria and bacteria provide strong evidence that mitochondria evolved from intracellular prokaryotic symbionts that took up residence in primitive eukaryotic cells.

10.4.2 MITOCHONDRIAL REDOX CARRIERS

Four membrane-bound complexes have been identified in mitochondria.[347] Each is an extremely complex transmembrane structure that is embedded in the inner membrane. Three of them are proton pumps. The structures are electrically connected by lipid-soluble and water-soluble electron carriers. The overall electron transport chain is as follows:

NADH → Complex I → Q → Complex III → Cytochrome *c* →
Complex IV → O_2
↑
Complex II

10.4.2.1 COMPLEX I

Complex I (NADH dehydrogenase, also called NADH: ubiquinone oxidoreductase; EC 1.6.5.3) removes two electrons from NADH and transfers them to a lipid-soluble carrier, ubiquinone (Q). The reduced product, ubiquinol (QH_2) is free to diffuse within the membrane. At the same time, Complex I moves four protons (H^+) across the membrane, producing a proton gradient. Complex I is one of the main sites at which premature electron leakage to oxygen occurs, thus being one of the main sites of production of a harmful free radical called superoxide.

The pathway of electron transfer occurs as follows:

NADH is oxidized to NAD^+, reducing flavin mononucleotide to $FMNH_2$ in one two-electron step. The next electron carrier is a Fe-S cluster, which can only accept one electron at a time to reduce the ferric ion into a ferrous ion. In a convenient manner, $FMNH_2$ can be oxidized in only two one-electron steps, through a semiquinone intermediate. The electron thus travels from the

$FMNH_2$ to the Fe-S cluster, then from the Fe-S cluster to the oxidized Q to give the free-radical (semiquinone) form of Q. This happens again to reduce the semiquinone form to the ubiquinol form, QH_2. During this process, four protons are translocated across the inner mitochondrial membrane, from the matrix to the intermembrane space. This creates a proton gradient that will be later used to generate ATP through oxidative phosphorylation.

10.4.2.2 COMPLEX II

Complex II (succinate dehydrogenase; EC 1.3.5.1) is not a proton pump. It serves to funnel additional electrons into the quinone pool (Q) by removing electrons from succinate and transferring them (via FAD) to Q. Complex II consists of four protein subunits: SDHA, SDHB, SDHC, and SDHD. Other electron donors (e.g., fatty acids and glycerol-3-phosphate) also funnel electrons into Q (via FAD), again without producing a proton gradient.

10.4.2.3 COMPLEX III

Complex III (cytochrome *bc*$_1$ complex; EC 1.10.2.2) removes two electrons from QH_2 at the Q_o site in a stepwise fashion and sequentially transfers them to two molecules of cytochrome *c*, a water-soluble electron carrier located within the intermembrane space. The two other electrons are sequentially passed across the protein to the Q_i site where quinone is reduced to quinol. A proton gradient is formed because it takes 2 quinol ($4H+4e^-$) oxidations at the Q_o site to form one quinol ($2H+2e^-$) at the Q_i site. (in total 6 protons; 2 protons reduce quinone to quinol and 4 protons are released from 2 ubiquinol). The *bc*$_1$ complex does not "pump" protons, it helps to build the proton gradient by an asymmetric absorption or release of protons.

When electron transfer is hindered (by a high membrane potential, point mutations, or respiratory inhibitors such as antimycin A), complex III may leak electrons to oxygen resulting in the formation of superoxide, a highly toxic species, which is thought to contribute to the pathology of a number of diseases, including aging.

10.4.2.4 COMPLEX IV

Complex IV (cytochrome *c* oxidase; EC 1.9.3.1) removes four electrons from four molecules of cytochrome *c* and transfers them to molecular oxygen

(O_2), producing two molecules of water (H_2O). At the same time, it moves four protons across the membrane, producing a proton gradient.

10.4.3 OXIDATIVE PHOSPHORYLATION

The proton gradient across the inner mitochondrial membrane is maintained by the action of electron transport chain.[348] The chain consists of the following six proteins associated with inner mitochondrial membrane:

- NADH dehydrogenase (complex I)
- Succinate coenzyme Q reductase (complex II)
- Coenzyme Q (CoQ) (also called ubiquinone)
- Cytochrome bc_1 complex (complex III)
- Cytochrome *c* (cytochrome *c*)
- Cytochrome oxidase (complex IV)

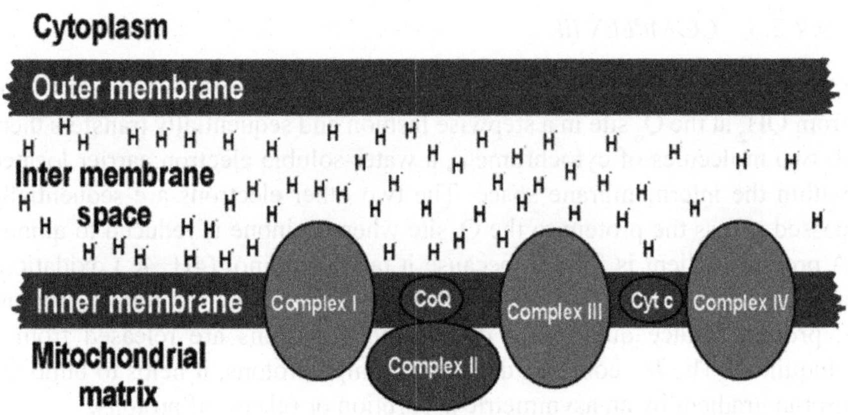

STEP I

NADH binds complex I and passes two electrons to a flavin mononucleotide (FMN) prosthetic group. The FMN is reduced to $FMNH_2$. Each electron is transferred with a proton. The electrons are then passed to iron-sulphur proteins (FeS) in complex I (this is nonheme iron). The electron is accepted by Fe^{3+}, which is reduced to Fe^{2+} (Fe^{3+} is reduced to Fe^{2+} by electrons).

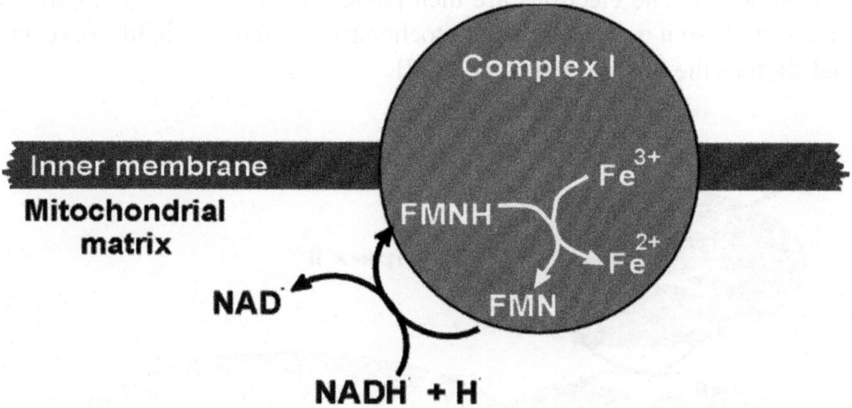

STEP II

Two electrons from the reduced FeS proteins are then passed to Co-Q along with two protons. The Co-Q is thus reduced to Co-QH_2 (ubiquinol) while the FeS proteins are oxidized back to Fe^{3+} state.

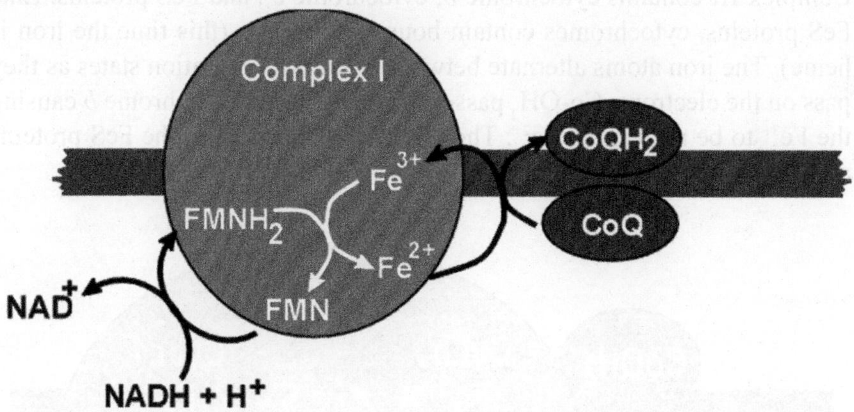

Complex II actually contains the enzyme succinate dehydrogenase that catalyses the conversion of succinate to fumarate. FAD oxidizes succinate to fumarate (FAD becoming reduced to $FADH_2$ as it picks up two electrons and two protons). Succinate dehydrogenase is actually associated with complex II. $FADH_2$ is oxidized back to FAD by passing the electrons to FeS proteins in complex II. The electrons are then passed to Co-Q. Co-Q is small and lipid soluble so it is mobile in the mitochondrial membrane; it diffuses easily and shuttles the electrons to complex III.

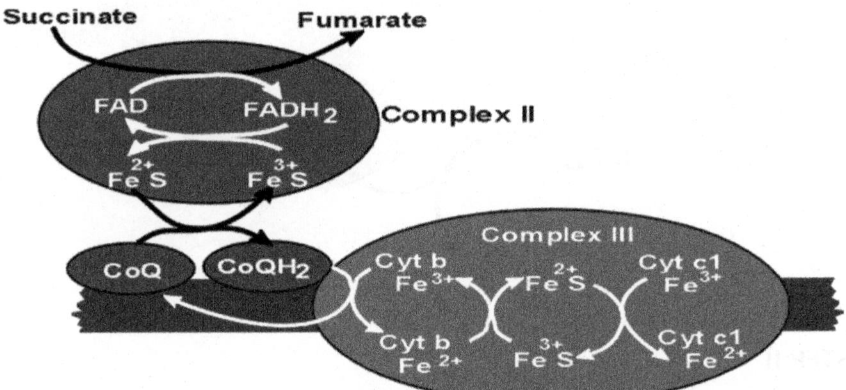

STEP III

Complex III contains cytochrome *b*, cytochrome c_1, and FeS proteins. Like FeS proteins, cytochromes contain bound iron atoms (this time the iron is heme). The iron atoms alternate between +3 and +2 oxidation states as they pass on the electrons. Co-QH_2 passes two electrons to cytochrome *b* causing the Fe^{3+} to be reduced to Fe^{2+}. The electrons are passed to the FeS proteins and then to cytochrome c_1.

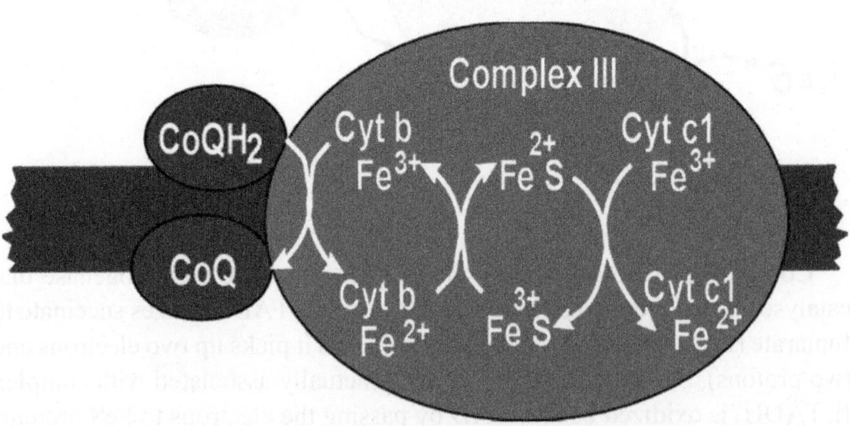

STEP IV

Cytochrome *c* is another small mobile protein. It accepts electrons from complex III (Fe^{3+} is reduced to Fe^{2+}) and shuttles them to the last electron transport protein in the chain (complex IV).

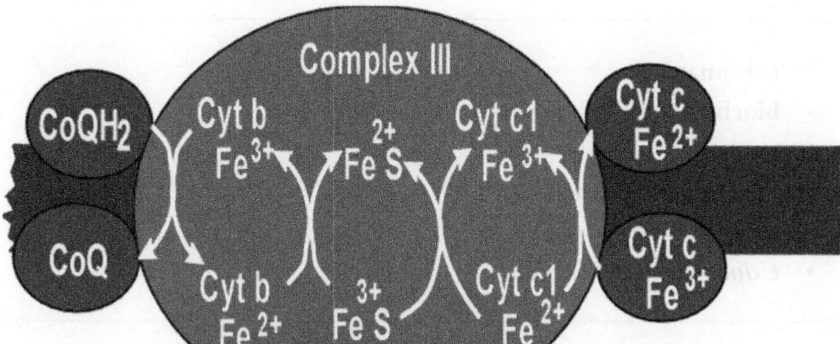

STEP V

Complex IV contains cytochrome *a* and cytochrome a_3 (both use Fe and Cu atoms to handle the electrons). Four cytochrome *c* molecules pass on four electrons to complex IV. These are eventually transferred with four H^+ to O_2 to form two water molecules.

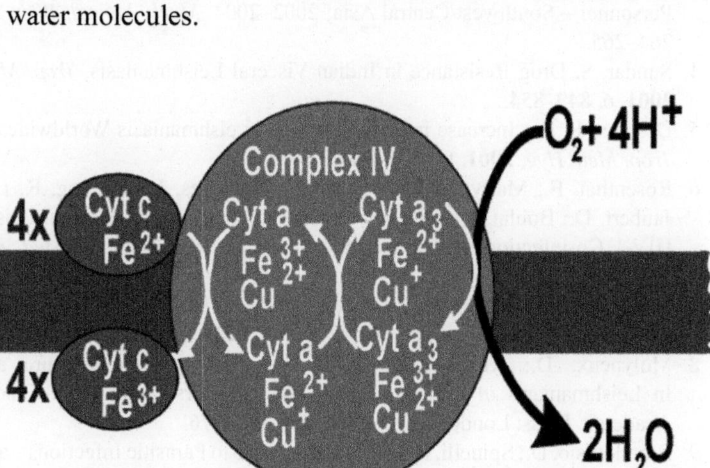

This is a complex reaction mechanism and no attempt has been made in the above diagram to explain how the four electrons from four cytochrome *c* are conveyed to the O_2 (it does not balance with respect to electrons).[347,348]

KEYWORDS

- **Leishmaniasis**
- **biochemical**
- **strain**
- **electron transport**
- ***Leishmania***
- ***L.donvani***

REFERENCES

1. Ashfold, R. W, Desjeux, P, Deraadt, P.Estimation of Population at Risk of Infection and Number of Cases of Leishmaniasis. *Parasitol. Today* **1991,** *8*, 104–105.
2. Rosypal, A. C.; Troy, G. C.; Zajac, A. M.; Duncun, R. B.; Waki Jr, K.; Chang, K. P.; Lindsay, D. S. Emergence of Zoonotic Canine Leishmaniasis in the United States: Isolation and Immunohistochemical Detection of *Leishmnia infantum* from Foxhounds from Virginia. *J. Eukaryot. Microbiol.* **2003,** *50*, 691–693.
3. Centers for Disease Control. Updates: Cutaneous Leishmaniasis in U.S. Military Personnel – Southwest/Central Asia; 2002–2004. *Morb. Mortal. Wkly. Rep.* **2004,** *53*, 264–265.
4. Sundar, S. Drug Resistance in Indian Visceral Leishmaniasis. *Trop. Med. Int. Health* **2001,** *6*, 849–854.
5. Desjeux, P. The Increase in Risk Factors of Leishmaniasis Worldwide. *Trans. R. Soc. Trop. Med. Hyg.* **2001,** *95*, 239–243.
6. Rosenthal, E.; Marty, P.; Poizot-Martin, I.; Reynes, J.; Pratlong, F., Lafeuillade, A.; Jaubert, D.; Boulat, O.; Dereure, J.; Gambarelli, F.; et al. Visceral Leishmaniasis and HIV-1 Co-infection in Southern France. *Trans. R. Soc. Trop. Med. Hyg.* **1995,** *89*, 159–162.
7. Desjeux, P. *Leishmania and HIV Co-infection in Southwestern Europe, 1990–1998, Retrospective Analysis of 965 Cases*; World Health Organization: Geneva, 2000.
8. Molyneux, D.; Killick-Kendrick, R. Morphology, ultrastructure and lifecycles. In Leishmaniasis *in Biology and Medicine*; Peters, W., Killick-Kendrick, R., Eds. Academic Press: London, 1987; Vol. 1, pp 121–176.
9. Brandonisio, D.; Spinelli, R. Immune Response to Parasitic Infections – an Introduction. *Curr. Drug. Target Immun. Endocr. Metabol. Disorder* **2002,** *2*, 193–199.

10. Herwaldt, B. L. Leishmaniasis. *Lancet* **1999,** *354*, 1191–1199.
11. Faraut-Gambbarelli, F.; Pioroux, R.; Deniau, M.; Giusiano, B.; Marty, G.; Faugere, B.; Dumon, H. *In vitro* Resistance of *Leishmania infantum* to Meglumine Antimoniate: A Study of 37 Strains Collected from Patients with Visceral Leishmaniasis. *Antimicrob. Agents Chemother.* **1997,** *41*, 827–830.
12. Lira, R.; Sunder, S.; Makharia, A.; Kenney, R.; Gam, A.; Saraiva, E.; Sack, D. Evidence that Incidence of Treatment Failure in Indian Kala-azar is due to the Emergence of Antimony Resistant Strains of *Leishmania donovani*. *J. Infect. Dis.* **1999,** *180*, 564–567.
13. Sundar, S.; More, D. K.; Singh, M. K.; Singh, V. P.; Sharma, S.; Makharia, A.; Kumar, P. C.; Murray, H. W. Failure of Pentavalent Antimony in Visceral Leishmaniasis in India: Report from the Center of the Indian Epidemic. *Clin. Infect. Dis.* **2000,** *31*, 1104–1106.
14. Mishra, M.; Biswas, U. K.; Jha, D. N.; Khan, A. B. Amphotericin Versus Pentamidine in Antimony-unresponsive Kalaazar. *Lancet* **1992,** *340*, 1256–1257.
15. Sundar, S.; Gupta, L. B.; Makharia, M. K.; Singh, M. K.; Voss, A.; Rosenkaimer, F.; Engel, J.; Murray, H. W. Oral Treatment of Visceral Leishmaniasis with Miltefosine. *Ann. Trop. Med. Parasitol.* **1999,** *93*, 589–597.
16. Perez-Victoria, F. J.; Castanys, S.; Gamarro, F. *Leishmania donovani* Resistance to Miltefosine Involves a Defective Inward Translocation of the Drug. *Antimicrob. Agents Chemother.* **2003,** *47*, 2397–2403.
17. Thakur, C. P.; Kanyok, T.P.; Pandey, A. K. Treatment of Visceral Leishmaniasis with Injectable Paromomycin (aminosidine). An Open-label Randomized Phase- II Clinical Study. *Trans. R. Soc. Trop. Med. Hyg.* **2000,** *94*, 432–433.
18. Armijos, R. X.; Weigel, M. M.; Calvopina, M. Comparison of the Effectiveness of Two Topical Paromomycin Treatments Versus Meglumine Antimoniate for New World Cutaneous Leishmaniasis. *Acta. Trop.* **2004,** *91*, 153–160.
19. Sundar, S.; Jha, T. K.; Thakur, C. P. Injectable Paromomycin for Visceral Leishmaniasis in India. *N. Engl. J. Med.* **2007,** *356*, 2571–2581.
20. el-On, J.; Halevy, S.; Grunwald, M. H. Topical Treatment of Old World Cutaneous Leishmaniasis Caused by *Leishmania major*: A Double-blind Control Study. *J. Am. Acad. Dermatol.* **1992,** *27*, 227–231.
21. Scott, J. A.; Davidson, R. N.; Moody, A. H. Aminosidine (Paromomycin) in the Treatment of Leishmaniasis Imported into the United Kingdom. *Trans. R. Soc. Trop. Med. Hyg.* **1992,** *86*, 617–619.
22. Jhingrana, A.; Chawlaa, B.; Saxenaa, S.; Barrett, M. P.; Madhubala, R. Paromomycin: Uptake and Resistance in *Leishmania donovani*. *Mol. Biochem. Parasitology* **2009,** *164*, 111–117.
23. Bera, T.; Lakshman, K.; Ghanteswari, D.; Pal, S.; Sudhahar, D.; Islam, N.; Bhuyan, N. R.; Das, P. Characterization of Redox Components of Transplasma Membrane Electron Transport System from *Leishmania donovani* Promastigotes. *Biochem. Biophys. Acta.* **2005,** *1725*, 314–326.
24. Biswas, S.; Haque, R.; Bhuyan, N. R.; Bera, T. Participation of Chlorobium Quinone in the Transplasma Membrane Electron Transport System of *Leishmania donovani* Promastigote: Effect of Near-ultraviolet Light on the Redox Reaction of Plasma Membrane. *Biochem. Biophys. Acta.* **2008,** *1780*, 116–127.
25. Chakraborty, B.; Biswas, S.; Mondal, S.; Bera, T. Stage Specific Developmental Changes in the Mitochondrial and Surface Membrane Associated Redox System of *Leishmania donovani* Promastigote and Amastigote. *Biochemistry* **2010,** *75*, 494–504.

26. Debrabant, A.; Joshi, M. B.; Pimenta, P. F.; Dwyer, D. Generation of *Leishmania donovani* Axenic Amastigotes: Their Growth and Biological Characteristics. *Int. J. Parasitol.* **2004,** *34*, 205–217.
27. Pelczar Jr, M. J.; Chan, E. C. S.; Krieg, N. R. *Microbiology*. Tata McGraw-Hill Education: Uttar Pradesh, 1993.
28. Kinnamon, K. E.; Loizeaux, P. S.; Waits, V. B.; Stick, E. A.; Hendrick, L. D.; Chapman, W. L.; Hanson, W. L. Leishmaniasis: Military Significance and New Hope for Treatment. *Mil. Med.* **1979,** *144*, 660–664.
29. WHO. *Tropical Diseases Today–The Challenge and the Opportunity*. World Health Organization: Geneva, 1975.
30. Neal, R. A. In *Recent Advances on Chemotherapy of* Leishmaniasis, Proceedings of Indo–U.K. Workshop on Leishmaniasis, Patna, Dec 6–10, 1982; Indian Council of Medical Research: New Delhi, 1983; pp 56–61.
31. WHO Expert Committee Report. *Control of* Leishmaniasis; Technical Report Series: Geneva, 1991; p 793.
32. Momen, H.; Cupolillo, E. Speculations on the Origin and Evolution of the Genus *Leishmania. Mem. Inst. Oswaldo Cruz.* **2000,** *95*, 583–588.
33. Noyes, H. A.; Morrison, D. A.; Chance, M. L.; Ellis, J. T. Evidence for a Neotropical Origin of *Leishmania. Mem. Inst. Oswaldo Cruz.* **2000,** *95*, 575–578.
34. Kerr, S. F. Palaearctic Origin of *Leishmania. Mem. Inst. Oswaldo Cruz.* **2000,** *95*, 75–80.
35. World Health Organisation. Communicable diseases surveillance and response. Leishmaniasis. 44(77), 365–372.
36. Houston Chronicle: Texas Doctors Find Skin Disease Moving North. Retrieved on 2007-09-15.
37. Al Jazeera English - CENTRAL/S. ASIA - Kabul: A city in intensive care.
38. e-Ariana - Todays Afghan News.
39. http://www.pdhealth.mil/downloads/Leishmaniasis_exsu_16Mar042.pdf.
40. *The American Heritage Dictionary of the English Language*; Houghton Mifflin: Boston, 1969.
41. Ryan, K. J.; Ray, C. G.. *Sherris Medical Microbiology;* McGraw Hill: New York, 2004; pp 749–754.
42. A Small Charity Takes the Reins in Fighting a Neglected Disease. *New York Times, July 31, 2006.*
43. Marinkelle, C. J. The Control of Leishmaniases. *Bull. World Health Organ.* **1980,** *58* (6), 807–818.
44. Rab, M. A.; Evans, D. A. *Leishmania infantum* in the Himalayas. *Trans. R. Soc. Trop. Med. Hyg.* **1995,** *89*, 27–32.
45. Sanyal, R. K.; Chang, K. P.; Bray, R. S. Leishmaniasis *in the Indian sub-continent*. Elsevier Science Publishers: Amsterdam, 1985; pp 443–467.
46. De Beer, P.; El-Harith, A.; Van Grootheest, M.; Winkler, A. Outbreak of Kala-azar in the Sudan. *Lancet* **1990,** *535*, 224.
47. Thakur, C. P.; Narayan, S.; Ranjan, A. Epidemiological, Clinical & Pharmacological Study of Antimony-resistant Visceral Leishmaniasis in Bihar, India. *Clin. Infect. Dis.* **2004,** *120*, 166–172.
48. Thakur, C. P.; Singh, R. K.; Hassan, S. M.; Kumar, R.; Narain, S.; Kumar, A. Amphotericin B Deoxycholate Treatment of Visceral Leishmaniasis with Never Modes of Administration and Precautions: A Study of 938 Cases. *Trans. R. Soc. Trop. Med. Hyg.* **1999,** *93*, 319–323.

49. Thakur, C. P.; Pandey, A. K.; Sinha, G. P.; Roy, S.; Behbehani, K.; Olliaro, P. Comparison of Three Treatment Regimens with Liposomal Amphotericin B (AmBisome) for Visceral Leishmaniasis in India: A Randomized Dose-finding Study. *Trans. R. Soc. Trop. Med. Hyg.* **1996,** *90,* 319–322.
50. Sundar, S.; Mehta, H.; Chhabra, A.; Singh, V.; Chauhan, V.; Desjeux, P.; Rai, M. Amphotericin B Colloidal Dispersion for the Treatment of Indian Visceral Leishmaniasis. *Clin. Infect. Dis.* **2006,** *42,* 608–613.
51. New Cure for Deadly Visceral Leishmaniasis (Kala-azar) approved by Government of India, *Institute for OneWorld Health Press Release*, Sept 8, 2006.
52. Peters, H. S.; Fish, D.; Golden, R.; Evens, D. A.; Bryceson, A. D. M.; Plenching, A. J. Visceral Leishmaniasis in HIV Infection and AIDS: Clinical Feature and Response to the Therapy. *O. J. Med.* **1990,** *77,* 1101–1111.
53. Pardes, R.; Munoz, J.; Diaz, I.; Domingo, P.; Gurgci, M.; Clotet, B. Leishmaniasis in HIV Infections. *J. Postgrad. Med.* **2003,** *49,* 39–49.
54. Sundar, S. Drug Resistance in Indian Visceral Leishmaniasis. *Trop. Med. Int. Health* **2001,** *6,* 849–854.
55. Guevin, P. J.; Olliaro, P.; Sundar, S.; Boelaert, M.; Craft, S. L.; Desjeux, P.; Wasunna, M. K.; Bryceson, A. D. Visceral Leishmaniasis: Current Status of Control, Diagnosis and Treatment and a Proposed Research and Development Agenda. *Lancet Infect. Dis.* **2002,** *2,* 494–501.
56. World Health Organization. *Leishmania*/HIV Co–infection. Epidemiological Analysis of 692 Retrospective Cases. *Wkly. Epidemiol. Rec.* **1997,** *72,* 49–54.
57. Cox Francis, E. G. *The Wellcome Trust Illustrated History of Tropical Diseases;* The Wellcome Trust: London, 1996; 206–217.
58. WHO: Leishmaniasis: background information. Retrieved on 2007-07-04, http://www.who.int/leishmaniasis/en/.
59. Cunningham, D. D. *On the Ppresence of Peculiar Parasitic Organisms in the Tissue of a Specimen of Delhi Boil;* Scientific Memoirs Officers Medical Sanitary Departments, Government of India, Printed by the Superintendent of Government Printing: Calcutta, India, 1885; pp 21–31.
60. Cox, F. E. History of Human Parasitology. *Clin. Microbiol. Rev.* **2002,** *15,* 595–612.
61. Lainson Shaw, J. J. Evaluation, classification and geographical distribution. In *The* Leishmaniasis *in Biology and Medicine*; Peters, W., Killick–Kendrick, R., Eds.; Academic Press: London., 1987; Vol. I, pp 1–20.
62. Baker, A. C. The Typical Epidemic Series. *Am. J. Trop. Med.* **1943,** *23,* 559–560.
63. Twining, W. *Clinical Illustrations of the More Important Diseases of Bengal, with a Result of an Enquiry into their Pathology and Treatment*; Baptist Mission Press: Calcutta, 1832.
64. Leishman, W. B. On the Possibility of the Occurrence of Trypanosomiasis in India. *Br. Med. J.* **1903,** *1,* 1252–1254.
65. Donovan, L. On the Possibility of the Occurrence of Trypanosomiasis in India. *Br. Med.* J. **1903,** *2,* 79.
66. Knowles, R.; Napier, L. E.; Smith, R. O. A. On a Herpetomonas Found in the Gut of the Sandfly, *Phlebotomus argentips*, Fed on Kala–azar Patients. *Ind. Med. Gaz.* **1924,** *59,* 593–597.
67. Gilles, H. M. *Protozoal Diseases*; Arnold publishers: London, 1999.
68. Manson, P. *Manson's Tropical Diseases: A Manual of the Diseases of Warm Climate,* 15th ed.; Manson–Bahr, P. H, Ed.; Cassell & Co.: London,1960.

69. Baker, J. R. *Parasitic Protozoa*. Hutchinson University Library: London, 1969.
70. Smyly, H. J.; Young, C. W. The Experimental Transmission of Leishmaniasis to Animals. *Proc. Soc. Expt. Biol. Med.* **1924,** *21*, 354–356.
71. Doflin F, Reichnow. (1929) Lehrbuclider Protozoan Kunde, Jena.
72. Ross, R. Note on the Bodies Recently Described by Leishman and Donovan. *Brit. Med. J.* 1903, 2, 1261–1262.
73. Lainson, R.; Shaw, J. J. Evolution, classification and geographical distribution. In *The* Leishmaniases *in Biology and Medicine*; Peters, W., Killick-Kendrick, R., Eds.; Academic Press: London, 1987; Vol. 1, pp 1–120.
74. Crumers, J.; Jadin, J. M. Study of the Ultrastructure and Biology of *Leishmania mexicana* Biagi 1953. I. The Modification which Occur at the Time of *Leishmania*-leptomonas Transformation. *Bull. Soc. Pathol. Exot.* **1967,** *60*, 53–58.
75. Pham, T. D.; Azar, H. A.; Moscovic, E. A.; Kurban, A. K. The Ultrastructure of *Leishmania tropica* in the Oriental Sore. *Ann. Trop. Med. Parasitol.* **1907,** *64*, 1–4.
76. Bray, R. S.; Ellis, D. S.; Bird, R. G. The Fine Structure of *Leishmania enriettii*. *Trans. Roy. Soc. Trop. Med. Hyg.* **1969,** *63*, 10–11.
77. Brun, R.; Krassner, S. M. Quantitative Ultra–structural Investigations of Mitochondrial Development in *Leishmania donovani* during Transformation. *J. Protozool.* **1976,** *23*, 493–497.
78. Akiyama, H. J.; McQuillen, N. K. Interaction and Transformation of *Leishmania donovani* within in vitro Cultured Cells. *Am. J. Trop. Med. Hyg.* **1972,** *21*, 873–879.
79. Sanyal, A. B.; Sengupta, P. C. Fine Structure of *Leishmania* in Dermal Leishmanoid. *Trans. Roy. Soc. Trop. Med. Hyg.* **1967,** *61*, 211–216.
80. Granham PCC, Bird RG. (1962) *Sci Rep 1st Super Santa* 2: 83.
81. Angelopoulas, E. Pellicular Microtubule in the Family Trypanosomatidae. *J. Protozool.* **1970,** *17*, 39–51.
82. Safjanova, V. M.; Avkyan, A. A.; Aliv, E. I.; Koshelev, B. A. *Progr. Protozoal.* **1973,** *17*, 358.
83. McAlpine, J. C. Electronic Cytochemical Demonstration of a Lysosome in *Leishmania donovani*. *Trans. Roy. Soc. Trop. Med. Hyg.* **1970,** *64*, 822–825.
84. Brun, R.; Krassner, S. M. Quantitative Ultrastructural Investigation of Mitochondrial Development in *Leishmania donovani* during Transformation. *J. Protozool.* **1976,** *23*, 493–497.
85. Chatterjee, S. N.; Sengupta, P. C. Ultrastructure of the Promastigotes of *Leishmania donovani*. *Ind. J. Med. Res.* **1970,** *58*, 70–76.
86. Cherepova N. (1970) *Izv Microbiol Inst Bulg Aknd Nauk* 21: 265.
87. Taylor, M. B.; Berghausen, H.; Heyworth, P.; Messenger, N.; Rees, L. J.; Gutteridge, W. E. Subcellular Localization of Some Glycolytic Enzymes in Parasitic Flagellated Protozoa. *Int. J. Biochem.* **1980,** *11*, 117–120.
88. Chang, K. P.; Dwyer, D. M. Multiplication of a Human Parasite (*Leishmania donovani*) in Phagolysosomes of Hamster Macrophages in vitro. *Science* **1976**, *193*, 678–680.
89. Rivas, L.; Chang, K. P. Intraparasitophorous Vacuolar pH of *Leishmania mexicana* Infected Macrophages. *Biol. Bull.* **1983,** *165*, 536–537.
90. Pearson, R. D, Harcus, J. L.; Symes, P. H.; Romito, R.; Donowitz, G. R. Failure of the Phagocytic Oxidative Response to Protect Human Monocyte Derived Macrophages from Infection by *Leishmania donovani*. *J. Immunol.* **1982,** *129*, 1282–1286.

91. Murray, H. W. Interaction of *Leishmania* with a Macrophage Cell Line. Correlation between Intracellular Killing and the Generation of Oxygen Intermediates. *J. Exp. Med.* **1981,** *153*, 1690–1695.
92. Murray, H. W. Cellular Resistance to Protozoal Infection. *Ann. Rev. Med.* **1986,** *37*, 61–69.
93. Kirk, R. Studies in Leishmaniasis in the Anglo–Egyptian Sudan. Part–I–Epidemiology and General Considerations. *Trans. Roy. Soc. Trop. Med. Hyg.* **1939,** *32*, 533–544.
94. Pampiglione, S.; Manson–Bahr, P. E. C.; Giunti, G.; Giungi, F.; Parenti, A.; Canestri Trotti, G. Studies on Mediterranean Leishmaniasis. 2. Asymptomatic Cases of Visceral Leishmaniasis. *Trans. Roy. Soc. Trop. Med. Hyg.* **1974,** *68*, 447–453.
95. Shujkina, E. E. Clinico–immunological Variants of Leishmaniasis. *Meditsinskaia Parazitologiia Parzitarnye Bolezni (Moskva)* 49: 75–81.
96. Bray, R.S. Leishmaniasis in the Old World. *Brit. Med. Bull.* **1972,** *28*, 39–43.
97. Bray, R. S. Zoonoses in Leishmaniasis. In *Parasitic Zoonoses*; Soulsby, E. J. L., Ed. Academic Press: New York, San Frasislo, London, 1974; pp 65–67.
98. WHO. Studies on leishmaniasis vectors/reservoirs and their control in the Old World. General review and parts I and II All Parts prepared by A.R. Zahar. Unpublished document WHO/VBC/79, 749.88PP, 1979.
99. Killick–Kendrick, R.; Rioux, J. A.; Baily, M. W.; Wilkes, T. J.; Guy, F. M.; Davidson, I.; Knechtli, R.; Ward, R. D.; Guilvard, E.; Perieres, J.; et al. Ecology of Leishmaniasis in the South of France. 20. Dispersal of *Phlebotomus ariasi* Tonnoir, 1921 as a Factor in the Spread of Visceral Leishmaniasis in the Cevennes. *Ann. Parasitol. Hum. Comp.* **1984,** *59*, 555–572.
100. Swaminath, C. S.; Shortt, H. E.; Anderson, L. A. Transmission of Indian Kala–azar to Man by the Bite of *P. argentipes*, ANN and BRUN. *Ind. J. Med. Res.* **1942,** *30*, 473–477.
101. Low, G. C.; Cooke, W. E. A Congenital Case of Kala–azar. *Lancet.* **1925,** *ii*, 1209–1211.
102. Loke, Y. Transmission of parasites across the placenta. In *Advances in Parasitology.* Academic Press: New York, 1982; Vol. 12, p 155.
103. Nuwayri–Salti, N.; Khanas, H. Direct Noninsect–Vector Transmission of *Leishmania* Parasites in Mice. *Int. J. Parasitol.* **1985,** *15*, 497.
104. Napier, L.; Gupta, C. D. Indian Kala-azar in a New Born. *Indian Med. Gazette* **1928,** *62*, 199.
105. Chung, H. L.; Chow, H. K.; Lu, J. P. The First Two Cases of Transfusion Kala–azar. *Chinese Med. J.* **1948,** *66*, 325.
106. Kostman, R.; Barr, M.; Bengtson, E.; Garnham, P. C. C.; Hult, G.In *Kala–azar Transferred by Exchange Blood Transfusion in two Swedish Infants*, Proceedings of the Seventh International Congress of Tropical Medicine and Malaria, Geneva, Switzerland, 1963; World Health Organization; Geneva, 1963; p 384.
107. Kager PA (1988). Visceral leishmaniasis. *Med Int 54*, 2235.
108. Walker, R. *Technical Manual*, 11th ed.; American Association of Blood Bank: Bethesda, MD, 1993; pp 1.
109. Forkner, C. E, Zia, L. S. Viable *Leishmaina donovani* in Nasal and Oral Secretions of Patients with Kala–azar and the Bearing of this Finding on the Transmission of the Disease. *J. Expt. Med.* **1934,** *59*, 491–499.
110. Shortt, H. E.; Craighead, A. C.; Smith, R. O. A.; Swaminath, C. S. The Infection of Hamsters with Kala–azar by the Oral Route. *Ind. J. Med. Res.* **1929,** *17*, 335–338.
111. Symmers, W. S. Leishmaniasis Acquired by Contagion: A Case of Marital Infection in Britain. *Lancet* **1960,** *1*, 127–132.

112. Terry, L. L.; Lewis Jr, J. L.; Sessons, S. M. Laboratory Infection with *Leishmaina donovani*: A Case Report. *Am. J. Trop. Med.* **1950,** *30*, 643–649.
113. Trager, W. Nutrition of Hemoflagellates (*Leishmania torentolae*) Having an Interchangeable Requirement of Choline or Pyroxal. *J. Protozool.* **1957,** *4*, 269–276.
114. Lemma, A.; Schiller, E. L. Extracellular Cultivation of Leishmanial Bodies of Species Belonging to the Protozoan Genus *Leishmania. Exp. Parasitol.* 1964, *15*, 503–513.
115. Krassner, S. M. Effect of Temperature on Growth and Nutritional Requirements of *Leishmania* in a Defined Medium. *J. Protozool.* **1965,** *12*, 73–79.
116. Trager, W. The Development of *Leishmania donovani* in vitro at 37°C. *J. Exptl. Med.* **1953,** *97*, 177–188.
117. Pan, C. J. Cultivation of the Leishmaniform Stage of *Trypanosoma cruzi* in Cell–free Media at Different Temperatures. *Am. J. Trop. Med. Hyg.* **1968,** *17*, 823–832.
118. Hawking, F. Growth of Protozoa in Tissue Culture. V. *Leishmania donovani*: *Trans. Roy. Soc. Trop. Med. Hyg.* **1948,** *41*, 545–554.
119. Lomy, L.; Sense, A.; Lamy, H.Installation, Multiplication and Maintenance of a *Leishmania donovani* Strain in Cell Culture. *Bull. Soc. Pathol. Exot. Filiales* **1964,** *57*, 16–21.
120. Vickerman, K. The Mechanism of Cyclical Development in Trypanosomes of *Trypanosoma brucei* Sub Group: A Hypothesis Based on Ultrastructural Observations. *Trans. Roy. Soc. Trop. Med. Hyg.* **1962,** *56*, 487–495.
121. Ristic, M.; Trager, W. Cultivation at 37°C of a Trypanosome (*Trypanosoma theileri*) from Cows with Depressed Milk Production. *J. Protozool.* **1958,** *5*, 146–148.
122. D'Alesandro, P. A. In vitro Studies of Ablastin, the Reproduction–inhibiting Antibody to *Trypanosoma lewisi*. *J. Protozool.* **1962,** *9*, 351–358.
123. Deane MP, Deane LM .(1961) *Rev Inst Med Trop Sao Panlo* 3: 149.
124. Desowitz, R. S. The Development and Survival of the Blood–stream Forms of *Trypanosoma conorhini* in Culture. *J. Protozool.* **1963,** *10*, 390–391.
125. Deane, M. P.; Kirchner, E. Life Cycle of *Trypanosoma conorhini*. Influence of Temperature and Other Factors on Growth and Morphogenisis. *J. Protozool.* **1963,** *10*, 391–400.
126. Trager, W. *The Cell*; Brachet, J., Mirsky, A. E., Eds. Academic Press: New York, 1960; Vol. 4, p 151.
127. Guttman, H. N.; Nallace, F. G. *Biochemistry and Physiology of Protozoa*; Hunter, S. H., Eds. Academic Press: New York and London, 1964; Vol. 3, p 459.
128. Roy, D. K.; Ghosh, D. K. *Leishmania donovani*: Effect of Temperature on RNA Metabolism. *Expt. Parasitol.* **1981,** *33*, 147–154.
129. Fong, D.; Chang, K. P. Tubulin Biosynthesis in the Development Cycle of a Parasitic Protozoan, *Leishmania mexicana*: Changes during Differentiation of Motile and Nonmotile Stages. *Proc. Natl. Acad. Sci. USA* **1981,** *78*, 7626–7628.
130. Vickirman, K.; Preston, T. M. *Biology of the Kinetoplastidae;* Lumsden, W. H., Evans, D. A., Eds. Academic Press: New York, 1972; Vol. 1, p 35.
131. Dwyer, D. M. Isolation and Partial Characterization of Surface Membranes from *Leishmania donovani* Promastigotes. *J Protozool.* **1980,** *27,* 176–182.
132. Simpson, L. The *Leishmania*–leptomonad Transformation of *Leishmania donovani*: Nutritional Requirements, Respiration Changes and Antigenic Changes. *J. Protozool.* 1988, 15, 201–207.

133. Morrow, D. C.; Flory, B.; Krassner, S. M. Polyamines in the Hemoflagellate, *Leishmania donovani*: Evidence for Spermine in the Amastigote Stage. *Comp. Biochem. Physiol.* **1980,** *66B*, 307–311.
134. Janory Jr, J. Respiratory Changes Accompanying *Leishmania* to Leptomonad Transformation in *Leishmania donovani*. *Exptl. Parasitol.* **1967,** *20,* 51–55.
135. Walter, R. D.; Buse, E.; Ebert, F. Effect of Cyclic AMP on Transformation and Proliferation of *Leishmania* cells. *Tropenmed. Parasitol.* **1978,** *29*, 439–442.
136. Hart, D. T.; Coombs, G. H. Morphological and Biochemical Studies of the in vitro Transformation of *Leishmania mexicana* Amastigotes to Promastigotes. *J. Protozool.* **1980,** *27*, 63A.
137. Brun, R.; Berens, R. L.; Krassner, S. M. Inhibition of *Leishmania donovani* Transformations by Hamster Spleen Homogenates and Active Human Lymphocytes. *Nature* **1976,** *262*, 689–691.
138. Krassner, S. M.; Morrow, C. D.; Flory, B. Inhibition of *Leishmania donovani* Amastigote–to–Promastigote Transformation by Infected Hamster Spleen Lymphocyte Lysates. *J. Protozool.* **1980,** *27*, 87–92.
139. Dwyer, D. M.; Langreth, S. G.; Dwyer, N. K. Evidence for a Polysaccharide Surface Coat in the Development stagesof *Leishmania donovani*: A Fine Structure-cytochemical Study. *Z. Parasitenkd.* **1974,** *43*, 227–249.
140. Dwyer, D. M. Antibody–induced Modulation of *Leishmania donovani* Surface Membrane Antigens. *J. Immunol.* **1976,** *117*, 2081–2091.
141. Konigk, E.; Putfarkau, B. Stage-specific Differences of a Perhaps Signal-transferring System in *Leishmania donovani*. *Tropenmed. Parasitol.* **1980,** *31*, 421–424.
142. Wallach, M.; Fong, D.; Chang, K. P. Post–transcriptional Control of Tubulin Biosynthesis during Leishmanial Differentiation. *Nature* **1982,** *299*, 650–652.
143. Steiger, R. F.; Mc Shnick, S. R. Amimo Acid and Glucose Utilization of *Leishmania donovani* and *Leishmania braziliensis*. *Trans. Roy. Soc. Trop. Med. Hyg.* **1977,** *71*, 441–443.
144. Steiger, R. F.; Steiger, E. Cultivation of *Leishmania donovani* and *Leishmania braziliensis* in Defined Media: Nutritional Requirements. *J. Protozool.* **1977,** *24*, 437–441.
145. Steiger, R. F.; Black, C. D. Simplified Defined Media for Cultivating *Leishamania donovani* Promastigotes. *Acta. Tropica.* **1980,** *37*, 195–198.
146. Novy, F. G.; Mc Neal, W. J.Trypanosomes and Bird Malaris. *Am. Med.* **1904,** *45*, 932–934.
147. Nicolle C. (1908) *Compt Rend* 146: 842.
148. Salle, A. J.; Schmidt, C.L. A. The Metabolism of *Leishmania tropica*. *J. Infect. Dis.* **1928,** *43*, 378–384.
149. Ray, J. C. Cultivation of Various *Leishmania parasites* on Solid Medium. *Ind. J. Med. Res.* **1932,** *20*, 355–367.
150. Lowfly M. (1933) *Am Inst Pasteur* 51: 55.
151. Lwoff A. (1934) *Zentr Bakt Pava Sitek Abst 9. Orig* 130: 448.
152. Lwoff M. (1938) *Compt Rend* 206: 540.
153. Lwoff M. (1938) *Compt Rend Soc Biol* 128: 241.
154. Goat H, Mova C. (1947) *Anals Soc Biol Bogota* 2: 188.
155. Guttman, H. N.; Eisenman, R. N. Cure of *Crithidia (Strigomonas) oncopelti* of its Bacterial Endosymbiote. *Nature* **1965,** *206*, 113–114.
156. Krassner, S. M.; Flory, B. Proline Metabolism is *Leishmania donovani* Promastigotes. *J. Protozool.* **1972,** *19*, 682–685.

157. Beach, D. H.; Holz Jr, G. G.; Anekwe, G. E. Lipids of *Leishmania* Promastigotes. *J. Parasitol.* **1979,** *65*, 203–216.
158. Krassner, S. M.; Flory, B. Essential Amino Acids in the Culture of *Leishmania torentolae*. *J. Parasitol.* **1971**, 57, 917–920.
159. Aaronsons, S.; Nathan, H. A. Utilization of Imidazole Counter Parts Purines in Microbial Systems. *Biochem. Biophys. Acta.* **1954,** *15*, 306–307.
160. Nathan, H. A.; Cowperthwaite, J. "Crithidia factor" – A New Member of the Folic Acid Group of Vitamins. *J. Protozool.* **1955,** *2*, 37−42.
161. Nathan, H. A. Purine Biosynthesis by the Trypanosomid flagellate, *Striogomonas oncopelti*. *J. Protozool.* **1958,** *5*, 194−195.
162. Kidder, G. W.; Dewey, I. C. *Biochemistry and Physiology of Protozoa;* Lowoff, A. Eds.; Academic Press: New York, 1951.
163. Von Brand, J. *Biochemistry and Physiology of Endoparasites,* 2nd ed.; Elsevier Science: North Holland, 1979.
164. Holz Jr, G. G.; Wagner, B.; Erwin, J.; Britt, J. J.; Block, K. Sterol Requirements of a Ciliate *Tetrahymena corlissi* Th-X. I. A Nutritional Analysis of the Sterol Requirements of *T. corlissi* Th-X. II. Metabolism of Titrated Lopohenol in *T. corlissi* Th-X. *Comp. Biochem. Physiol.* **1966,** *2*, 202–217.
165. Holz, G. G., Jr.; Erwin, J.; Wagner, B.; Rosenbaum, N. The Nutrition of *Terrahymena setifera* Hz–1: Sterol and Alcohol Requirements. *J. Protozool.* **1962,** *9,* 359–363.
166. Rey, L.; Fernandes, J. F. Nucleotide and Polynucleotide Synthesis in *Trypanosoma cruzi*. VII. Precurssors of the Pyrimidine Nucleotide. *Exptl. Parasitol.* **1962,** *12*, 55–60.
167. Wonde, T.; Honigberg, B. M. Morphology and Infectivity of *Leishmania donovani* Cultivated in Nonliving Media at Elevated Temperatures. *Am. J. Trop. Med. Hyg.* **1971,** *20*, 828–838.
168. Von Brand, T. *Biochemistry and Physiology of Protozoa;* Lwoff, A., Ed.; Academic Press: New York, 1951.
169. Von Brand, T. *Biochemistry of Parasites*; Academic Press: New York, 1966.
170. Chang, S. L. Studies on Hemoflagellates. IV. Observations Concerning Some Biochemical Activities in Culture and Respiration of Three Species of *Leishmania* and *Trypanosoma cruzi*. *J. Infect. Diseases* **1948,** *82*, 109–118.
171. Mukherjee, R. Ph.D. Thesis, Department of Pharmaceutical Technology, Jadavpur University, Kolkata, India, 1975.
172. Fulton, J. D.; Joyner, L. P. Studies on Protozoa. Part 1. The Metabolism of *Leishmania donovani* Bodies and Flagellates of *Leishmania donovani*. *Trans. Roy. Soc. Trop. Med. Hyg.* **1949,** *43*, 273–286.
173. Bowman, I. B. R. Intermediary metabolism of pathogenic flagellates. In *Trypanosomiasis and* Leishmaniasis *with Special References to Chagas Disease*, Ciba Foundation Symposium No. 20 (New Series), Associated Scientific Publishers: Amsterdam, 1974; pp 255–284.
174. Chattejee, T.; Datta, A. G. Anaerobic Formation of Succinate from Glucose and Bicarbonate in Resting Cells of *Leishmania donovani. Exp. Parasitol.* **1973,** *33*, 138–146.
175. Berens, R. L.; Deutsch–king, L. C.; Marr, J. J. *Leishmania donovani* and *Leishmania braziliensis*: Hexokinase, Glucose–6–Phosphate Dehydrogenase and Pentose Phosphate Shunt Activity. *Exp. Parasitol. 1980*, *49*, 1–8.
176. Mukkada, A. J. Tricarboxylic Acid and Glyoxylate Cycles in *Leishmaniae*. *Acta. Tropica.* **1977,** *34*, 167–175.

177. Simon, M. W.; Martin, E.; Mukkada, A. J. Evidence for a Functional Glyoxylate Cycle in *Leishmaniae*. *J. Bacteriol.* **1978,** *135*, 895–899.
178. Martin, E.; Mukkada, A. J. Respiratory Chain Components of *Leishmania tropica* Promastigotes. *J. Protozool.* **1979,** *26*, 138–142.
179. Ryley, J. F. Studies on the Metabolism of Protozoa. 9. Comparative Metabolism of Blood–Stream and Culture forms of *Trypanosoma rhodesiense*. *Biochem. J.* **1962,** *85*, 211–223.
180. Ghosh, D. K. D Phil Thesis, Calcutta University, Calcutta, 1967.
181. Small, J. V.; Herzog, M. *Cell Biology: A Laboratory Hand book*; Celis, J. E., Ed.; Academic Press: New York, 1994; Vol. 2, pp 135–139.
182. Opperdoes, F. R.; Borst, P. Localization of Nine Glycolytic Enzymes in a Microbody–like Organelle in *Trypanosoma brucei*: The Glycosome. *FEBS. Lett.* **1977,** *80*, 360–364
183. Visser, N.; Opperdoes, F. R.; Borst, P. Subcellular Compartmentation of Glycolytic Intermediates in *Trypanosoma brucei*. *Eur. J. Biochem.* **1981,** *118*, 521–526.
184. Mackenzie, N. E.; Seed, J. R.; Scott, A. L. Carbon 13 Nuclear – Magnetic Resonance Studies on Glucose Catabolism by *Trypanosoma brucei gambiense*. *Eur. J. Biochem.* **1982,** *121*, 657–661.
185. Njogu, R. M.; Nyindo, M. Presence of Peculiar Pathway of Glucose Metabolism in Infective Forms of *Trypanosoma brucei* Cultured from Salivary Glands of Tsetse Flies. *J. Parasitol.* **1981,** *67*, 847–851.
186. Roberts, W. L.; Rainey, P. M. Antileishmanial Activity of Sodium Stibogluconate Fractions. *Antimicrob. Agents Chemother.* **1993,** *37*, 1842–1846.
187. Myler, P. J.; Fasel, N. *Leishmania: After the Genome*; Caister Academic Press/Horizon Scientific Press:United Kingdom, 2008.
188. Rosen, B. P. Transport and Detoxification Systems for Transition Metals, Heavy Metals and Metalloids in Eukaryotic and Prokaryotic Microbes. *Comp. Biochem. Physiol. A. Mol. Integr. Physiol.* **2002,** *133*, 689–693.
189. Shaked-Mishan, P.; Ulrich, N.; Ephros, M.; Zilberstein, D. Novel Intracellular SbV Reducing Activity Correlates with Antimony Susceptibility in *Leishmania donovani*. *J. Biol. Chem.* **2001,** *276*, 3971–3976.
190. Denton, H.; McGregor, J. C.; Coombs, G. H. Reduction of Antileishmanial Pentavalent Antimonial Drugs by a Parasite-specific Thiol Dependent Reductase TDR1. *Biochem. J.* **2004,** *381*, 405–412.
191. Berman, J. D.; Gallalee, J. V.; Hansen, B. D. *Leishmania mexicana*: Uptake of Sodium Stibogluconate (Pentostam) and Pentamidine by Parasite and Macrophages. *Exp. Parasitol.* **1987,** *64*, 127–131.
192. Croft, S. L.; Neame, K. D.; Homewood, C. A. Accumulation of ^{125}Sb Sodium Stibogluconate by *Leishmania mexicana amazonensis* and *Leishmania donovani in vitro*. *Comp. Biochem. Physiol. C.* **1981,** *68C*, 95–98.
193. Brochu, C.; Wang, J.; Roy, G.; Messier, N.; Wang, X. Y.; Saravia, N. G.; Ouellette, M. Antimony Uptake Systems in the Protozoan Parasite *Leishmania* and Accumulation Differences in Antimony-resistant Parasites. *Antimicrob. Agents Chemother.* **2003,** *47*, 3073–3079.
194. Roberts, W. L.; Berman, J. D.; Rainey, P. M. *In vitro* Antileishmanial Properties of Tri- and Pentavalent Antimonial Preparations. *Antimicrob. Agents Chemother.* **1995,** *39*, 1234–1239.

195. Sereno, D.; Lemesre, J. L. Axenically Cultured Amastigote Forms as an *in vitro* Model for Investigation of Antileishmanial Agents. *Antimicrob. Agents Chemother.* **1997,** *41*, 972–976.
196. Sereno, D.; Cavaleyra, M.; Zemzoumi, K.; Maquaire, S.; Ouaissi, A.; Lemesre, J. L. Axenically Grown Amastigotes of *Leishmania infantum* Used as an *in vitro* Model to Investigate the Pentavalent Antimony Mode of Action. *Antimicrob. Agents Chemother.* **1998,** *42*, 3097–3102.
197. Callahan, H. L.; Portal, A. C.; Devereaux, R.; Grogl, M. An Axenic Amastigote System for Drug Screening. *Antimicrob. Agents. Chemother.* **1997,** *41*, 818–822.
198. Ephros, M.; Bitnun, A.; Shaked, P.; Waldman, E.; Zilberstein, D. Stage-specific Activity of Pentavalent Antimony against *Leishmania donovani* Axenic Amastigotes. *Antimicrob. Agents Chemother.* **1999,** *43*, 278–282.
199. Carrio, J.; de Colmenares, M.; Riera, C.; Gallego, M.; Arboix, M.; Portus, M. *Leishmania infantum*: Stage-specific Activity of Pentavalent Antimony Related with the Assay Conditions. *Exp. Parasitol.* **2000,** *95*, 209–214.
200. Ferreira Cdos, S.; Martins, P. S.; Demicheli, C.; Brochu, C.; Ouellette, M.; Frezard, F. Thiol-induced Reduction of Antimony (V) into Antimony (III): A Comparative Study with Trypanothione, Cysteinyl-glycine, Cysteine and Glutathione. *Biometals* **2003,** *16*, 441–446.
201. Basselin, M.; Denise, H.; Coombs, G. H.; Barrett, M. P. Resistance to Pentamidine in *Leishmania mexicana* Involves Exclusion of the Drug from the Mitochondrion. *Antimicrob. Agents Chemother.* **2002,** *46*, 3731–3738.
202. Mukherjee, A.; Padmanabhan, P. K.; Sahani, M. H.; Barrett, M. P.; Madhubala, R. Roles for Mitochondria in Pentamidine Susceptibility and Resistance in *Leishmania donovani. Mol. Biochem. Parasitol.* **2006,** *145*, 1–10.
203. Lux, H.; Heise, N.; Klenner, T.; Hart, D.; Opperdoes, F. R. Ether--lipid (Alkylphospholipid) Metabolism and the Mechanism of Action of Ether--lipid Analogues in *Leishmania. Mol. Biochem. Parasitol.* **2000,** *111*, 1–14.
204. Rakotomanga, M.; Blanc, S.; Gaudin, K.; Chaminade, P.; Loiseau, P. M. Miltefosine Affects the Lipid Metabolism in *Leishmania donovani* Promastigotes. *Antimicrob. Agents Chemother.* **2007,** *51*, 1425–1430.
205. Sundar, S.; Murray, H. W. Availability of Miltefosine for the Treatment of Kala-azar in India. *Bull. World Health Organ.* **2005,** *83*, 394–395.
206. Davis, B. D. Mechanism of Bactericidal Action of Aminoglycosides. *Microbiol. Rev.* **1987,** *51*, 341–350.
207. Gillin, F. D.; Diamond, L. S. Inhibition of Clonal Growth of *Giardia lamblia* and *Entamoeba histolytica* by Metronidazole, Quinacrine, and Other Antimicrobial Agents. *J. Antimicrob. Chemother.* **1981,** *8*, 305–316.
208. Flanigan, T. P.; Ramratnam, B.; Graeber, C. Prospective Trial of Paromomycin for Cryptosporidiosis in AIDS. *Am. J. Med.* **1996,** *100*, 370–372.
209. Davies, J.; Wright, G. D. Bacterial Resistance to Aminoglycoside Antibiotics. *Trends Microbiol.* **1997,** *5*, 234–240.
210. Maarouf, M.; Lawrence, F.; Croft, S. L. Ribosomes of *Leishmania* Are a Target for the Aminoglycosides. *Parasitol. Res.* **1995,** *81*, 421–425.
211. Maarouf, M.; de Kouchkovsky, Y.; Brown, S. *In vivo* Interference of Paromomycin with Mitochondrial Activity of *Leishmania. Exp. Cell. Res.* **1997,** *232*, 339–348.
212. Maarouf, M.; Lawrence, F.; Brown, S. Biochemical Alterations in Paromomycin Treated *Leishmania donovani* Promastigotes. *Parasitol. Res.* **1997,** *83*, 198–202.

213. Myler, P. J.; Fasel, N. Chapter 7, The metabolic repertoire of *Leishmania* and implications for drug discovery. In *Leishmania: After the Genome*; Opperdoes, F. R., Michels, P. A. M., Eds.; Caister Academic Press/Horizon Scientific Press: United Kingdom, 2008.
214. Hart, D. T.; Coombs, G. H. *Leishmania mexicana*: Energy Metabolism of Amastigotes and Promastigotes. *Exp. Parasitol.* **1982,** *54*, 397–409.
215. Coombs, G. H.; Tetley, L.; Moss, V. A.; Vickerman, K. Three Dimensional Structure of the *Leishmania amastigote* as Revealed by Computer-aided Reconstruction from Serial Sections. *Parasitology* **1986,** *92*,13–23.
216. Tetley, L.; Vickerman, K. The Glycosomes of Trypanosomes: Number and Distribution as Revealed by Electron Spectroscopic Imaging and 3-D Reconstruction. *J. Microsc.* **1991,** *162*, 83–90.
217. Mottram, J. C.; Coombs, G. H. *Leishmania mexicana*: Enzyme Activities of Amastigotes and Promastigotes and Their Inhibition by Antimonials and Arsenicals. *Exp. Parasitol.* **1985,** *59*, 151–160.
218. Mottram, J. C.; Coombs, G. H. *Leishmania mexicana*: Subcellular Distribution of Enzymes in Amastigotes and Promastigotes. *Exp. Parasitol.* **1985,** *59*, 265–274.
219. Bringaud, F.; Riviere, L.; Coustou, V. Energy Metabolism of Trypanosomatids: Adaptation to Available Carbon Sources. *Mol. Biochem. Parasitol.* **2006,** *149*,1–9.
220. Burchmore, R. J.; Hart, D. T. Glucose Transport in Amastigotes and Promastigotes of *Leishmania mexicana mexicana. Mol. Biochem. Parasitol.* **1995,** *74*, 77–86.
221. Burchmore, R. J.; Landfear, S. M. Differential Regulation of Multiple Glucose Transporter Genes in *Leishmania mexicana. J. Biol. Chem.* **1998,** *273*, 29118–29126.
222. Rodriguez-Contreras, D.; Feng, X.; Keeney, K. M.; Bouwer, H. G.; Landfear, S. M. Phenotypic Characterization of a Glucose Transporter Null Mutant in *Leishmania mexicana. Mol. Biochem. Parasitol.* **2007,** *153*, 9–18.
223. Chen, M.; Zhai, L.; Christensen, S. B.; Theander, T. G.; Kharazmi, A. Inhibition of Fumarate Reductase in *Leishmania major* and *L. donovani* by Chalcones. *Antimicrob. Agents Chemother.* **2001,** *45*, 2023–2029.
224. Ralton, J. E.; Naderer, T.; Piraino, H. L.; Bashtannyk, T. A.; Callaghan, J. M.; McConville, M. J. Evidence that Intracellular Beta1-2 Mannan Is a Virulence Factor in *Leishmania* parasites. *J. Biol. Chem.* **2003,** *278*, 40757–40763.
225. Darling, T. N.; Blum, J. J. D-Lactate Production by *Leishmania braziliensis* Through the Glyoxalase Pathway. *Mol. Biochem. Parasitol.* **1988,** *28*, 121–127.
226. Irsch, T.; Krauth-Siegel, R. L. Glyoxalase II of African Trypanosomes Is Trypanothione-dependent. *J. Biol. Chem.* **2004,** *279*, 22209–22217.
227. Van Hellemond, J. J.; Opperdoes, F. R.; Tielens, A. G. Trypanosomatidae Produce Acetate via a Mitochondrial Acetate: Succinate CoA Transferase. *Proc. Natl. Acad. Sci. USA.* **1998,** *95*, 3036–3041.
228. Riviere, L.; Van Weelden, S. W.; Glass, P.; Vegh, P.; Coustou, V.; Biran, M.; Van Hellemond, J. J, Bringaud, F.; Tielens, A. G.; Boshart, M. Acetyl: Succinate CoA-Transferase in Procyclic *Trypanosoma brucei*. Gene Identification and Role in Carbohydrate Metabolism. *J. Biol. Chem.* **2004,** *279*, 45337–45346.
229. Bochud-Allemann, N.; Schneider, A. Mitochondrial Substrate Level Phosphorylation is Essential for Growth of Procyclic *Trypanosoma brucei. J. Biol. Chem.* **2002,** *277*, 32849–32854.
230. Sacks, D. L. Metacyclogenesis in *Leishmania* Promastigotes. *Exp. Parasitol.* **1989,** *69*, 100–113.

231. Chang, K. P. Cellular and Molecular Mechanisms of Intracellular Symbiosis in Leishmaniasis. *Int. Rev. Cytol. Suppl.* **1983,** *14*, 267–305.
232. Sacks, D. L.; Perkins, P. V. Identification of an Infective Stage of *Leishmania* Promastigotes. *Science* **1984,** *223*, 1417–1419.
233. Handman, E.; Schnur, L. F.; Spithill, T. W.; Mitchell, G. F. Passive Transfer of *Leishmania* Lipopolysaccharide Confers Parasite Survival in Macrophages. *J. Immunol.* **1986,** *137*, 3608–3613.
234. Pearson, R. D.; Wilson, M. E. Host defences against prototypical intracellular protozoans, the *Leishmania*. In *Parasitic Infections in the Compromised Host*; Walzer, P. D.;Genta, R. M.; Eds.; Mercel Dekker, Inc.: New York, 1989; pp 31–81.
235. Ephros, M.; Bitnun, A.; Shaked, P.; Waldman, E.; Zilberstein, D. Stage-specific Activity of Pentavalent Antimony against *Leishmania donovani* Axenic Amastigotes. *Antimicrob. Agents Chemother.* **1999,** *43*, 278–282.
236. Ramos, H.; Milhaud, J.; Cohen, B. E.; Bolard, J. Enhanced Action of Amphotericin B on *Leishmania mexicana* Resulting from Heat Transformation. *Antimicrob. Agents Chemother.* **1990,** *34*, 1584–1589.
237. Chen, M.; Christensen, S. B.; Blom, J.; Lemmich, E.; Nadelmann, L.; Fich, K.; Theander, T. G.; Kharazmi, A. Licochalcone A, a Novel Antiparasitic Agent with Potent Activity against Human Pathogenic Protozoan Species of *Leishmania. Antimicrob. Agents Chemother.* **1993,** *37*, 2550–2556.
238. Glew, R. H.; Saha, A. K.; Das, S.; Remaley, A. T. Biochemistry of the *Leishmania* Species. *Microbiol. Rev.* **1988,** *52*, 412–432.
239. Joshi, M.; Dwyer, D. M.; Nakhasi, H. L. Cloning and Characterization of Differentially Expressed Genes from in vitro-grown 'amastigotes' of *Leishmania donovani. Mol. Biochem. Parasitol.* **1993,** *58*, 345–354.
240. Rainey, P. M.; MacKenzie, N. E. A Carbon-13 Nuclear Magnetic Resonance Analysis of the Products of Glucose Metabolism in *Leishmania pifanoi* Amastigotes and Promastigotes. *Mol. Biochem. Parasitol.* **1991,** *45*, 307–315.
241. Zilberstein, D.; Shapira, M. The Role of pH and Temperature in the Development of *Leishmania* Parasites. *Annu. Rev. Microbiol.* **1994,** *48*, 449–470.
242. Gupta, N.; Goyal, N.; Rastogi, A. K. *In vitro* Cultivation and Characterization of Axenic Amastigotes of *Leishmania. Trends Parasitol.* **2001,** *17*, 150–153.
243. Barak, E.; Amin-Spector, S.; Gerliak, E.; Goyard, S.; Holland, N.; Zilberstein, D. Differentiation of *Leishmania donovani* in Host-free System: Analysis of Signal Perception and Response. *Mol. Biochem. Parasitol.* **2005,** *141*, 99–108.
244. Krobitsch, S.; Clos, J. A Novel Role for 100 kD Heat Shock Proteins in the Parasite *Leishmania donovani. Cell Stress Chaperones* **1999,** *4*, 191–198.
245. Bente, M.; Harder, S.; Wiesgigl, M.; Heukeshoven, J.; Gelhaus, C.; Krause, E.; Clos, J.; Bruchhaus, I. Developmentally Induced Changes of the Proteome in the Protozoan Parasite *Leishmania donovani. Proteomics* **2003,** *3*, 1811–1829.
246. Bates, P. A. The Developmental Biology of *Leishmania* Promastigotes. *Exp. Parasitol.* **1994,** *79*, 215–218.
247. Shapira, M.; McEwen, J. G.; Jaffe, C. L. Temperature Effects on Molecular Processes Which Lead to Stage Differentiation in *Leishmania. EMBO. J.* **1988,** *7*, 2895–2901.
248. Harder, S.; Bente, M.; Isermann, K.; Bruchhaus, I. Expression of a Mitochondrial Peroxiredoxin Prevents Programmed Cell Death in *Leishmania donovani. Eukaryot. Cell* **2006,** *5*, 861–870.

249. Mottram, J. C.; Coombs, G. H. Purification of Particulate Malate Dehydrogenase and Phosphoenolpyruvate Carboxykinase from *Leishmania mexicana mexicana*. *Biochim. Biophys. Acta.* **1985,** *827*, 310–319.
250. Paulin, J. J. The Chondriome of Selected Trypanosomatids. A Three-dimensional Study Based on Serial Thick Sections and High Voltage Electron Microscopy. *J. Cell Biol.* **1975,** *66*, 404–413.
251. Stinson, S.; Sommer, J. R.; Blum, J. J. Morphology of *Leishmania braziliensis*: Changes during Reversible Heat-induced Transformation from Promastigote to an Ellipsoidal form. *J. Parasitol.* **1989,** *75*, 431–440.
252. Rudzinska, M. A.; D Alesandro, P. A.; Trager, W. The Fine Structure of *Leishmania donovani* and the Role of the Kinetoplast in the Leishmani-leptomonad Transformation. *J. Protozool.* **1964,** *11*, 166–191.
253. Hill, G. C. Electron Transport Systems in Kinetoplastida. *Biochim. Biophys. Acta.* **1979,** *456*, 149–193.
254. Vercesi, A. E.; Bernardes, C. F.; Hoffmann, M. E.; Gadelha, F. R.; Docampo, R. Digitonin Permeabilization Does Not Affect Mitochondrial Function and Allows the Determination of the Mitochondrial Membrane Potential of *Trypanosoma cruzi in situ*. *J. Biol. Chem.* 1991, *266*, 14431–14434.
255. Angelopoulos, E. Pellicular Microtubules in the Family Trypanosomatidae. *J. Protozool.* **1970,** *17*, 39–51.
256. Martin, E.; Mukkada, A. J. Identification of the Terminal Respiratory Chain in Kinetoplast. Mitochondrial Complexes of *Leishmania tropica* Promastigotes. *J. Biol. Chem.* **1979,** *254*, 12192–12198.
257. Kusel, J. P.; Storey, B. T. Evidence for the Presence of Two Phosphorylation Sites in Mitochondria Isolated from the Trypanosomatid Hemoflagellate, *Crithidia fasciculata*. *Biochem. Biophys. Res. Commun.* **1972,** *46*, 501–507.
258. Santhamma, K. R.; Bhaduri, A. Characterization of the Respiratory Chain of *Leishmania donovani* Promastigotes. *Mol. Biochem. Parasitol.* **1995,** *75*, 43–53.
259. Bermúdez, R.; Dagger, F.; D'Aquino, J. A.; Benaim, G.; Dawidowicz, K. Characterization of Mitochondrial Electron-transfer in *Leishmania mexicana*. *Mol. Biochem. Parasitol.* **1997,** *90*, 43–54.
260. Iverson, T. M.; Chavez, C. L.; Cecchini, G.; Rees, D. C. Structure of the *Escherichia coli* Fumarate Reductase Respiratory Complex. *Science* **1999,** *284*, 1961–1966.
261. Peschek, G. A.; Kurz, M. A.; an Erber, W. W. A. Impermeant Electron Acceptors and Donors to the Plasma Membrane of Intact Cynobacterium *Anacystis nidulans* in the Dark. *Physiol. Plant* **1988,** *73*, 175–181.
262. Robertson, R. N. *Oxidoreduction at the Plasma Membrane: Relation to Growth and Transport*; Crane, F. L., Morre, D. J., Low, H., Eds.; CRC Press: Boca Ranton, 1991; Vol. II, pp 1–20.
263. Williams, L. T. Signal Transduction by the Platelet Derived Growth Receptor. *Science* **1989,** *243*, 1564–1566.
264. Mikchell, B. The Lethal Oxidase of Leukocytes. *Trends Biochem. Sci.* **1983,** *8*, 117–118
265. Tritsch, G. L.; Niswander, P. W. Modulation of Macrophage Superoxide Release by Purine Metabolism. *Life Sci.* **1983,** *32*, 1359–1364.
266. Chmelar, M.; Giacobino, J. P. Comparison of Plasma Membranes and Endoplasnic Reticulum Fractions Obtained from Whole White Adipose Tissue and Isolated Adipocytes. *Int. J. Biochem.* **1976,** *7*, 159–163.

267. Henderson, L. M.; Chappell, J. B.; Jones, O. T. G. Internal pH Changes Associated with the Activity of NADPH Oxidase of Human Neutrophils. Further Evidence for the Presence of an H^+ Conducting Channel. *Biochem. J.* **1988,** *251*, 563–568.
268. Kant, J. A.; Steck, T. L. Cation Impermeable Inside – Out and Right Side Out Vesicles from Human Erythrocyte Membranes. *Nature* **1972,** *240*, 26–28.
269. Ramirez, J. M. *Redox Functions in the Eukaryotic Plasma Membrane*; Consejo superiour de investigaciones cientificas: Madrid, 1987.
270. Crane, F. L.; Morre, D. J.; Low, H. *Plasma Membrane Oxido Reductiases in Control of Animal and Plant Growth*; Plenum Press: New York, 1988; pp 1–443.
271. Crane, F. L.; Morre, D. J.; Low, H. *Oxidoreduction at the Plasma Membrane Relation to Growth and Transport*; CRC Press: Boca Raton, 1990; Vol. I, p 318.
272. Dahse, I.; Bernstein, M.; Muller, E.; Petzold, U. On the Possible Function of Electron Transport in the Plasmalemma of Plant Cells. *Biochem. Physiol. Pflanzen.* **1989,** *185*, 145–180.
273. Morre, D. J.; Vigil, E. L.; Frantz, C.; Goldenberg, H.; Crane, F. L. Cytochemical Demonstration of Glutaraldelyde–resistant NADH–ferricyanide Oxidoreductase Activities in Rat Liver Plasma Membranes and Golgi Apparatus. *Eur. J. Cell. Biol.* **1978,** *18,* 213.
274. Morre, D. J.; Auderset, G.; Penel, C.; Canut, H. Cytochemical Localization of NADH-Ferricyanide Oxido-reductase in Hypocotyl Segments and Isolated Membrane Vesicles of Soybean. *Protoplasma* **1987,** *140*, 130–140.
275. Sun, I. L.; Navas, P.; Crane, F. L.; Morre, D. J.; Low, H. NADH Differric Transferrin Reductase in Liver Plasma Membrane. *J. Biol. Chem.* **1987,** *262*, 15915–15921.
276. Bottger, M. *Plant Membrane Transport*; Dainty, J., De Michelis, M. L., Marre, E., Rasi–Caldogno, F., Eds.; Elsevier: Amsterdam, 1987; pp 50–60.
277. Askerlund, P. Redox Processes of Plant Plasma Membrane. Ph.D. Thesis, University of Lund, Sweden, 1990.
278. Hassidim, M.; Rubinstein, B.; Lerner, H.; Reinhold, L. Generation of Membrane Potential and Electron Transport in Plasmalemma-enriched Vesicles of Cotton and Raddish. *Plant Physiol.* **1987,** *85*, 872–875.
279. Morre, D. J.; Navas, P.; Crane, F. L. *Redox Functions of the Eukaryotic Plasma Membrane*; Ramirez, J. M., Ed.; Consejo superior de investigaciones Cicntificas: Madrid, 1987; pp 92–116.
280. Grebing, C.; Crane, F. L.; Low, H.; Hall, K. A Transmembranous NADH–dehydrogenase in Human Erythrocyte Membrane. *J. Bienerg. Biomembr.* **1984,** *16*, 517–534.
281. Morre, D. J.; Brightman, A.; Wang, J.; Barr, R.; Crane, F. L. *Plasma Membrane Oxido Reductase in Control of Animal and Plant Growth;* Crane, F. L., Morre, D. J., Low, H., Eds.; Plenum Press: New York, 1988; pp 45–56.
282. Moller, I. M.; Lin, W. Membrane–bound NADPH Dehydrogenases in Higher Plant Cells. *Ann. Rev. Plant Physiol.* **1986,** *37*, 309–334.
283. Navas, P.; Sun, I. L.; Morre, D. J.; Crane, F. L.*Plasma Membrane Oxido Reductase in Control of Animal and Plant Growth*; Crane, F. L., Morre, D. J., Low, H., Eds.; Plenum Press: New York, 1988; p 339.
284. Goldenberg, H.; Grebing, C.; Low, H. NADH–Monodehydroascorbate Reductase in Human Erythrocyte Membrane. *Biochem. Int.* **1983,** *6*, 1–9.
285. Low, H.; Crane, F. L.; Morre, D. J.; Sun, I. L. *Oxido Reduction at the Plasma Membrane: Relation to Growth and Transport*; Crane, F. L., Morre, D. J., Low, H., Eds.; CRC Press: Boca Raton, 1990; pp 29–66.

286. Crane, F. L.; Sun, I. L.; Clark, M. G.; Grebing, C.; Low, H. Transplasma Membrane Redox Systems in Growth and Development. *Biochim. Biophys. Acta.* **1985,** *811*, 233–264.
287. Gayda, D. P.; Crane, F.; Morre, D. J.; Low, H. Hormone Effect on NADH – Oxidizing Enzymes of Plasma Membranes of Rat Liver. *Proc. Indiana Acad. Sci.* **1977,** *86*, 385–390.
288. Morre, D. J.; Crane, F. L.*Oxidoreduction at the Plasma Membrane: Relation to Growth and Transport*; Crane, F. L., Morre, D. J., Low, H., Eds.; CRC Press: Boca Raton, 1990; Vol. I, pp 67–84.
289. Crane, F. L.; Low, H.; Clark, M. G. *The Enzymes of Biological Membranes*; Martonose, A. N., Ed.; Plenum Press: New York, 1985; Vol. 4, pp 465–510.
290. Thorstensen, K.; Aisen, P. Release of Iron from Diferric Transferrin in the Presence of Rat Liver Plasma Membrane: No Evidence of a Plasma Membrane Diferric Transferrin Reductase. *Biochim. Biophys. Acta.* **1990,** *1052*, 29–35.
291. Crane, F. L.; Sun, I. L.; Barr, R.; Law, H. Electron and Proton Transport Across the Plasma Membrane. *J. Bioenerg. Biomembr.* **1991,** *23*, 773–803.
292. Sun, F. L.; Navas, P. *Redox Functions of the Eukanriotic Plasma Membrane*; Ramirez, J. M., Ed.; Consejo Superior de Investigaciones Cientificas: Madrid, 1987; pp 65–89.
293. Fry, M. Diferric Transferrin Reductase in *Plasmodium falciparum* – Infected Erythrocytes. *Biochim. Biophys. Res. Commun.* **1989,** *158*, 469–473.
294. Bates, G. W.; Workman, E. F., Jr.; Schlabach, M. R. Does Transferrin Exhibit Ferro Oxidase Activity? *Biochem. Biophys. Res. Commun.* **1973,** *50*, 84–90.
295. Low, H.; Sun, I. L.; Navas, P.; Grebing, C.; Crane, F. L.; Morre, D. J. Transplasmalemma Electron Transpart from Cells Is Part of a Diferric Transferrion Reductase System. *Biochem. Biophys. Res. Commun.* **1986,** *139*, 1117–1123.
296. Low, H.; Gvebing, C.; Lindgreen, A.; Tally, M.; Sun, I. L.; Crane, F. L. Involvement of Transferrin in the Reduction of Iron by the Transplasma Membrane Electron Transport System. *J. Bioenerg. Biomembr.* **1987,** *19*, 535–549.
297. Goldenberg, H.; Eder, M.; Pumm, R.; Dodel, B.*Plasma Membrane Oxido Reductases in Control of Animal and Plant Growth;* Crane, F. L., Morre, D. J., Low, H. Eds.; Plenum Press: New York, 1988; pp 131–152.
298. Sun, I. L.;, Crane, F. L. Effect of Anthracyline Compounds on Transmembrane Redox Function of Cultured HeLA Cells. *Proc. Indiana. Acad. Sci.* **1984,** *93*, 267–274.
299. Crane, F. L.; Low, H.; Sun, I. L.; Morre, D. J.; Faulk, W. P. *Growth Factor from Genes to Clinical Applications*; Sara, V., Hall, K., Low, H., Eds.; Raven Press: New York, 1990; pp 129–140.
300. Trinder, D.; Morgan, E. H.; Baker, E. The Effect of an Antibody to the Rat Transferrin Receptor and of Rat Serum Albumin on the Uptake of Diferric Transferrin by Rat Hepatocytes. *Biochim. Biophys. Acta.* **1988,** *943*, 440–446.
301. White, S.; Teatle, R.; Seligman, P. A.; Rutherford, M.; Trowbridge, I. S. Combination of Antitransferrin Receptor Monoclonal Antibodies Inhibit Human Tumor Cell Growth *in vitro* and *in vivo*: Evidence for Synergestic Antiproliferative Effects. *Cancer Res.* **1990,** *50*, 6295–6301.
302. Moller, I. M.; Crane, F. L. *The Plant Plasma Membrane;* Larson, C., Moller, I. M., Eds.; Springer–verlag: Berlin, 1990; pp 93–126.
303. Yamamoto, Y.; Niki, E.; Eguchi, J.; Kamiya, Y.; Shimasaki, H. Oxidation of Biological Membranes and Its Inhibition Free Radical Chain Oxidation of Erythrocyte Ghost Membranes by Oxygen. *Biochim. Biophys. Acta.* **1985,** *819*, 29–36.

304. Kalen, A.; Norling, B.; Appelkvist, E. L.; Dallner, G. Ubiquinone Biosynthesis by the Microsomal Fraction from Rat Liver. *Biochim. Biophys. Acta.* **1987,** *926*, 70–78.
305. Crane, F. L.; Sun, I. L.; Sun, E.; Morre, D. J. *Biomedical and Clinical Aspects of Coenzyme Q*; Folkers, K., Littaru, G. P., Eds.; Elsevier: Amsterdam, 1991; Vol. 6, pp 59–70.
306. Sun, I. L.; Crane, F. L. *Oxidoreduction at the Plasma Membrane: Relation to Growth and Transport*; Crane, F. L., Morre, D. J., Low, H., Eds.; CRC Press: Boca Raton, 1990; Vol. I, pp 257–280.
307. Norling, B.; Glazek, E.; Nelson, B. D.; Eranster, L. Studies with Ubiquinone – depleted Submitochandrial Particles. Quantitative Incorporation of Small Amounts of Ubiquinone and its Effects on NADH and Succinate Oxidase Activity. *Eur. J. Biochem.* **1974,** *47*, 475–482.
308. Crane, F. L.; Sun, I. L.; Sun, E. E.; Brightman, A.; Morre, D. J.; Low, H. Growth Control by Transferrin Stimulated Transplasma Membrane Electron Transport Requires Coenzyme Q. *J. Cell Biol.* **1990,** *111*, 231 a.
309. Lenaz, G. *Coenzyme Q*; Wiley: Chichester, 1985.
310. Trumpower, B. L. *Function of Quinones in Energy Coupling Systems*; Academic Press: New York, 1982.
311. Hall, C.; Wu, M.; Crane, F. L.; Takahashi, H.; Tamura, S.; Folkers, K. Piericidin A: A New Inhibition of Mitochandrial Election Transport. *Biochim. Biophys. Commun.* **1966,** *25*, 373–377.
312. Clerk, M. G.; Patrick, E. J.; Patter, G. S.; Crane, F. L.; Low, H.; Grebing, C. Evidence for Extracellular Reduction of Ferricyanide by Rat Liver: A Tranplasma Membrane Redox System. *Biochem. J.* **1981,** *200*, 565–572.
313. Barr, R.; Craing, T. A.; Crane, F. L. Transmembrane Ferricyamide Reduction in Carrot Cells. *Biochim. Biophys. Acta.* **1985,** *812*, 49–54.
314. Crane, F. L. *Highlights in Ubiquinone Research*; Lenaz, G., Barnabei, O., Rabbi, A., Battino, M., Eds.; Taylor and Francis: London, 1990; pp 3–20.
315. Low, H.; Crane, F. L. Redox Function in Plasma Membrane *Biochim. Biophys. Acta.* **1978,** *515*, 141–161.
316. Toole–Simms, W.; Sun, I. L.; Morre, D. J.; Crane, F. L. Tansplamembrane Electron and Proton Transport Is Inhibited by Chloroquine. *Biochem. Int.* **1990,** *21*, 761–769.
317. Sun, I. L.; Crane, F. L.*Plasma Membrane Oxidoreductase in Control of Animal and Plant Growth*;Crane, F. L., Morre, D. J., Low, H., Eds.; Plenum Press: New York, 1988; pp181–190.
318. Sun, I. L.; Crane, F. L.; Chou, J. Y. Modification of Transmembrane Electron Tranport Activity in Plasma Membrane of Simian Virus 40 Transformed Pineal Cells. *Biochim. Biophys. Acta.* **1986,** *886*, 327–336.
319. Sun, I. L.; Toole-Simms, W.; Crane, F. L.; Morre, D. J.; Low, H.; Chou, J. Y. Transformation with SV 40 Virus Prevents Retinic Acid Inhibition of Plasma Membrane NADH Differric Transferrin Reductase in Rat Liver Cells. *J. Bioenerg. Biomembr.* **1988,** *20*, 383–391.
320. Faulk, W. P.; Torry, D. S.; Harats, H.; Mc Intyre, J. A.; Taylor, C. *Plasma Membrane oxidoreductase in control of Animal and Plant Growth*; Crane, F. L., Morre, D. T., Low, H., Eds.; Plenum Press: New York, 1988; pp 173–180.
321. Faulk, W.P.; Hanats, H.; Crane, F.; Sun, I. L.9th International Conference on Proteins of iron transport, Brisbane, 1989; Abstracts, p 53.

322. Faulk WP, Harats Mc Intyre JA, Berezi A, Sun IL, Crane FL. Recent Advances in Cancer Research: Drug Targeting without the Use of Monoclonal Antibodies. *Am. J. Reprod. Immunol.* **1990,** *21,* 151–154.
323. Dormandy, T. L.; Zarday, Z. The Mechanism of Insulin Action: The Immediate Electrochemical Effects of Insulin on Red-Cell Systems. *J. Physiol.* **1965,** *180*, 684–707.
324. Sun, I. L.; Crane, F. L.; Grebing, C.; Low, H. Properties of a Transplasma Membrane Electron Transport System in HeLa Cells. *J. Bioenerg. Biomembr.* **1965,** *16*, 583–595.
325. Sun, I. L.; Crane, F. L. Bleomycin Control of Transplasma Membrane Redox Activity and Proton Movement in HeLa Cells. *Biochem. Pharmacol.* **1985,** *34*, 617–622.
326. Toole-Simms, W. Regulation of Protein Release from HeLa Cells by Ferric Reductase. Ph.D. Thesis, Purdue University, West Lafayette, 1988.
327. Wikstrom, M. *Mitochondria and Microsomes;* Lec, C. P., Schatz, G., Dallner, Eds.;. Addison–Welsley, Reading: Massachusetts, 1981; pp 249–269.
328. Wikstrom, M.; Krab, K. Proton–Pumping Cytochrome C Oxidase. *Biochim. Biophys. Acta.* 1979, *549*, 177–222.
329. Wikstrom, M.; Krab, K.; Saraste, M. Proton – translocating of Cytochrome Complexes. *Annu. Rev. Biochem.* **1981,** *50*, 623–655.
330. Garcia-Canero, R.; Diaz-Gil, J. J.; Guevva, M. A. *Redox Functions of the Eukaryotic Plasma Membrane*; Ramirez, J. M., Ed; Consejo superior de Investigaciones Cientficas: Madrid, 1987; pp 42–47.
331. Sun, I. L.; Garcia-Canero, R.; Liu, W.; Toole-Simms, W.; Crave, F. L.; Morre, D. J.; Low, H. Diferric Transferrin Reduction Stimulates Na^+/H^+ Antiport of He La Cells. *Biochem. Biophys. Res. Commun.* **1987,** *145*, 467–473.
332. Fuhrmann, G. F.; Fehlan, R.; Schneider, H.; Knauf, P. A. The Effect of Ferricyanide with Iodoacetale in Calcium-free Solution on Passive Cation Permeability in Human and Red Cells: Comparison with the Gardos – Effect and with the Influence of PCMBS on Passive Cation Permeability. *Biochim. Biophys. Acta.* **1982,** *183*, 179–185.
333. Low, H.; Lindgreen, A.; Crane, F. L.; Sun, I. C.; Toole-Simms, W.; Morre, D. J. *Plasma Membrane Oxidoreductase in Control of Animal and Plant Growth;* Crane, F. L., Morre, D.J., Low, H., Eds.; Plenum Press: New York, 1988; pp 152–153.
334. Sun, I. C.; Toole–Simms, W.; Crane, F. L.; Morre, D. J.; Low, H.; Chou, J. Y. Reduction of Deferric Transferrin by SV 40 Transformed Pineal Cells Stimulates Na^+/H^+ Antiport Activity. *Biochim. Biophys. Acta.* **1988,** *938*, 17–23.
335. Golub, E. S.; Diaz de Pagan, T.; Sun, I.; Crane, F. L. *Plasma Membrane Oxidoreductase in Control of Animal and Plant Growth*; Crane, F. L., Morre, D. J., Low, H., Eds.; Plenum Press: New York, 1988; pp 313–321.
336. Ladoux, A.; Cragoe, E. J., Jr.; Gery, B.; Abita, J. P.; Frelin, C. Differentiation of Human Promyelocytic HL 60 Cells by Retinic Acid Is Accompanied by an Increase in the Intracellular pH. The Role of the Na^+/H^+ Exchange System. *J. Biol. Chem.* **1987,** *262*, 811–815.
337. Sun, I. L.; Sun, E. E.; Crane, F. L.; Morre, D. J.; Lindgren, A.; Low, H. Requirement for Coenzyme Q in Plasma Membrane Electron Transport. *Proc. Natl. Acad. Sci. USA.* **1992**, *98*,11126–11130.
338. Grinstein, S.; Rotin, D.; Mason, M. J. Na^+/H^+ Exchange and Growth Factor–Induced Cytosolic pH Changes. Role in Cellular Proliferation. *Biochim. Biophys. Acta.* **1989,** *988*, 73–97.
339. Boniface, J.; Reichert, L. Evidence for a Novel Thioredoxin– Like Catalytic Property of Gonadotrophic Hormones. *Science* **1990,** *247*, 61–64.

340. Sardet, C.; Counillon, L.; Franchi, A.; Pouyssegur, J. Growth Factors Induced Phosphorylation of the Na^+/H^+ Antiporter, a Glycoprotien of 110 KD. *Science* **1990,** *247*, 723–726.
341. Gopalkrishna, R.; Anderson, W. B. Ca^{+2} and Phospholipid–independent Activation of Protein Kinsase C by Selective Oxidative Modification of the Regulatory Domain. *Proc. Natl. Acad. Sci. USA.* **1989,** *86*, 6758–6762.
342. Koshio, O.; Akanuma, Y.; Kasuga, M. Hydrogen Peroxide Stimulates Tyrosine Phophorylation of the Insulin Receptor and its Tyrosine Kinase Activity in Intact Cells. *Biochem. J.* **1998,** *250*, 95–101.
343. Ramasarma, T.; Swaroop, A.; Mc Kellar, W.; Crane, F. L. Generation of Hydrogen Peroxide on Oxidation of NADH by Hepatic Plasma Membranes. *J. Bienerg. Biomembr.* **1981,** *13*, 241–253.
344. Anderson, J. M.; Andersson, B. The Dynamic Photosynthetic Membrane and Regulation of Solar Energy Conversion. *Trends Biochem. Sci.* **1988,** *13*, 351–355.
345. Dilley, R. A.; Chiang, G. G. *Plasm Membrane Oxidoreductase in Control of Animal and Plant Growth*; Crane, F. L.; Morre, D. J.; Low, H., Eds.; Plenum Press: New York, 1988; pp 199–208.
346. Heyworth, P. G.; Badway, J. A. Protein Phosphorylation Associated with the Stimulation of Neutrophils. Modulation of Superoxide Production by Protien Kinase C and Calcium. *J. Bioenerg. Biomembr.* **1990,** *22*, 1–26.
347. en.wikipedia.org/wiki/Electron_transport_chain.
348. http://www.dentistry.leeds.ac.uk/biochem.

INDEX

B

O

Q